FITNESS FOR LIFE
An Individualized Approach

Fourth Edition

FITNESS FOR LIFE
An Individualized Approach

Philip E. Allsen
Brigham Young University

Joyce M. Harrison
Brigham Young University

Barbara Vance
Brigham Young University

ωcb
Wm. C. Brown Publishers
Dubuque, Iowa

Book Team

Editor *Chris Rogers*
Developmental Editor *Sue Pulvermacher-Alt*
Designer *Teresa E. Webb*
Production Editor *Carla J. Aspelmeier*
Photo Research Editor *Mary Roussel*

wcb group

Chairman of the Board *Wm. C. Brown*
President and Chief Executive Officer *Mark C. Falb*

wcb

Wm. C. Brown Publishers, College Division

President *G. Franklin Lewis*
Vice President, Editor-in-Chief *George Wm. Bergquist*
Vice President, Director of Production *Beverly Kolz*
Vice President, National Sales Manager *Bob McLaughlin*
Director of Marketing *Thomas E. Doran*
Marketing Communications Manager *Edward Bartell*
Marketing Information Systems Manager *Craig S. Marty*
Marketing Manager *Kathy Law Laube*
Manager of Visuals and Design *Faye M. Schilling*
Production Editorial Manager *Julie A. Kennedy*

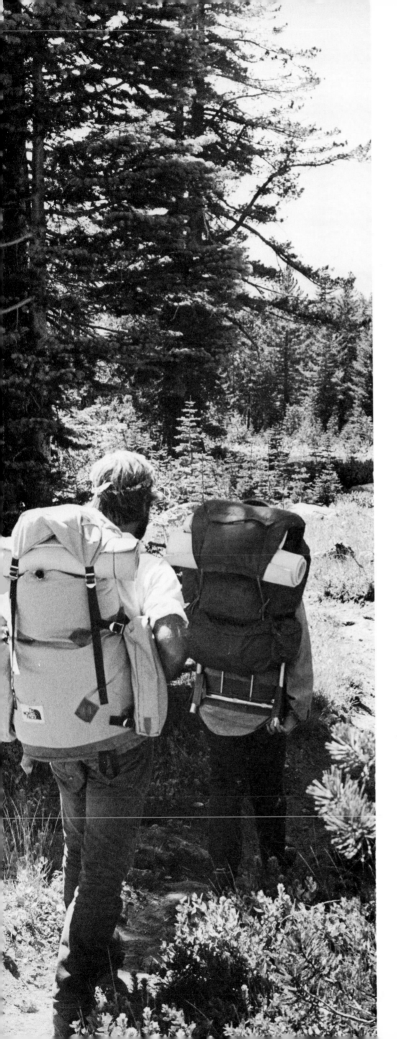

CONTENTS

10

APPLYING A FLEXIBILITY PROGRAM

11

WRITING AND APPLYING A RELAXATION PROGRAM

12

WHERE DO WE GO FROM HERE?

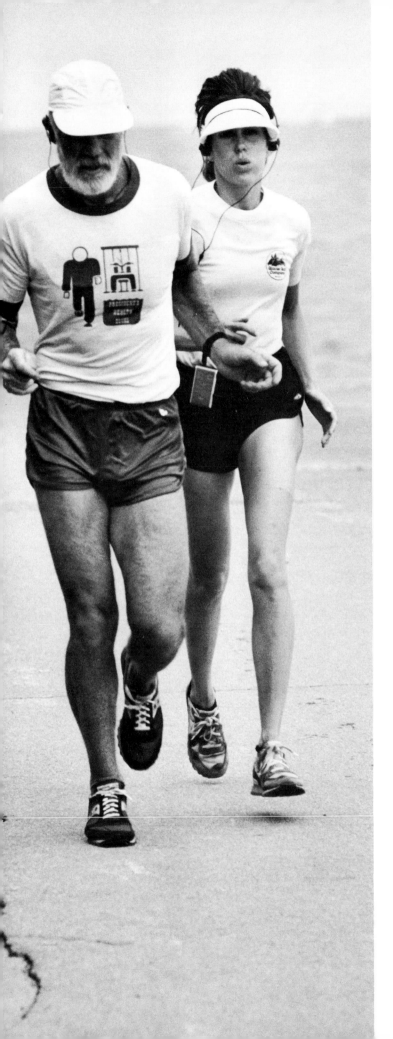

PREFACE

Attempting to reach the goal of physical fitness can be compared with preparing to take a journey. If you were driving from Los Angeles to New York City, you would first obtain a road map in order to determine the route to follow. The journey to physical fitness is very similar, but most people are not familiar with, or do not know where to obtain, a road map to fitness.

Fitness for Life: An Individualized Approach is intended to provide such a road map. It takes people from their current levels of fitness toward increased cardiovascular endurance, proper weight control, increased strength and flexibility, and the ability to relax.

The individualized approach to physical fitness in this text is designed to do more than teach the principles of cardiovascular endurance, weight control, strength, flexibility, and relaxation. Individuals will also apply what they learn by writing and engaging in their own personalized fitness programs.

Too often people are placed in a required physical fitness program where all of the decisions are made for them by the instructor. When people leave such an organized program, they are unable to carry on the program by themselves, and they start on the road to poor physical fitness. We are convinced that it is possible to teach correct principles of physical fitness. These principles can be utilized every day to make the right choices and decisions that will enable people to become and remain physically fit for their entire lives.

It should be emphasized that physical fitness should be an on-going endeavor for a lifetime. By using the information contained in this text, you will be able to write programs for yourself and for others. The testing program can be used for a variety of ages and the information can be used to develop physical fitness programs for any age group.

We wish to emphasize that this textbook is geared to the needs of the average person, and is not a book on exercise physiology. Too often books on exercise include a lot of information concerning in-depth physiology and the use of sophisticated equipment and facilities that is not pertinent to the planning of an individualized exercise program. Suggested reading sources are included at the end of some chapters for those readers who wish to obtain this kind of information.

This fourth edition of *Fitness for Life* features changes that should be of help in writing physical fitness programs.

All of the chapters have been reorganized to make the presentation of the material easy to follow in planning individualized training programs.

In this new edition, it should be possible to start with the beginning of a program and proceed in an orderly fashion to the goal of physical fitness. The work sheets in Appendix C that can be used in writing a personalized fitness program are frequently filled out as sample cases within the chapters. It should be pointed out that permission has been given by the publisher to make photocopies of the blank work sheets in the appendix for use as handouts by the teacher or for multiple use by the student.

The material in this textbook has been used and evaluated in a "class-testing" situation involving thousands of students at Brigham Young University and other schools. Follow-up studies were conducted to determine whether these students had the ability to write and engage in fitness programs after leaving the university setting. The results of this research indicate that it is possible for people to learn how to write programs of exercise for themselves so that they can achieve and maintain high levels of physical fitness.

SUPPLEMENTARY MATERIALS

Instructor's Manual

The Instructor's Manual available with *Fitness for Life* offers variable approaches to instruction, a variety of course schedules, a course overview, helpful hints on administering and grading fitness tests, and instructions for constructing quizzes using the TestPak program.

TestPak

wcb TestPak is a computerized system that enables you to make up customized exams quickly and easily. Test questions can be found in the Test Item File, which is printed in your instructor's manual or as a separate packet. For each exam you may select up to 250 questions from the file and either print the test yourself or have **wcb** print it.

Printing the exam yourself requires access to a personal computer—an IBM that uses 5.25- or 3.5-inch diskettes, an Apple IIe or IIc, or a Macintosh. TestPak requires two disk drives and will work with any printer. Diskettes are available through your local **wcb** sales representative or by phoning Educational Services at 319–588–1451. The package you receive will contain complete instructions for making up an exam.

If you don't have access to a suitable computer, you may use **wcb**'s call-in/mail-in service. First determine the chapter and question numbers and any specific heading you want on the exam. Then call Pat Powers at 800–351–7671 (in Iowa, 319–589–2953) or mail information to: Pat Powers, Wm. C. Brown Publishers, 2460 Kerper Blvd., Dubuque, IA 52001. Within two working days, **wcb** will send you via first-class mail a test master, student answer sheet, and an answer key.

GradePak

wcb GradePak is a computerized service available free to qualifying adopters of *Fitness for Life*. GradePak makes calculating and reporting your students' grades an easy task! A single disk holds data for classes of up to 500 students with room for 60 scores per student. GradePak calculates class averages on all scores and overall class averages. Plus, it gives you a grade profile report showing what each student requires to earn an A, B, C, or D for the term. GradePak allows numeric input as well as letter grades. It is available for the Apple® II+, IIe, and IIc, and for the IBM PC.

Profile Disk

The profile disk available with *Fitness for Life* is an IBM-compatible diskette that contains a program that automatically constructs a personal fitness appraisal profile from data input by the student including cardiovascular endurance, recommended body weight, and strength and flexibility. Based on the appraisal, the program can then personalize a cardiovascular endurance or weight control program for the student.

Audiovisual Presentations

wcb audiovisual presentations are a series of fourteen lessons for the various fitness programs associated with the *Fitness for Life* program. This is a service available free to qualifying adopters of *Fitness for Life*.

These presentations can be utilized as classroom lectures or made available to students who have questions and need to review any material covered in the textbook.

LIST OF REVIEWERS

We gratefully acknowledge the invaluable assistance of the following reviewers in the development and preparation of the text:

LIST OF REVIEWERS

We gratefully acknowledge the invaluable assistance of the following reviewers in the development and preparation of the text:

Jeanne M. Herman, PhD *Gustavus Adolphus College*
C. Douglas Clinger *Slippery Rock University*
Janet E. Demars *Worcester State College*
Nikki A. Assman *Ball State University*
Ronald T. Mulder, EdD *Westmont College*
Wade L. Anderson *Ricks College*
Dr. Nancy Macnamara *Broward Community College South*
Mark Adams *Western Oregon State College*
Lori Richards *Utah Valley Community College*

ACKNOWLEDGMENTS

The textbook plan and the material included in it are the result of many hours of work and the help of many people. We are grateful to our colleagues at Brigham Young University for their support throughout the book's development.

We wish to thank Tammy Boyd, Mark Bradley, Danny Frazier, and Gina Hansen who served as models for the exercise photographs. Thanks are also given to Walter Cryer who was the photographer for all of the photographs in this new edition.

We extend our special thanks to the Division of Instructional Research, Development, and Evaluation at Brigham Young for helping us put together what we feel is a concise and instructionally sound program for physical fitness.

Philip E. Allsen
Joyce M. Harrison
Barbara Vance

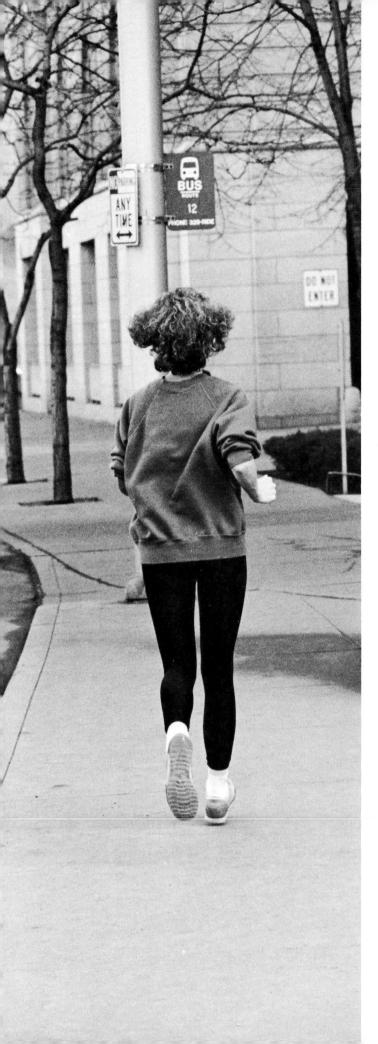

1

INTRODUCTION TO FITNESS FOR LIFE

Objectives

After study of this chapter you should be able to

1. understand the need for physical fitness;
2. correctly define physical fitness;
3. know the effects of a healthy life-style;
4. understand the specific objectives for physical fitness.

It was a beautiful spring day in Centerville. The sun was shining, a light breeze was blowing, and there was excitement in the air. It had been a long, cold winter, and this was one of those beautiful sunny spring days, just right for the first high school track meet of the year. There was a special excitement for the Mason family because Johnny, who was in his first year of high school, was running the high hurdles. The whole family was there to watch him.

Johnny's father, Ed, had been one of the best high hurdlers in that part of the country. He won the high school state championship when he was at Centerville High. He had beaten everyone in the state, even the hurdlers from the big city high schools. Ed went to college on a track scholarship and won the conference championship in the high hurdles.

After college, he returned to Centerville, married, and took a job at the bank. Now, many years later, his oldest son was going to run the high hurdles in competition for the first time. Ed had let the coach do the coaching, so he had never seen Johnny run.

In the high hurdle event, Johnny finished in third place behind two seniors, one from his school and one from the opponent's school. It was not a bad showing for his first time. But Ed, watching the race, knew how Johnny could have run a better race and perhaps could have won. He decided to give Johnny some lessons after the meet.

As soon as the last race had ended, Ed went down on the track and found Johnny. He tried to explain a better way to clear the hurdles but Johnny did not understand. Caught up in the excitement of the day, Ed decided to show Johnny what he meant.

With a job and a family, Ed had not kept up his track training schedule after college. Instead he had been playing golf every Saturday morning hoping to keep in shape.

As he came out of the blocks, his stride did not quite live up to his memory, but it wasn't too bad for a man his age. Then, as he tried to clear the first hurdle, his back leg caught on the hurdle and tripped him. He slid face first along the cinder track, breaking his glasses and cutting himself from head to toe. There was total silence. What could he say? What could anyone say? Ed Mason was not what he used to be, but what a way to find out.

This incident was told to the authors by a former graduate student, Jim Hesson. As he pointed out, if Ed had continued a fitness training program, he would either have been able to run the hurdles or would have known that he could not run the hurdles. In this case, however, he was totally unaware of what his body could and could not do.

In the United States, we live in an age of disposable products and containers. There are bottles, cans, and cartons for nearly everything. We use the contents, then throw away the containers. This has become such an acceptable practice in our lives that we do the same thing with people—many times including our athletes. You don't believe it? Think about it. What do we do for our athletes after the last basket is made and the last race is run? Do we provide them with a sound fitness program so that they can maintain a high level of fitness and health for the rest of their lives? The answer in most cases is *no!*

The primary reason that this happens is that most of us, including athletes, have never been taught how to be responsible for our own physical fitness. After the competiton ends, there may be a handshake and a wish for "good luck in the big world," but that is the end of physical activity. The next time activity is considered is after the first heart attack at the age of forty.

Thus, there is a great need for a personalized fitness program for people of all ages. It should be one that is not based on competition where only one person or one team can emerge victorious, but a program in which everyone can be a winner. The program should be the type from which a person can select many activities as dictated by personal needs and likes.

The ordinary tasks of daily living no longer provide individuals with enough vigorous exercise to develop and maintain good muscle tone, recommended body weight, or cardiovascular fitness. Yesterday's man and woman were engaged in a constant hand-to-hand combat with the environment, and our ancestors needed a strong body just to stay alive. Their typical day consisted of twelve to fourteen hours of hard labor. We have the same kind of body as that created for ancient people—one designed for physical activity. Unfortunately our world no longer demands fitness, and inactivity, together with poor personal health practices on the part of many Americans, have resulted in a massive national physical fitness problem.

In homes, factories, and farms, machines now supply the power for most jobs. They have virtually eliminated the necessity of walking, running, lifting, or climbing. One modern machine—television—holds people in captive idleness for an average of twenty-one hours a week.

It has been estimated that children spend more time in front of the television set than they spend in school. Research conducted at Tufts University and Harvard Medical School examined the relationship between excess body fat in children and the amount of television they watch. The results revealed that the more television watched, the greater the amount of body fat. It was also found that the earlier a person begins to watch television, the greater the problem. When more than two thousand children were followed into adolescence, it was discovered that the children who watched the most television at a younger age had the greatest amount of fat as teenagers.

It has been stated that watching television not only requires no skills, it develops no skills. No one can get better at watching television by watching more of it.

The U.S. Department of Health and Human Services conducted a survey on health habits, health knowledge, and physical activity. The results of the survey indicated that only 42 percent of the adult population exercise on a regular basis and only 25 percent of this population have done so for five or more years.

A study of children ages six through seventeen conducted by the Institute of Social Research of the University of Michigan indicated that the physical fitness of American public school children hasn't shown an improvement in the last ten years and, in some cases, has greatly deteriorated.

Similar results were found in another study conducted by the Institute for Aerobics Research in Dallas, Texas. This study indicated that today's students generally have more body fat and perform more poorly in cardiovascular endurance events than students in the past. Only seventeen states have mandatory physical education classes and only 36.3 percent of students in grades 5–12 take physical education classes on a daily basis.

Dr. Kenneth Cooper, director of the institute, stated, "It's discouraging and I'm afraid that as these kids grow up, we will see all the gains made against heart disease in the last twenty years wiped out in the next twenty years."

Many people are older than their years would indicate. Dr. Thomas Cureton, outstanding researcher in exercise at the University of Illinois, states that middle age for the average person begins at age twenty-six, because at that age he or she has the physical capacity that our ancestors had when they were forty. By the time we are sixty-five we are told to retire, and we think we have to take it easy, when what we really need is exercise.

One of the amazing stories concerning exercise is that of Eula Weaver in California.

At the age of sixty-seven, Eula had a severe heart attack. She survived but, at age seventy-five, she was hospitalized with congestive heart failure, arthritis, high blood pressure, angina, atherosclerosis, and claudication. Claudication is a condition that prevents adequate blood flow in the extremities. Eula could walk only about one hundred feet and wore gloves in the summer for warmth. She also was taking fifteen to twenty pills a day for all of her ailments.

At the age of eighty-one she began a special diet and exercise program. It started out with walking and then progressed to a jogging and running regime. When she was eighty-five, Eula won two gold medals in the Senior Olympics in the 880 and mile run! She repeated these gold medals at age eighty-six and eighty-seven. She ran one to two miles daily and also rode a stationary bike each day. Eula is living proof that we are never too old or too out of shape to accomplish something with our bodies.

Seneca's adage, "Man does not die, he kills himself," is more true now than when the words were written nineteen centuries ago. Medical science has conquered the diseases of former times, such as diphtheria, influenza, polio, and tuberculosis. Today our lives are far more likely to be imperiled by our own conduct: by smoking, alcohol, fatty foods, obesity, and lack of exercise. For this reason, heart disease and lung cancer are sometimes referred to as "diseases of choice." The gravity of America's physical fitness problem can be gauged by the following facts and figures:

1. More than 50 percent of the deaths in the United States result from cardiovascular diseases, many of which are associated with obesity and inactivity. Heart attacks alone cost industry approximately 132 million workdays annually (4 percent of the gross national product) in addition to a loss of output by those who are stricken. More than a hundred thousand people, many of them at the pinnacle of their value to the companies employing them, will die of heart attacks this year.

   Many people think that heart disease is an old person's problem, but nothing could be farther from the truth. A study conducted during the Korean and Vietnam conflicts revealed that approximately 70 percent of the twenty-two-year-old or younger servicemen killed had the beginning stages of atherosclerosis. In a study of eight- to twelve-year-old children in California, it was found that 37 percent were obese, 20 percent had increased blood cholesterol levels, 8 percent had increased blood fat levels, and some were even showing indications of abnormal electrocardiograms. We start to develop heart disease at an early age and it reaps its toll of death as we become older.

2. Obesity is a major health hazard. If all deaths from cancer could be eliminated, two years would be added to a person's life span. If all deaths related to obesity could be prevented, it is estimated that the life span would increase seven years! Some authorities indicate that life expectancy decreases approximately 1 percent for each pound of excess fat carried by an individual between the ages of forty-five and fifty.

3. The common backache, far less dramatic than a heart attack, is usually a result of physical degeneration. Once again, the price is high. According to the National Safety Council, backache costs American industry $1 billion annually in lost goods and services and another $225 million in worker's compensation.

   Dr. Lawrence Friedmann, head of rehabilitation medicine at the Nassau County Medical Center, indicates that most backache cases result from "either inelastic muscles or weak muscles." One study in two New York hospitals found that 81 percent of the patients with back pain had no underlying organ problems such as damaged vertebrae, ruptured discs, or arthritis.

4. Chronic tiredness is one of the frequently heard complaints of modern life. In many people this is the result of the body's gradual deterioration due to a lack of physical activity. It is known that continual inactivity results in

a loss of muscle tissue, which causes an individual to lose the strength and endurance to do daily tasks with ease and efficiency.

5. In the past few years a new term has been coined to describe the effects of inactivity. **"Hypokinetic disease"** is the term given to a disease that is related to, or caused by, a lack of regular physical activity. Such diseases as coronary heart disease, high blood pressure, lower-back problems, increased body fat, and joint disorders are some of the so-called hypokinetic diseases.

6. The stress of modern-day living has brought about an increase in two undesirable psychological states known as "anxiety" and "depression." **Anxiety,** or the feeling of uncertainty and apprehension, can bring about confusion and distorted perceptions that can interfere with thinking and other normal mental processes. **Depression** is associated with feelings of hopelessness and a reduction of the mental processes and other body functions. Some experts in the field of mental health estimate that more than 50 percent of all patients who are in hospitals because of emotional illness are suffering from various depressive disorders. It is reported by some medical doctors that approximately 70 percent of the pseudo-physical ailments in patients are illnesses that have an origin in emotional causes.

7. One of every six children in the United States is so weak, uncoordinated, or generally inept that he or she is classified as physically underdeveloped by the standards of the President's Council on Physical Fitness and Sports. Such a child is likely to become a sedentary adult with all of the added health risks associated with poor physical fitness.

WHAT IS PHYSICAL FITNESS?

Physical fitness means different things to different people. The American Alliance for Health, Physical Education, Recreation, and Dance and the President's Council on Physical Fitness and Sports report that physical fitness is a state of physical well-being with attributes that contribute to: (1) performing daily activities with vigor; (2) having minimal risk of health problems that are related to lack of exercise; and (3) providing a fitness base for participation in a variety of physical activities.

In more meaningful personal terms, it is a reflection of the ability to work with vigor and pleasure without undue fatigue, with energy left for enjoying hobbies and recreational activities, and for meeting unforeseen emergencies. It relates to how you feel mentally as well as physically. Physical fitness is many-faceted. Basic to it are proper nutrition, adequate rest and relaxation, good health practices, and good medical and dental care. But these are not enough. An essential element of fitness is physical activity—exercise for a body that needs it.

Using the benefits of physical fitness as guidelines, we concluded that the evidence of research indicates that physical fitness is built upon a foundation of five major factors—cardiovascular endurance, strength, flexibility, proper body weight and body composition, and relaxation. If these objectives can be accomplished, a person is well on the way to achieving optimal physical fitness. By achieving physical fitness, an individual can engage in a life-style that produces health and happiness.

WHAT DO YOU KNOW ABOUT EXERCISE?

Now that we have come to a common definition of physical fitness, let me ask you the question, "What do you really know about exercise?" Bill Maness, editor of the Aviation Medical Bulletin, has prepared a quiz that determines what one knows about fitness. This information helps to separate truth from fallacy and removes some of the confusion from the burgeoning world of exercise advice.

1. The best way to reduce the midsection is to do abdominal exercises. (true or false)

   The statement would appear to be true. Many people believe that when certain muscles are exercised, the fatty tissues in the immediate area are "burned up." In other words, if you bend at the waist often enough, you'll trim down your midsection.

   Several years ago, however, a team of doctors studied a number of tennis players to see if the "spot" theory of fat reduction was fact. The subjects chosen for the study played tennis an average of six or more hours a week. The playing arm of each was subjected to more exercise than the other arm. The doctors expected to find the working limb larger because the muscles were more developed, and that is what they found. When the amount of fat was measured, however, it was the same on both arms for all the subjects.

Compared with a group of similar non-tennis playing individuals, however, the players had less fat in both arms than their more sedentary peers. The conclusion is that exercise causes fat to be burned from all over the body and not from one specific area, regardless of the type of exercise.

So the statement is false. Despite claims to the contrary, "spot reducing" doesn't work. It is impossible to reduce the amount of fat in a particular area without affecting the amount in other parts of the body.

2. To maintain an adequate level of physical fitness, one needs to exercise at least _____ days a week. (fill in the blank)

No one denies that a sedentary life leads to physical deterioration, but until recently scientists were unable to pinpoint specific bodily changes. The advent of space travel, however, has changed all that. Studies conducted by NASA scientists show that muscles that are not exercised regularly deteriorate at a phenomenal rate. For example, for every three days that a person is immobile, he loses one-fifth of his maximal muscle strength. Other findings are equally disturbing. Immobility adversely affects the circulatory system, the respiratory system, the digestive system, and even the nervous system. While the changes brought about by sedentary living are not as dramatic as those demonstrated in the NASA laboratories, they are no less real. The difference is only in degree. Fortunately, exercising reverses the degenerative changes. Muscles quickly return to normal and metabolic systems respond positively.

What does this mean to you?

After extensive testing, NASA scientists concluded that, while daily exercise is desirable, three nonconsecutive days of programmed activity each week will maintain an adequate level of physical fitness. Just as the body cannot store certain vitamins but must have them regularly, it likewise cannot store certain conditioning effects of exercise. After forty-eight to seventy-two hours, one must use the muscles again to reestablish the desirable physical effects. You therefore should exercise at least three days a week. Of course, you can use a daily schedule.

3. The amount of perspiration indicates your level of fitness. (true or false)

Frequently people say they want to "work up a good sweat" when they exercise. In fact, some of them even don special rubber suits that make them perspire more profusely.

While exercising, we produce extra heat—in proportion to the amount of muscle activity. The body's temperature could easily rise as much as 10°F or more if this energy wasn't dissipated. Fortunately, the body is designed to keep itself from overheating. Warm blood is brought to the skin where it loses heat to the surrounding air. The sweat glands begin to secrete water and the body is further cooled by evaporation of the perspiration. In cool weather, heat is given off easily, but when the environmental temperature rises, the body must work harder to cool itself and sweating becomes more profuse. Sweating, however, doesn't do anything other than lower body temperature: it does not help you reduce. You may weigh less immediately after a workout, but this is a result of water loss. Replace the lost liquid and you'll regain the weight. Sweating does not "clean the pores" either—there is no evidence that it is of any value in removing toxic materials from the body. Perspiration does not promote fitness. Fitness is developed by exercising the muscles of the body, not the sweat glands. The statement above is false.

4. You burn more calories jogging one mile than walking the same distance. (true or false)

Work is defined as the energy required to move a given weight through a given distance. A 120-pound woman expends equal amounts of energy (i.e., does the same amount of work) traveling one mile, whether she walks or jogs.

So the statement is false.

Remember, of course, that you can jog a mile faster than you can walk it. If you jog rather than walk for thirty minutes you'll cover more distance and, consequently, burn more calories.

5. If your breathing doesn't return to normal within ten minutes after you finish exercising, you've exerted yourself too much. (true or false)

Exercise does not have to be strenuous to be beneficial. In fact, if it is too difficult, it can prove harmful. A good rule of thumb is that your breathing should return to normal within ten minutes after you've finished your routine. This statement is true.

There are some other guidelines to help you determine if you are working too hard. Ten minutes after exercising you shouldn't feel your heart pounding in your chest nor should you be "all pooped out." In fact, you should begin to experience a "comeback" sensation. Too much exercise may make sleeping difficult and can produce fatigue into the next day. Exercise should not be strenuous, unpleasant, and exhausting; it should be moderate, enjoyable, and refreshing.

6. Walking is one of the best exercises. (true or false)

Physical anthropologists say human bone structure makes us the perfect walkers—ever notice how long your legs are in proportion to the rest of your body? But you don't see many people walking anymore. The "Don't Walk" light on busy street corners is not just a warning to pedestrians. It has become a sign of our times—that pedestrians are on the way out. That is too bad because walking is one of the best exercises known. It helps circulation of blood throughout the body and thus has a direct effect on your overall feeling of well-being. This statement is true.

7. Vigorous stretching exercises keep muscles flexible. (true or false)

Flexibility comes from stretching the muscles and tendons that move the joints. This elasticity produces a smooth and graceful carriage—straight back, full gait, square shoulders. The look is easy to achieve if you do the proper exercises the correct way. Most people choose the right activities; the problem is that they don't practice them properly.

For example, if you want to stretch the hamstrings—the muscles that run up the back of your thighs—you should sit on the floor, legs flat in front of you, and bend forward. Most people, anxious to "get on with it," will start bouncing and bobbing in an attempt to stretch out those tight hamstrings. What they are actually doing, however, is defeating the purpose. The muscles will become tighter, not more flexible.

Stretching exercises should be done slowly, deliberately, and carefully, allowing the muscles to relax and let go. So the statement is false. Vigorous training encourages tightness. When doing stretching exercises, move slowly; when the first sign of pain occurs, hold that position for several seconds, then relax. Repeat the exercise several times.

8. It is possible to get enough exercise from one's ordinary daily activities. (true or false)

Exercise used to be commonplace. People didn't go around touching their toes or doing push-ups, but before the industrial revolution, most work was physical. It entailed movement and exercise. Today we use machines to do many tasks, and to do all the "exercising" involved. You can mow your lawn while sitting down, and brush your teeth without moving your arm, and "let your fingers do the walking" in the telephone directory. Unless your job involves manual labor, it's almost impossible to find an opportunity to exercise in the course of an ordinary day. So although the question is debatable, usually the answer is false.

Granted there are still those who walk when they could ride, climb steps instead of taking the elevator, and hang clothes on the line instead of tossing them in the dryer, but do *you* know anyone who does? The conveniences are just too convenient for most of us to forgo.

Years ago people were trying to find ways to do less exercise. Now they are trying to find ways to do more. If you find it easy to program exercise into your daily routine, then, by all means, do so. If you're like most people, however, you are going to have to set aside some time for regular exercise.

9. The minimum amount of time you should spend exercising is
1 3 5 10 15 20 30 60 minutes.
(circle your answer)

There are more than four hundred skeletal muscles in the body. They are responsible for movement of the joints, maintenance of posture, support of body weight, circulation of blood, and for respiration and elimination. When muscles are used they stay firm, strong, supple, and shapely. When they are not used they become limp, weak, inflexible, and shapeless.

An exercise program should involve all of the muscles. It should put the joints through their full range of motion. Some joints, such as the knee and elbow, are "hinge" joints; they basically move in only one plane—straightening and bending the limbs. Other joints allow a wider range of motion. The hip joint, a ball-socket type, permits movement forward, backward and to the sides, as well as in a rotating motion. The spine, which is really a series of joints, also facilitates movement in three planes. One can twist the trunk, and bend forward, backward, and to either side.

In addition, all skeletal muscles work in pairs—in opposition to one another. While one muscle moves a joint, another relaxes to permit the movement to take place. For example, when you bend your arm, the biceps contract while the triceps relax. When you straighten your arm, the reverse occurs.

A good exercise routine should contract and stretch all the major muscle groups, and this simply cannot be done with four or five exercises in five minutes. Research indicates about fifteen minutes or more is the minimum amount of time needed for an adequate workout.

10. It takes 7   14   21   30   60   120 days to become physically fit. (circle your answer)

How long it takes you to become physically fit depends on how fit or unfit you are when you start. If you're out of condition, you certainly can't shape up in twenty-one days, as one book claims. You can, however, make significant progress in three weeks and be well on the way to becoming physically fit in time.

The question is really moot, because shaping up does not do any good unless you plan to stay in shape, and that means exercising—from now on. Don't think in terms of how long it will take you to get in shape, but rather in terms of a life plan to keep that way.

EFFECTS OF A HEALTHY LIFE-STYLE

The human body is a marvelous and intricate machine. From two cells, contributed by the mother and father, develop millions of cells that make up the blood, bone, muscle, nerves, skin, and other systems and organs.

We start to grow old at an early age. Physical vitality begins to decrease at about age twenty, and then at a more rapid rate, depending on the changing habits of individuals as they grow older.

Mankind has always tried to find ways to increase the length of life. According to Dr. Walter Bortz of Stanford University, the human body may have the capacity to live 120 years. His contention is that by abusing this wonderful machine, we create conditions that bring about death around the age of seventy.

The evidence is clear that we don't have to die at this age if we are willing to use preventive medicine as a means to bring about a longer, more productive, and healthier life. It may be that the time has come for mankind to shift from a curative to a preventive approach to medicine. This is not a new consideration. Thomas Jefferson, more than two-hundred years ago, stated: "The doctor of the future will give no medicine, but will interest his patients in the care of the human body in diet and in the causes and prevention of disease." No pill, vaccine, or injection can completely offset the diseases brought on by an unhealthy life-style. In order to bring about positive results, it is necessary to change our life-styles.

The question that arises is What changes should I consider if I want to live longer and have a better quality of life? Some answers have been produced by a five-and-one-half-year study that was conducted by the UCLA School of Public Health in Alameda County in northern California. The study consisted of some seven thousand adults and was designed to determine what daily practices might result in an increase in life expectancy. As a result of this research, some basic health practices are found among people who live longer and healthier lives and are missing among people who suffer from degenerative diseases earlier in life.

Following are some basic health practices that were found to contribute to longevity.

1. Healthy people maintain a normal body weight. Dr. Jeremiah Stamler, who co-authored the book *Your Heart Has Nine Lives,* states, "The overweight man—depending on the amount of blubber—is two to three times more susceptible to heart disease than his neighbor of normal weight."

   Compared with persons of proper weight, people with excess body fat have a higher risk of developing cancer, hypertension, diabetes, diseases of the heart and circulatory system, and many types of bone and joint diseases.

   Some research indicates that a child who is obese when entering adolescence has only one chance in four of ever achieving normal weight and those who leave adolescence in an obese state have only one chance in twenty-eight of ever achieving proper weight.

   The late Dr. Paul Dudley White, a noted heart specialist, may have been right when he said, "Intemperance in food may be more dangerous than intemperance in alcohol or tobacco."

2. Another common practice among longer-living people was that they ate breakfast.

   A survey has revealed that almost half the adults in the United States don't eat breakfast. A study conducted at the University of Iowa indicated that people who skip breakfast are less efficient, less attentive, and more clumsy when compared to those who eat breakfast. The approximate twelve-hour time span since the last meal may deprive a person of essential nutrients needed for good performance.

Sometimes people who are trying to lose weight skip breakfast. A study at the University of Minnesota revealed that dieters placed on a diet of 2,000 calories per day and told to eat all 2,000 calories in only one meal lost significantly more weight when the calories were consumed during the breakfast meal.

This advice might be true: "Eat breakfast like a king, eat lunch like a prince, but eat dinner like a pauper."

3. Healthy people tend to sleep no more than seven to eight hours each night.

According to Dr. Ernest Hartmann of Boston State Hospital's Sleep Laboratory, people who regularly need more than nine hours of sleep are likely to be rebellious, opinionated, critical, chronic worriers, insecure, anxious, and indecisive.

Dr. Allen Rechtschaffen of the University of Chicago has stated that people who sleep nine or more hours a night are more prone to strokes and heart disease than short sleepers.

4. Another contributor to longevity was not smoking.

Smoking contributes to heart disease, cancer, emphysema, ulcers, and chronic bronchitis. Pregnant women who smoke increase the risk of miscarriage, birth defects that might be fatal, and complications during labor.

It has been estimated that on the average, cigarette smokers remove nearly eight and one-half years from their life.

The sad fact is that not only smoking, but continual exposure to someone else's smoke can be hazardous to your health. Dr. Peter Fong of Emory University contends that nonsmokers who are in frequent contact with tobacco smoke run the risk of losing three years of their life. He stated, "The point is, nuclear energy accidents or just radiation in general, account for a trivially small number of deaths compared to cigarette smoke, but everyone makes a tremendous fuss over that. No one pays much attention to whether cigarette smoke is present in the air."

5. People who live longer exercise regularly.

The human body was designed to be exercised. When we become inactive, the joints stiffen, the muscles weaken, the circulatory system is affected by increased fats, the heart loses strength, and thus, we become more prone to injury and disease.

It is possible to add years to your life, according to Dr. Ralph Paffenbarger, Jr., of the Stanford University School of Medicine. A study conducted by himself and other researchers of 16,936 Harvard alumni found that men who exercised regularly increased their lifespans by one to more than two years when compared to their sedentary counterparts.

The optimum expenditure of energy in exercise seems to be about 3,500 calories per week. Moreover, it may be that a lifetime of engaging in exercise could reduce the negative health effects of cigarette smoking or high blood pressure. It may even partly offset an inherited tendency toward early death. Paffenbarger makes the point that the years of life gained through exercise are comparable to the amount gained if a cure for cancer could be found. A regular exercise program not only improves the quality of life, but also its length.

The late Dr. Paul Dudley White has called the span from age twenty to forty the critical years in a person's life. During these years, we settle into a certain life-style that may very well determine our physical condition when we reach fifty and sixty.

Thus, it is important that we look at the life-style we lead and, if necessary, make the changes needed to bring about a longer and happier life.

Research indicates that engaging in vigorous exercise can partially retard physical deterioration and bring about the following benefits:

1. Physically active individuals are less likely than those who are sedentary to experience a heart attack or other form of cardiovascular disease. An active person who does suffer a coronary attack will probably have a less severe form and will be more likely to survive the experience.

2. Physical activity is as important as diet in maintaining proper weight. Being overweight is more than a matter of individual discomfort; it is related to several chronic diseases, shortened life expectancy, and emotional problems. Medical authorities now recommend that weight reduction be accomplished by a reasonable increase in daily physical activity supplemented, if

necessary, by proper dietary controls. Jean Mayer, one of the world's foremost nutritionists, has reported that he is "convinced that inactivity is the most important factor explaining the frequency of 'creeping' overweight in modern societies."

3. Most medical authorities support the belief (and most active people will testify to it) that exercise helps a person look, feel, and work better. Various organs and systems of the body are stimulated through activity and, as a result, function more effectively. Proper exercise that increases the tone of supporting muscles can also improve posture. This not only improves appearance but also can decrease the frequency of lower-back pain and disability.

4. Increased physical fitness is worth money to you. Did you know that being overly fat can lower your chances of getting a job or winning a promotion? One research report involving 50,000 executive positions estimated that excess fat can cost an executive ten thousand dollars a year in potential salary. A California utility company recently gave its overweight employees six months to reduce or face unemployment One large southwestern city is even stricter. It refuses to hire anyone who is 15 percent overweight.

   The National Aeronautics and Space Administration conducted a study with its employees that showed the physical condition of workers brings back dollar dividends. After one year of participating in an exercise program, it was found that more than 60 percent of the people had improved work performance and had more positive attitudes toward their jobs.

   Dr. Roy Shepard, internationally known physician and exercise physiologist from Canada, states that through the use of an appropriate fitness program it is possible to improve the working capacity of people by at least 15 to 20 percent.

5. People who are habitual exercisers usually state that one of the reasons they exercise is that they "feel better" as a result of engaging in vigorous physical activity. It appears that physical activities provide an opportunity for the individual to enjoy a feeling of success that, in turn, may reinforce a positive self-concept and body image.

There is some current research that supports this fact. The body has the capacity to produce a substance called **beta-endorphins.** They have a characteristic similar to that of morphine, and can act as painkillers by binding the nerve receptor sites to prevent the transmission of pain.

Exercise appears to stimulate the release of these body chemicals and thus reduces the onset of the pain stimulus. Laboratory studies have shown that runners are less sensitive to pain while they are running.

Two St. Louis University researchers, Dr. Thomas Forrester and Dr. Alexander R. Lind, report that exercise may release extremely small amounts of the chemical adenosine triphosphate (ATP). This in turn causes the blood vessels to dilate and bring circulation in the brain to near the maximum possible level.

It may be that this release of ATP and beta-endorphins may lead to the sensation that many exercisers feel and describe as euphoria: it makes them feel better and think more clearly.

The relationship between participation in physical activity and a sense of well-being has yet to be scientifically proven. The important factor is that people state they feel better as a result of exercise and they perform better when faced by physical demands.

Roger Bannister states these feelings in his book *First Four Minutes*. He explains how he felt as a barefoot boy on the sand of the beach.

In this supreme moment I leapt in sheer joy. I was startled and frightened by the tremendous excitement that so few steps could create. I glanced around uneasily to see if anyone was watching. A few more steps—self-consciously now and firmly gripping the original excitement. The earth seemed almost to move with me. I was running now, and a fresh rhythm entered my body. No longer conscious of my movement I discovered a new unity with nature. I had found a new source of power and beauty, a source I never dreamt existed. From intense moments like this, love of running can grow. . . . This attempt at explanation is of course inadequate, just like any analysis of the things we enjoy—like the description of a rose to someone who has never seen one."[1]

6. Perhaps the greatest benefit of maintaining physical fitness is the degree of independence it affords. Research indicates that a fit person

1. Roger Bannister, *First Four Minutes* (London: Corgi Special, 1957), pp. 11–12.

uses less energy for any given movement or task than a flabby or weak person. This is an asset to be most prized in one's later years when energy levels may be lower.

If people don't engage in some sort of an exercise program, it is estimated that they will lose about 1 percent of their muscle mass every year. This means that by the age of seventy, the limit of endurance might be on the order of approximately three miles per hour. As the thigh muscles become weakened, the average eighty-year-old is taxed to the limit when attempting to get up from a sitting position. Because of the weakened condition of the muscles of the body, it is impossible for many older people to cross the street in the time allotted by the traffic signals. It has been estimated that if we increase the strength of the thigh muscles by only 10 percent, we can postpone the day of losing our independence by ten to twenty years.

Exercise that at one time was considered too strenuous and even dangerous for older persons is now being prescribed as a form of preventive medicine. The positive results seem to indicate that a proper training program can help ward off the effects of aging and improve both physical and mental well-being. Dr. Frederick Swartz, a spokesperson for the American Medical Association, reported to a Senate subcommittee that poor fitness is the elderly's greatest health problem and that exercise could have a tremendous impact on reducing morbidity and mortality rates.

There is great psychological and financial advantage in knowing that you can plan and carry out activities without depending upon relatives, friends, or hired help. To drive your own car, to succeed with do-it-yourself projects rather than trying to find and pay someone else for the service, to come and go as you please, to be an asset rather than a liability in emergencies—these are forms of personal freedom well worth the effort.

A PERSONALIZED FITNESS PROGRAM

Many people realize that there is a need for exercise but are confused by the question of how much is needed and what type is best. People should be prepared to accept the responsibility for their own physical well-being and that of their families. People should have the knowledge to select those activities that will be of value in meeting immediate and future fitness needs.

When you have completed your study of this text, you will be able to write a program for males or females of any age, using an exercise plan that has been scientifically developed.

In learning to write and engage in fitness programs, you will be able to improve your own and your family's physical condition by using a variety of exercises suitable to various temperaments and inclinations. No longer will the questions "How much?" and "What type of exercise?" be a puzzle. The objective of this text is to help you learn to maintain your own physical fitness so that you can enjoy a longer, happier, healthier, and more productive life.

OBJECTIVES FOR FITNESS

The average individual lacks the knowledge of how to increase or maintain cardiovascular endurance, control body weight, develop an adequate amount of strength and flexibility, or write a relaxation program.

You can realize definite fitness objectives by utilizing a *Fitness for Life* program.

Cardiovascular Endurance Objectives

1. You will be able to administer cardiovascular endurance tests correctly and interpret the results.
2. Given a person's age, weight, fitness category, and exercise preference, you will be able to write a personalized cardiovascular endurance program.
3. As a result of engaging in a personalized program, you will be able to increase and/or maintain your own cardiovascular endurance level.

Weight-Control Objectives

1. You will be able to administer and interpret tests correctly to determine proper body weight.
2. Given a person's sex, current weight, desired target weight, and activity preference, you will be able to write a personalized weight-control program.
3. As a result of engaging in a personalized weight-control program, you will be able to reach your proper weight and maintain the preferred level.

Strength Objectives

1. You will be able to administer a strength test correctly and interpret the results.
2. Given a person's choice of strength exercises, you will be able to write a personalized strength program.

3. As a result of engaging in a personalized strength program, you will be able to increase your own strength levels.

Flexibility Objectives

1. You will be able to administer flexibility tests correctly and interpret the results.
2. Given a person's choice of flexibility exercises, you will be able to write a personalized flexibility program.
3. As a result of engaging in a personalized flexibility program, you will be able to increase your own flexibility levels.

Relaxation Objectives

1. You will be able to evaluate your life-style to determine how vulnerable you are to stress and tension.
2. You will be able to write a personalized relaxation program.
3. As a result of engaging in a personalized relaxation program, you will be able to apply relaxation techniques to combat stress and tension.

SELF-CHECKS

At the end of most chapters there are self-checks to enable you to determine if you understand the material contained in the chapter, and to determine whether further practice is needed on the case studies included for that program. It is suggested that you pass these self-checks before proceeding to the next chapter.

SUGGESTIONS FOR FURTHER READING

1. American Heart Association. 1983 Heart Fact Reference Sheet. Dallas: American Heart Association, 1983.
2. Bartley, Dianne A. R., and Faye Z. Belgrave. "Physical Fitness and Psychological Well-being in College Students." *Health Education* 18 June–July (1987): no. 3, p. 57.
3. Bennett, J. "Effect of a Program of Physical Exercise on Depression in Older Adults." *Physical Educator* 39 March (1982):21.
4. Booth, G. M., R. E. Seegmiller, S. S. Zimmerman, and M. L. Lee. *Toward A Healthier Lifestyle.* Creative Publications: Orem, Utah, 1986.
5. Bortz, W. "The Runner's High." *Runner's World* 17 April (1982): no. 4, p. 58.
6. Folkins, C. H., S. Lynch, M. L. Pollock, and N. N. Cordner. "Psychological Fitness as a Function of Physical Fitness." *Archives of Physical Medicine and Rehabilitation* 53(1972):503.
7. Gettman, L. R., J. J. Ayres, M. L. Pollock, and A. Jackson. "The Effect of Circuit Weight Training on Strength, Cardiorespiratory Function, and Body Composition of Adult Man." *Medicine and Science in Sports* 10(1978): no. 3, p. 171.
8. Gilliam, T. G. "Exercise Programs for Children: A Way to Prevent Heart Disease?" *The Physician and Sports Medicine* 10 September (1982): no. 9, p. 96.
9. Goodman, C. E. "Low Back Pain in the Cosmetic Athlete." *The Physician and Sports Medicine* 15 August (1987): no. 8, p. 97.
10. Hanson, J. S., and W. H. Nedde. "Long-term Physical Training Effect in Sedentary Females." *Journal of Applied Physiology* 37(1974):112.
11. Hutchinson, P. L. "Metabolic and Circulatory Responses to Running during Pregnancy." *The Physician and Sports Medicine* 9 August (1981): no. 8, p. 55.
12. Kannel, W. B., and P. Sorlie. "Some Health Benefits of Physical Activity: The Framingham Study." *Archives of Internal Medicine* 139(1979):857.
13. Kraus, H., and W. Roab. *Hypokinetic Disease.* Springfield, Illinois: Charles C. Thomas, 1961.
14. Leon, A. S. "Age and Other Predictors of Coronary Heart Disease." *Medicine and Science in Sports and Exercise* 19 April (1987): no. 2, p. 159.
15. Maness, B. "What Do You Really Know About Exercise?" *Today's Health* 53(1975):14.
16. McCunney, R. J. "Fitness, Heart Disease, and High-Density Lipoproteins: A Look at the Relationships." *The Physician and Sports Medicine* 15 February (1987): no. 2, p. 67.
17. Paffenbarger, R. S., R. T. Hyde, A. L. Wing, and C. Hsieh. "Physical Activity, All-Cause Mortality, and Longevity of College Alumni." *New England Journal of Medicine* 314(1986): no. 10, p. 605.
18. Seefeldt, V.; Editor. *Physical Activity and Well-being.* Reston, Virginia: AAHPERD, 1986.
19. Shangold, M. M. "Sports and Menstrual Function." *The Physician and Sports Medicine* 8 August (1980): no. 8, p. 66.
20. Sharkey, B. J. "Functional vs. Chronologic Age." *Medicine and Science in Sports and Exercise* 19 April (1987): no. 2, p. 174.
21. Shepard, R. J. "Human Rights and the Older Worker: Changes in Work Capacity with Age." *Medicine and Science in Sports and Exercise* 19 April (1987): no. 2, p. 168.
22. Shepard, R. J. *Economic Benefits of Enhanced Fitness.* Champaign, Illinois: Human Kinetics, 1986.
23. Simon, D. G., and J. G. Travell. "Myofascial Origins of Low Back Pain." *Postgraduate Medicine* 73(1983):66.

24. Snow-Harter, C. "Biochemical Changes in Postmenopausal Women Following a Muscle Fitness Program." *The Physician and Sports Medicine* 15 August (1987): no. 8, p. 90.

25. Stewart, K. J., and B. Gutin. "Effects of Physical Training on Cardiorespiratory Fitness in Children." *The Research Quarterly* 47 (1976):110.

26. *The Health Letter,* "Status of Preventing Heart Attacks and Strokes." Volume 30, No. 6, September 25, 1987.

27. *The Physician and Sports Medicine,* "Physiological Adaptations to Chronic Endurance Exercise Training in Patients with Coronary Artery Disease—A Round Table." Volume 15, No. 9, September, 1987, p. 128.

28. Thompson, P. D., and A. Burfoot. "The Heart of the Matter." *Runners World* 21 August (1986): no. 8, p. 30.

29. Thornberry, O. T., and P. Golden. "Health Promotion and Disease Prevention: Provisional Data from the National Health Interview Survey—United States, January–June 1985." Advance Data from Vital and Health Statistics of National Center Health Sciences, Hyattsville, Maryland.

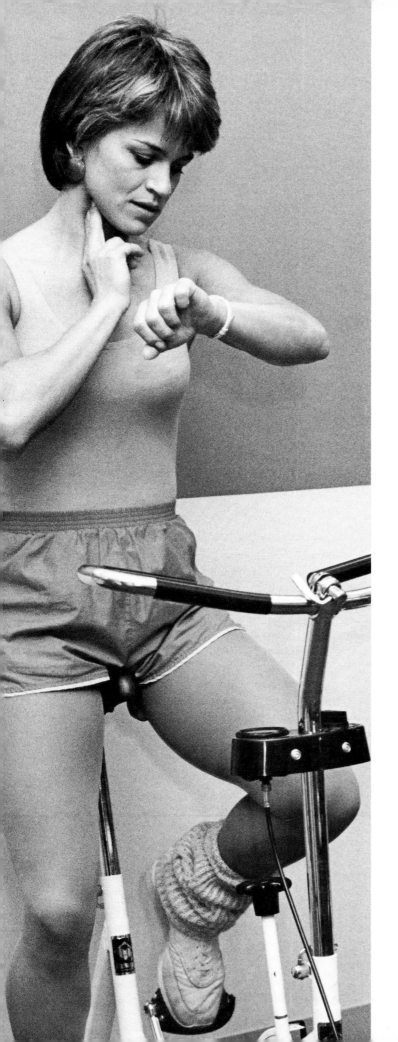

2

FITNESS APPRAISAL

Objectives

After study of this chapter you should be able to

1. administer and correctly interpret tests for
   a. cardiovascular endurance
   b. body weight
   c. strength
   d. flexibility;
2. pass a multiple-choice mastery check involving the selection of appropriate results of tests of
   a. cardiovascular endurance
   b. body weight
   c. strength
   d. flexibility;
3. evaluate your life-style to determine how vulnerable you are to stress and tension.

Ask average American automobile owners about their cars, and they will be able to tell you about miles per gallon, the proper oil weight, amount of air in the tires, and a flood of other information. Ask them about their physical fitness, however, and they will be hard pressed for an answer. What is worse, they probably will not know how to obtain this information.

In order to plan a trip, whether it is a journey to New York City or a journey to obtain improved physical fitness, you must know where you are starting and where you are going. Then you must have some means of knowing whether you have reached your destination or goal. The tests selected for the *Fitness for Life* program were chosen for ease of administration and for the valid and reliable information that can be obtained from each test. If you are serious about the objectives of physical fitness, you must attempt to evaluate them in order to determine your current status, your needs, and the effectiveness of your selected programs.

In this chapter you will be able to test correctly and interpret the results for

1. cardiovascular endurance;
2. body weight;
3. strength;
4. flexibility; and
5. stress and tension.

BASIC MEDICAL PREREQUISITES

Before starting any fitness program, you should consider some basic medical requirements. Under certain circumstances, exercise can be a risk; but do not forget that the hazards of sedentary living are far greater than most risks associated with exercise. Any problems that you might encounter in beginning a fitness program can be prevented in most cases by following some basic medical guidelines.

The Connecticut Mutual Life Insurance Company has compiled a screening questionnaire for people who are considering exercise programs. If you answer *yes* to any of the following questions, then you should check with your doctor. There is a possibility that a medical problem could hamper your fitness program. Remember, an ounce of prevention is worth a pound of cure!

1. Have you ever had pains or a sensation of pressure in your chest that occurred with exertion, lasted a few minutes, and then subsided with resting?
2. Do you get chest discomfort when climbing stairs, walking against a cold wind, or during any physical or emotional activity?
3. Does your heart ever beat unevenly or irregularly or seem to flutter or skip beats?
4. Do you have sudden bursts of very rapid heart action or periods of very slow heart action without apparent cause?
5. Do you take any prescription medicine on a regular basis?
6. Has your electrocardiogram at rest or during exercise ever been abnormal?
7. Do you have any respiratory problems such as emphysema, asthma, wheezing, chronic bronchitis, or do you experience an unusual breathlessness or exertion that is more than that experienced by others doing the same thing?
8. Do you have arthritis, rheumatism, gout, or any condition affecting your joints?
9. Do you have any orthopedic problems affecting your feet, ankles, knees, or hips that cause pain or limit your motion in any way?
10. Do you have a bad back, a sacroiliac or a disc problem?
11. Do you have any known cardiac condition that might prohibit an exercise program?
12. Are you aware of any risk factors, such as high blood pressure (**hypertension**), overweight (by more than 30 percent), diabetes, or high blood-fat levels? Are you a heavy smoker? Do your relatives have a history of heart disease?

One of the tests that your doctor might suggest is an **EKG** or **electrocardiogram.** This is a graphic tracing of the electric current produced by the contraction of your heart muscle. Your doctor, by examining this tracing taken during exercise, can determine any abnormalities that might indicate whether or not you are qualified to engage in an exercise program.

Some general guidelines concerning medical checkups follow.

Under 30: Medical checkup within the past year
30–39: Medical checkup with resting EKG
40 and above: Medical checkup with exercise EKG

By observing these basic medical requirements you can safely participate in a fitness program.

CARDIOVASCULAR ENDURANCE

Cardiovascular endurance is defined as the ability of the heart, lungs, and circulatory system to provide the cells of the body with the substances necessary to perform work for long periods of time. One of the best and most accurate measures of an individual's cardiovascular endurance is the maximum amount of oxygen the body can use. This can be measured very accurately in a laboratory, using a treadmill or bicycle ergometer. The gases drawn in from the atmosphere and the gases expired from the lungs are collected and analyzed to determine the body's ability to use oxygen during activity.

Obviously, such detailed laboratory procedures are too time consuming and impractical for mass use. Dr. Kenneth Cooper of the Institute for Aerobics Research has developed a simple test that correlates very well with laboratory measurements. The test involves measuring the time spent in running 1.5 miles. The time needed to cover the 1.5 miles is then used to determine the fitness category of the individual. Despite its simplicity and ease of administration, this field test is almost as accurate and reliable as laboratory measurements of a gas analysis obtained in tests on a treadmill. The test is easy to administer and easy to interpret. Individuals can very quickly assess their own cardiovascular endurance fitness category for themselves or for anyone else. Periodic evaluation of progress can also be determined by comparing fitness categories over specific lengths of time.

If a person cannot participate in the 1.5-mile test, there is an excellent alternative method to determine cardiovascular endurance fitness levels. This is the 3-mile walk test and it is a submaximal test that is easy to administer and doesn't place a great amount of stress on the individual. The same steps would be utilized in administering and interpreting this test as are explained in the following section concerning the 1.5-mile test.

ADMINISTERING AND INTERPRETING CARDIOVASCULAR ENDURANCE TESTS

The purpose of this unit is to provide you with a simple and safe method of measuring your cardiovascular endurance or that of someone else. By using the Cardiovascular Endurance Work Sheet in Appendix C, administering and interpreting a cardiovascular endurance test is a simple three-step process.

Step 1. Fill out the test form.
Step 2. Plan and administer the fitness test.
Step 3. Interpret the test correctly.

To help you become familiar with these procedures, we will go through them step-by-step, using a sample case.

CASE
Sally Harrison

Sally is nineteen years old. She has been a regular exerciser for the past six months. She had a medical examination two months ago and was considered to be in good health. Sally would like to take the cardiovascular endurance test.

Step 1: Filling out the test form

Item 1. Fill in Sally's name, sex, and age.

Item 2. Since Sally had a medical checkup two months ago and was given a clean bill of health, check *No Restrictions*. If she had not had a medical clearance, you would check the blank next to *Restrictions* and skip immediately to item 4.

Item 3. Sally has been a regular exerciser for the past six months, so check *Conditioned Beginner*. A **conditioned beginner** is defined as an individual who has been engaging in a continuous, large muscle activity for fifteen or more minutes and for three or more days per week for at least four weeks. If your subject had not been exercising regularly, you would check *Unconditioned Beginner*.

Item 4. Now you must determine whether your subject does or does not have clearance to take a cardiovascular endurance test. Use the chart in item 4 to help you find your subject's physical condition. To the right of these, in the *Test Clearance* column, you will find either a

Yes (indicating that the person does have test clearance) or a *No* (indicating that the person does not have test clearance). The *Suggestion* column will tell you what the subject must do to gain test clearance.

Sally is a conditioned beginner, so check the blank next to *Yes* for test clearance. If you check the *No* blank for a person, then you must determine whether it is necessary to get a medical examination or complete the beginner's program. An explanation of the beginner's program will be given in chapter 3, "Writing a Cardiovascular Endurance Program."

Item 5. Sally selects the 1.5-mile run as the test to be utilized. Check the blank next to 1.5-mile run.

Item 6. Fill in the time and place where the test will be administered. Sally will run on the high school track at 4:00 P.M. on Tuesday.

Step 2: Planning and administering the cardiovascular endurance test

Before administering the test you must do the following:

1. Determine the length of the testing area. Most school tracks are one-fourth mile in length.
2. Have a clock or stopwatch available to time your subject.

3. Have your subject warm up just before testing (i.e., walking, calisthenics, stretching, or slow jogging).

4. Give instructions to Sally, the person being tested: "You should cover the 1.5-mile distance in the fastest time you can. If you experience nausea during the test, *stop* immediately, and do not attempt the test again until you have completed the beginner's cardiovascular endurance program."

Item 7. At the conclusion of the test, enter the test time in the blank next to item 7. Remember, do not allow Sally to sit or lie down immediately after the test. Be sure she cools down slowly by walking or jogging slowly for about five minutes. (Sally's time for the 1.5-mile run was 13:23.)

Step 3: Interpreting the test correctly

At the bottom of the work sheet use the chart to locate Sally's age and sex category. Look down the 13–19 age column for women until you find the time range in which Sally's time of 13:23 is contained (12:30–14:30). Then, by tracing your finger to the left along the row of numbers, you will find in the extreme left column Sally's fitness category *(IV—Good)*.

Item 8. Now that you have determined that Sally's fitness category is *IV—Good,* make a check by the proper category in item 8. Once you know Sally's fitness category you can use this information as a guide in writing a cardiovascular endurance program for her. When you have completed Sally's Cardiovascular Endurance Test Work Sheet, check your copy with the completed work sheet in figure 2.1.

MASTERY CHECK INSTRUCTIONS

PART I

Instructions: Information follows about two people who would like to take a cardiovascular endurance test. Study each case and answer the questions.

A. Susan Young is twenty-eight years old. She had a medical examination two months ago, with a resting EKG, and was considered to be in good health. Since that time, she has been exercising regularly three days a week. She would like to take the 1.5-mile test.
1. Does the person requesting the test have medical clearance?
   a. Yes
   b. No
2. In what physical condition is the person requesting the test?
   a. Unconditioned beginner
   b. Conditioned beginner
3. What should your decision be?
   a. Suggest a beginner's program.
   b. Suggest a proper medical examination prior to testing.
   c. Administer a cardiovascular endurance test.

B. Jack Jacobsen, age forty-two, had a physical examination with an exercise EKG last week and was considered to be in good health. He has been inactive for some time but would like to take the 1.5-mile run.
1. Does the person requesting the test have medical clearance?
   a. Yes
   b. No
2. In what physical condition is the person requesting the test?
   a. Unconditioned beginner
   b. Conditioned beginner
3. What should your decision be?
   a. Suggest a beginner's program.
   b. Suggest a proper medical examination prior to testing.
   c. Administer a cardiovascular endurance test.

Cardiovascular Endurance Test Work Sheet

1. Name _Sally Harrison_ _____ Sex _Female_ Age _19_

2. Medical Clearance: No Restrictions ____X____ Restrictions _____

3. Physical Condition: Unconditioned Beginner _____
   Conditioned Beginner ____X____

4. **Physical Condition**   **Test Clearance**   **Suggestion**

Physical Condition	Test Clearance	Suggestion
No medical clearance	No	Get medical examination
Unconditioned beginner	No	Complete beginner's program
Conditioned beginner	Yes	

Test Clearance: Yes ____X____ No _____
If no: Subject must have a medical exam _____
Subject must complete beginner's program _____

5. Test: 1.5-mile run ____X____ 3-mile walk _____

6. When test will be held _Tuesday, 4:00 PM_ Where _High School Track_

7. Time for 1.5-mile run ___13:23___ Time for 3-mile walk _____

8. Fitness Category: _____ I. Very Poor   _____ III. Fair   _____ V. Excellent
                    _____ II. Poor   __X__ IV. Good   _____ VI. Superior

(These tables give times in minutes and seconds.)

1.5-Mile Run Test

Age (years)

Fitness Category		13–19	20–29	30–39	40–49	50–59	60+
I. Very Poor	(men)	>15:31*	>16:01	>16:31	>17:31	>19:01	>20:01
	(women)	>18:31	>19:01	>19:31	>20:01	>20:31	>21:01
II. Poor	(men)	12:11–15:30	14:01–16:00	14:44–16:30	15:36–17:30	17:01–19:00	19:01–20:00
	(women)	16:55–18:30	18:31–19:00	19:01–19:30	19:31–20:00	20:01–20:30	20:31–21:00
III. Fair	(men)	10:49–12:10	12:01–14:00	12:31–14:45	13:01–15:35	14:31–17:00	16:16–19:00
	(women)	14:31–16:54	15:55–18:30	16:31–19:00	17:31–19:30	19:01–20:00	19:31–20:30
IV. Good	(men)	9:41–10:48	10:46–12:00	11:01–12:30	11:31–13:00	12:31–14:30	14:00–16:15
	(women)	12:30–14:30	13:31–15:54	14:31–16:30	15:56–17:30	16:31–19:00	17:31–19:30
V. Excellent	(men)	8:37– 9:40	9:45–10:45	10:00–11:00	10:30–11:30	11:00–12:30	11:15–13:59
	(women)	11:50–12:29	12:30–13:30	13:00–14:30	13:45–15:55	14:30–16:30	16:30–17:30
VI. Superior	(men)	< 8:37	< 9:45	<10:00	<10:30	<11:00	<11:15
	(women)	<11:50	<12:30	<13:00	<13:45	<14:30	<16:30

3-Mile Walking Test (No Running)

Age (years)

Fitness Category		13–19	20–29	30–39	40–49	50–59	60+
I. Very Poor	(men)	>45:00*	>46:00	>49:00	>52:00	>55:00	>60:00
	(women)	>47:00	>48:00	>51:00	>54:00	>57:00	>63:00
II. Poor	(men)	41:01–45:00	42:01–46:00	44:31–49:00	47:01–52:00	50:01–55:00	54:01–60:00
	(women)	43:01–47:00	44:01–48:00	46:31–51:00	49:01–54:00	52:01–57:00	57:01–63:00
III. Fair	(men)	37:31–41:00	38:31–42:00	40:01–44:30	42:01–47:00	45:01–50:00	48:01–54:00
	(women)	39:31–43:00	40:31–44:00	42:01–46:30	44:01–49:00	47:01–52:00	51:01–57:00
IV. Good	(men)	33:00–37:30	34:00–38:30	35:00–40:00	36:30–42:00	39:00–45:00	41:00–48:00
	(women)	35:00–39:30	36:00–40:30	37:30–42:00	39:00–44:00	42:00–47:00	45:00–51:00
V. Excellent	(men)	<33:00	<34:00	<35:00	<36:30	<39:00	<41:00
	(women)	<35:00	<36:00	<37:30	<39:00	<42:00	<45:00

Figure 2.1. From *The Aerobics Way* by Kenneth H. Cooper, M.D. Copyright 1977 by Kenneth H. Cooper. Reprinted by permission of the publisher, M. Evans and Company, Inc., New York, New York.

PART II

Instructions: The following are the cases of three people who took cardiovascular endurance tests and received their results. Circle the cardiovascular endurance fitness category for each individual. You may use your textbook to assist you.

1. Dale, age forty-one, ran the 1.5-mile run in seventeen minutes. What is his fitness category?
    a. I
    b. II
    c. III
    d. IV
    e. V

2. Phyllis, age thirty-three, ran the 1.5-mile test in eleven minutes. What is her fitness category?
    a. II
    b. III
    c. IV
    d. V
    e. VI

3. Linda, age twenty-one, completed the 3-mile walk test in forty-one minutes. What is her fitness category?
    a. I
    b. II
    c. III
    d. IV
    e. V

Answers:

Part I	A.	1. a	B.	1. a	Part II	1. b
		2. b		2. a		2. e
		3. c		3. a		3. c

If you responded correctly to each item, you are ready to proceed with the next unit.

METHODS OF DETERMINING RECOMMENDED BODY WEIGHT

Most people depend on height/weight charts to determine proper body weight. Research indicates that in many cases this type of measurement is incorrect. For example, the so-called ideal weight within any one category of these tables can vary by as much as 22 pounds. The important factor is not only the body weight, but how much of the total body weight is fat. It is not unusual for a person to meet the criteria on the height/weight tables while actually carrying from 15 to 30 pounds of excess fat.

The optimal weight and percent body fat for an individual is that which is most conducive to health. The term **percent body fat** refers to the amount of fat in the body, expressed as a percentage of the total body weight. Unfortunately, scientists are not yet able to predict exactly what these optimal values are for a given individual. Certainly, it is undesirable to weigh a great deal more or less than the average weight of the population, but between these two extremes there is a fairly wide range of individual "desirable weights." The height/weight tables generally used provide a range of values for three different sizes of body frames. Unfortunately,

no accepted method has been devised for determining which type of frame an individual has. Furthermore, an increase in weight may represent muscle development rather than increased fat.

Many of the same problems exist in determining an optimal percentage of body fat. The percent fat of an apparently healthy person can be estimated, but it would not be known for certain whether it is really the best percentage of fat for that individual's optimal health. An estimate of from 10 to 15 percent body fat for men and 15 to 22 percent body fat for women has been used as a generally desirable goal.

The most reliable and accurate method of determining body composition is by chemical analysis, but it is necessary to destroy the organism to do this. Laboratory techniques utilizing the method of **hydrostatic (or underwater) weighing** also give very good indications of the amount of body fat. This method is very time consuming, and expensive equipment is necessary.

Located underneath the skin is a layer of fat (subcutaneous fat). By measuring these skinfolds at selected sites, charts indicating percent body fat have been developed that are correlated with hydrostatic weighing. The thickness of the skinfold reflects the percentage of body fat and is measured with a **skinfold**

caliper. By using these procedures it is fairly easy to obtain an estimate of body composition.

If you do not have access to a skinfold caliper, you can contact a physical education department at most colleges or universities and they will have one available. Following is a list of some of the various calipers available.

Caliper	Company	Cost
Lange	Cambridge Scientific Industries Cambridge, MD 21613	$125.00+
Harpenden	Quinton Instruments Company 2121 Terry Avenue Seattle, WA 98121	125.00+
Lafayette	Lafayette Instrument Company P.O. Box 5729 Lafayette, IN 47403	125.00+

There are cheaper skinfold calipers available and research indicates that measurements using this type of caliper are highly correlated with measurements using an expensive skinfold caliper. Figure 2.2 contains an illustration of such a caliper.

Caliper	Company	Cost
Fat-O-Meter	Health Education Services Corporation 714015 York Road Bensenville, IL 60106	Less than $15.00

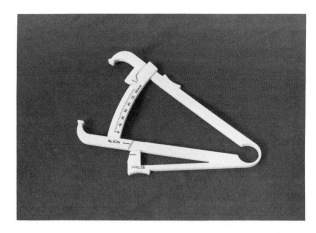

Figure 2.2. An inexpensive caliper to determine skinfold thickness.

Slim Guide	Creative Health Products 9135 General Court Plymouth, MI 48170	Less than $15.00
Fat Control	Fat Control, Inc. P.O. Box 10117 Towson, MD 21204	Less than $15.00

Another means of estimating percentage of body fat is to use body measurements. This is an easy method that anyone can use without special training or having to obtain expensive measuring equipment. All that is needed is a tape measure.

DETERMINING RECOMMENDED BODY WEIGHT

The *Fitness for Life* program uses **skinfold measurements** or body measurements to obtain an indication of body composition. This information is used to determine an estimate of what someone's body weight should be. A person can decide then if it is necessary to engage in a weight-control program.

By using the Body Weight Work Sheet, located in Appendix C, determining recommended body weight is a simple three-step process.

Step 1. Take measurements and record information.

Step 2. Compute the measurements to determine the percentage of body fat and compare with the percent body fat rating scale.

Step 3. Compute the measurements to determine estimated **target weight.**

To help you become familiar with these steps, we will determine the percent fat and the target weight for a sample case.

CASE
Bob Groves

Bob has asked you to determine his percent body fat and his estimated target weight. He is twenty-five years old and currently weighs 185 pounds.

Step 1: Taking measurements and recording information on the work sheet

Item 1. Using the Body Weight Work Sheet in Appendix C, fill in Bob's name, sex, and date.

Item 2. Weigh Bob on an accurate scale and write his current weight (185 pounds) to the right of item 2. He should be weighed without a lot of clothing. Also record his age (twenty-five years) in item 2.

Item 3. Skinfold measurements are a good indication of the amount of fat contained within the body. Studies have shown that there is a high relationship between the fat beneath the skin and the fat inside the body. As fat is lost within the body, it will also be lost at these skinfold sites. An estimation of total body composition, therefore, will help you decide what weight you want to be.

Procedures for Obtaining Skinfolds

The following procedures should be followed to obtain the best measurements. Make all of the skinfold measurements on the right side of the body. All measurements are taken in millimeters. The skinfold is picked up between the thumb and index finger. In order to include two thicknesses of skin and subcutaneous fat without any muscle tissue, have the subject contract the muscle involved and then relax it. Apply the calipers about one centimeter from the fingers holding the skinfold, and at a depth about equal to the thickness of the fold. Take all measurements with the skinfold vertical, except where natural folding of the skin is in opposition. Repeat the entire procedure three times and average the measurements for each site. Release and re-grasp the skinfold for each measurement.

Precautions

Differences between the measurements taken by two people of the same person may vary. The movement of body fluids, as in dehydration, may significantly affect the skinfold measurements. It would be best, therefore, to have all measurements made in the morning. Since this may not always be possible, measurements should be made by the same person at the same time of day.

The following sites should be used for determining percent body fat.

1. Triceps. Locate a point halfway between the tip of the acromial process (bony projection on top of shoulder) and the tip of the olecranon process (tip of elbow) with the elbow at a 90-degree angle. Then measure the skinfold with the arm relaxed and hanging in extension.
2. Chest. Locate a point over the outside edge of the pectoralis major muscle, just medial to the armpit. The skinfold will run diagonally between the shoulder and the opposite hip.

3. Abdomen. Locate a point adjacent to the umbilicus and use a vertical skinfold.
4. Thigh. Locate a point in the anterior midline of the thigh, midway between the hip and knee joints. Place the body weight on the opposite leg so that the thigh muscle is in a relaxed state, and use a vertical skinfold.
5. Iliac crest. Locate a point over the top of the hip at the mid-axillary line (middle of armpit) and use a skinfold that is in the diagonal plane.
6. Subscapula. This skinfold is taken at the tip of the scapula on a diagonal plane.

Different skinfold sites are used for different groups of people. Following are the sites utilized for the selected population groups:

Males (9–16 years)
1. Triceps
2. Subscapula
Males (15–60 years)
1. Chest
2. Abdomen
3. Thigh
Females (9–16 years)
1. Triceps
2. Subscapula
Females (15–60 years)
1. Triceps
2. Thigh
3. Iliac Crest

Bob has the following skinfold measurements: chest–14, abdomen–26, and thigh–23. Record these measurements in the blanks in item 3. Add the skinfold measurements together and record the total of 63 in item 3.

Item 4 If you do not have the use of a skinfold caliper, then body measurements are a good indication of the amount of fat contained within the body.

Procedures for Obtaining Body Measurements

In order to determine percent body fat, you measure the following:

Men—body weight and waist circumference
Women—height and hip circumference

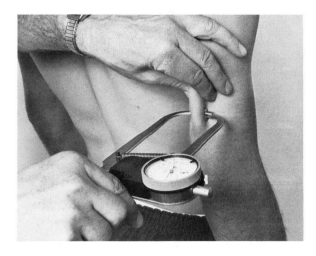

Figure 2.3. Triceps skinfold.

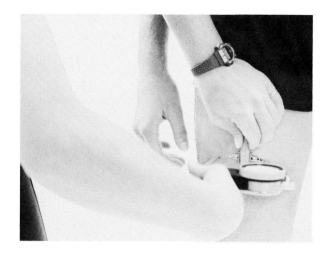

Figure 2.6. Thigh skinfold.

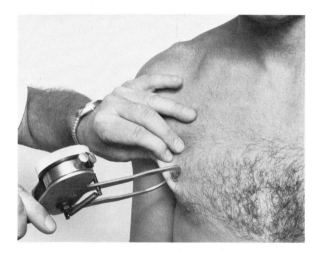

Figure 2.4. Chest skinfold.

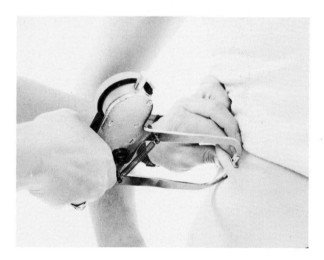

Figure 2.7. Iliac crest skinfold.

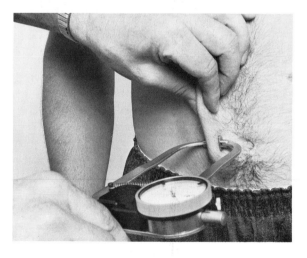

Figure 2.5. Abdomen skinfold.

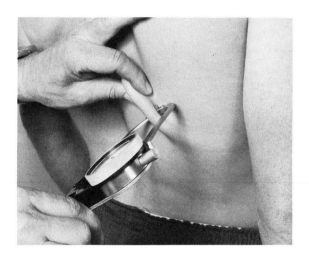

Figure 2.8. Subscapula skinfold.

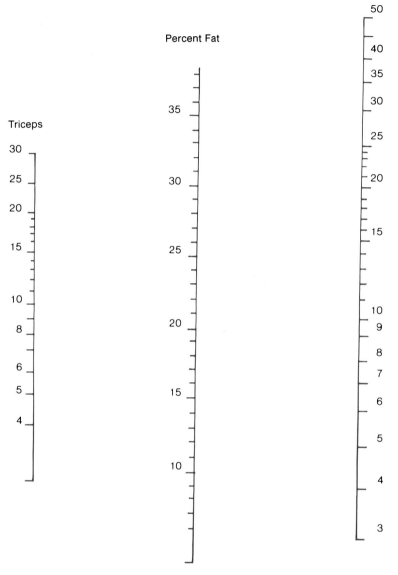

Figure 2.9. Nomogram for the determination of percent body fat from the values of the triceps and subscapula skinfolds in boys 9–12 years old. *(Adapted with permission from "Total Body Fat and Skinfold Thickness in Children," by Jana Parizkova, Metabolism—Clinical and Experimental, vol. 10, 1961, pp. 802–805.)*

The following procedures should be followed to obtain the best measurements.

1. Body Weight. Weigh the person on an accurate scale with very little clothing. Make sure you always have the shoes removed.
2. Body Height. Measure the person, without shoes, in inches.
3. Hip Circumference. The circumference of the hips is measured at the widest point.
4. Waist Circumference. Measure the waist at the level of the navel.

Bob has the following body measurements: body weight—185 pounds, and waist circumference—35 inches. Record these measurements in the blanks in item 4.

Skinfolds for 13–16-Year-Old Boys

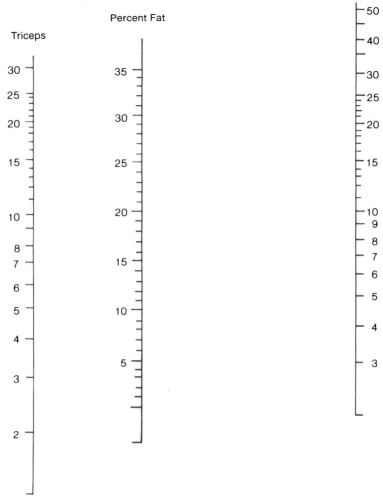

Figure 2.10. Nomogram for the determination of percent body fat from the values of the triceps and subscapula skinfolds in boys 13–16 years old. *(Adapted with permission from "Total Body Fat and Skinfold Thickness in Children," by Jana Parizkova,* Metabolism—Clinical and Experimental, *vol. 10, 1961, pp. 802–805.)*

Step 2: Computing the measurements to determine percent body fat

Item 5. In order to determine percent body fat it is necessary to use one of the following charts. Four are for age sixteen and below, and one is for age fifteen years and above.

Skinfolds for Children— Sixteen Years and Below

Use the triceps and subscapula skinfold measurements to determine the percent fat for children. Check the following charts for the desired age and sex and then, with a straight edge, align the triceps value in the first column with the subscapula value in the third column. Now you can obtain the percent fat value by reading where the straight edge crosses the middle column. In figure 2.10, for example, you will learn that a fourteen-year-old boy with a triceps skinfold of 4 and a subscapula skinfold of 6, would have approximately 9.2 percent body fat.

Skinfolds for Individuals— Fifteen Years and Above

You can find the percent body fat by finding the sum of three skinfolds. For males you use the chest, abdomen, and thigh measurements and for females the

Skinfolds for 9–12-Year-Old Girls

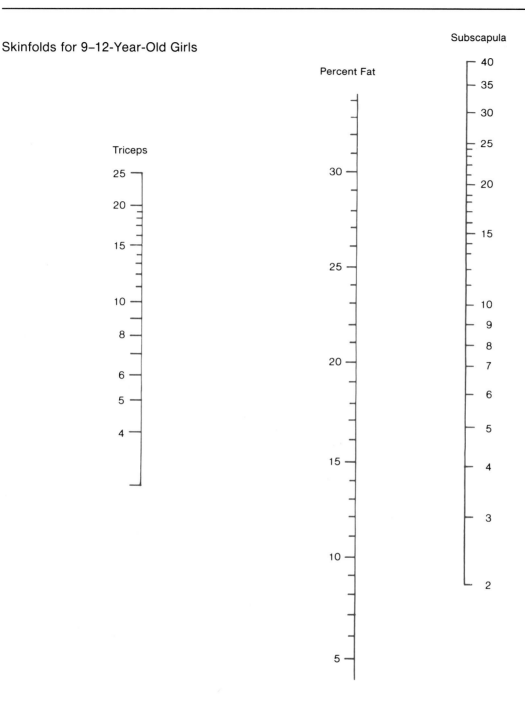

Figure 2.11. Nomogram for the determination of percent body fat from the values of the triceps and subscapula skinfolds in girls 9–12 years old. *(Adapted with permission* *from "Total Body Fat and Skinfold Thickness in Children," by Jana Parizkova,* Metabolism—Clinical and Experimental, *vol. 10, 1961, pp. 802–805.)*

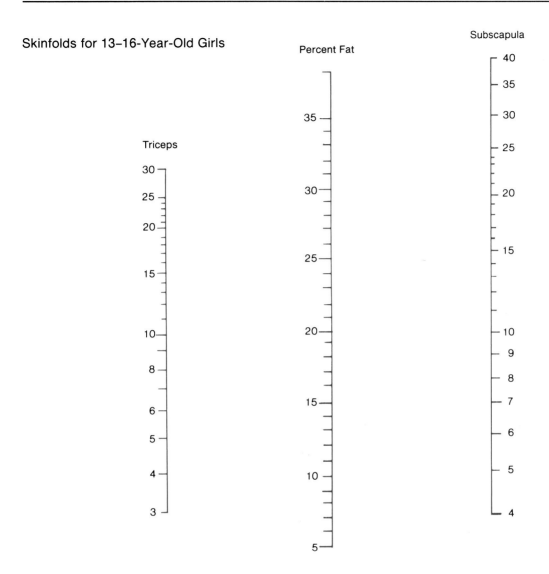

Skinfolds for 13–16-Year-Old Girls

Figure 2.12. Nomogram for the determination of percent body fat from the values of the triceps and subscapula skinfolds in girls 13–16 years old. *(Adapted with permission from "Total Body Fat and Skinfold Thickness in Children," by Jana Parizkova,* Metabolism—Clinical and Experimental, *vol. 10, 1961, pp. 802–805.)*

Skinfolds for Individuals Fifteen Years and Above

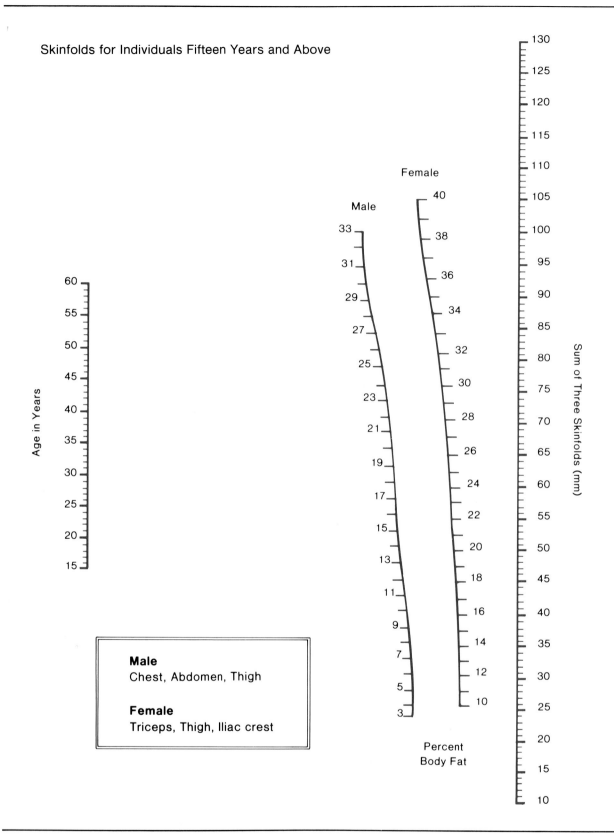

Figure 2.13. Nomogram for the determination of percent body fat for the sum of the chest, abdomen, and thigh skinfolds of males 15 years of age and above, and for the sum of the triceps, thigh, and iliac crest skinfolds of females 15 years of age and above. *(Adapted from "A nomogram for the estimate of percent body fat from generalized equations" by W. B. Baun, M. R. Baun, and P. B. Raven, Research Quarterly for Exercise and Sport, vol. 52, 1981, pp. 380–384. Reprinted by permission.)*

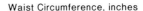

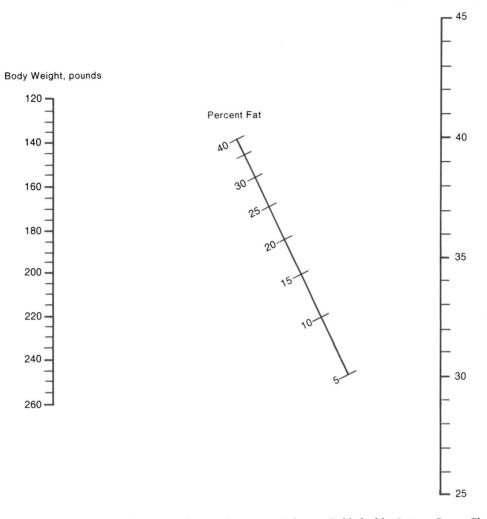

Figure 2.14. Estimation of relative fat in men from body weight and abdominal or waist circumference. *(Adapted with permission from* Sensible Fitness, *by Jack H.* *Wilmore. Published by Leisure Press, Champaign, Illinois, 1986.)*

triceps, thigh, and iliac crest measurements. Percent fat is then estimated by placing a straightedge on the nomogram that connects the individual's age (left axis) with the skinfold sum value (right axis) and reading the value from the appropriate percent body fat scale with respect to sex.

Bob has a sum total for his skinfolds of 63. This is a percent body fat of 18. Record this number in item 5.

In order to determine percent body fat using body measurements, it is necessary to use one of the charts in figure 2.14 or 2.15. One chart is for males and one is for females. Use a straight edge to align the body measurement values in the various columns. You can determine the percent fat value by reading where the straight edge crosses the middle column.

Bob had a waist circumference measurement of 35 inches and weighed 185 pounds. This is a percent body fat of 18 percent. Record this number in item 5.

Item 6. Although it is not possible to determine exactly what percent of the body should be fat in order to ensure good health, the "Percent Body Fat Rating Scale" in item 6 provides an estimate that can prove helpful. Bob's 18 percent body fat would place him in the *Fat* category, and he may want to consider seriously a program to reduce his body fat.

Step 3: Computing the measurements to determine estimated target weight

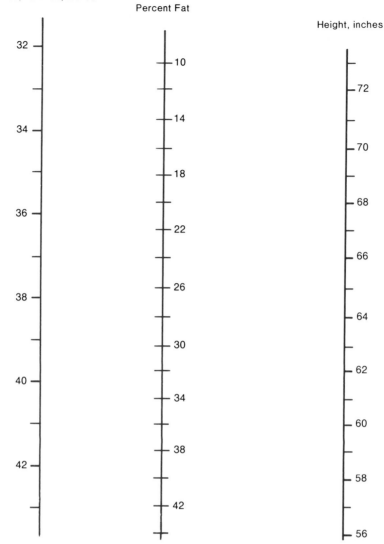

Hip Circumference, inches

Percent Fat

Height, inches

Figure 2.15. Estimation of relative fat in women from height and hip circumference. *(Adapted with permission* *from* Sensible Fitness, *by Jack H. Wilmore. Published by Leisure Press, Champaign, Illinois, 1986.)*

To estimate Bob's recommended target weight, you must know his current weight, his current fat weight, his current **lean body weight,** and his desired percent body fat.

Item 7. To find Bob's current fat weight you take his current weight from item 2 (185 pounds) and multiply it by his current percent body fat in item 5 (18%). Remember to change the percent to a decimal (.18). When rounded to the nearest whole number, the answer is 33 pounds. Record this in the blank next to item 7.

Item 8. In order to determine Bob's current lean body weight, you must subtract his fat weight in item 7 (33) from his current weight located in item 2 (185). This gives you an answer of 152. Record this number next to the blank in item 8.

Item 9. As indicated before, it is not possible to determine the optimal percent body fat for any individual. After reading the rating in the "Percent Body Fat Rating Scale" in item 6, however, Bob decides he would like to obtain a percent body fat of 10 percent, which would place him in the *Very Lean* category. Remember to record 10 percent as a decimal (.10) in the blank next to item 9.

Item 10. To determine an estimate of Bob's target weight subtract item 9 (.10) from 1.0. The number you obtain will be .9. You now divide item 8 (152) by .9 and round the answer to the nearest whole number. You will obtain a figure of 169. This is the estimated target weight that Bob should achieve. Even though it is not possible to predict the target weight exactly, this weight is a good indication of what Bob should weigh.

Item 11. In order to determine the number of pounds Bob should gain or lose, subtract item 10 (169) from his current weight in item 2 (185). This indicates that Bob should lose 16 pounds.

Once you know Bob's estimated target weight, you can use the information as a guide in writing a weight-control program for him.

When you have completed the Body Weight Work Sheet that you filled out for Bob, check your copy with the completed work sheet in figure 2.16.

MASTERY CHECK INSTRUCTIONS

Instructions: The following cases contain information about body measurements. Read each case carefully, then answer the multiple-choice items. There is only one correct answer for each question. You may use the Body Weight Work Sheet to determine the correct answers.

1. Tom, age twenty-two, has the following skinfold measurements: chest 10, abdomen 25, and thigh 18. His estimated percent body fat is
   a. 21.5.
   b. 15.
   c. 17.
2. Sally, age thirty-six, has the following skinfold measurements: triceps 15, thigh 19, iliac crest 10. Her estimated percent body fat is
   a. 19.
   b. 14.
   c. 22.

3. Janet has a hip circumference of 38 inches and a height of 68 inches. Her estimated percent body fat is
   a. 24.
   b. 27.
   c. 32.
4. John, age ten, has a triceps skinfold of 4 and a subscapula skinfold of 7.5. His estimated percent body fat is
   a. 10.
   b. 13.
   c. 15.
5. Phil has a percent body fat of 12.5. This percent body fat would be rated as
   a. lean.
   b. acceptable.
   c. fat.
6. Kathy weighs 140 pounds and has a percent body fat of 26. She would like to have a percent body fat of 18. Her estimated target weight is
   a. 104.
   b. 132.
   c. 127.

Answers:

1. b	4. c
2. a	5. a
3. a	6. c

Body Weight Work Sheet

1. Name __Bob Groves_____ Sex _Male__ Date _____

2. Current Weight __185_____ Age _25_

3. Skinfold Measurements

    Children: Triceps _____ Subscapula _____

    Men: Chest _14___ Abdomen _26___ Thigh _23_____

    Women: Triceps _____ Thigh _____ Iliac Crest _____

    Sum of Skinfolds _63_____

4. Body Measurements

    Men: Weight _185____ Waist _35____

    Women: Hip _____ Height _____

5. Percent Body Fat _18_____

6. Percent Body Fat Rating Scale

		Men (%)	Women (%)
_____	Very Lean	10 and below	13 and below
_____	Lean	11–14	14–17
_____	Moderate Fat	15–17	18–23
__X____	Fat	18–21	24–28
_____	High Fat	22+	29+

Determining Selected Target Weight

7. Current fat weight (current body weight × item 5) _____33_____
   (Round to nearest whole number.)

8. Current lean body weight (current body weight − item 7) _____152_____

9. Desired percent body fat (select from item 6) _____.10_____

10. Estimated target weight [item 8 ÷ (1.00 − item 9)] ___169_____
    (Round to nearest whole number.)

11. Estimated pounds to gain or lose (item 2 − item 10) ___16_____

Figure 2.16.

Strength is defined as the ability to exert force against resistance. In our society, many people think that strength is necessary only for athletes and others who are required to do hard muscular work. This is a false assumption. The average person who works in business or in the home would be better prepared to meet the rigors of everyday living if he or she had a sufficient amount of strength.

Although it is impossible to determine exactly the amount of strength each individual might require to do a given job, it is possible to estimate strength fitness ratings by a series of simple tests.

Using the Strength Appraisal Work Sheet in Appendix C, administering and interpreting muscular strength tests is a simple three-step process:

Step 1. Fill out the work sheet.
Step 2. Plan and administer the strength test.
Step 3. Interpret the strength test correctly.

To help you become familiar with these procedures, we will use a sample case and go through the process step-by-step.

CASE
John Jefferson

John has asked you to administer a strength test to determine his fitness category.

Step 1: Filling out the work sheet

Item 1. Fill in John's name and sex.

Item 2. Weigh John on an accurate scale and write his weight (150 lbs.) to the right of item 2 on the work sheet.

Step 2: Planning and administering the strength test

Item 3. Determine the recommended weight for each of the exercises by taking a fraction of John's current body weight. Since John weighs 150 pounds, he would do 50 pounds in the arm curl. This was found by multiplying .35 by 150. The answer is 52.5 pounds, but since most weights come in 5-pound increments, you always round down to the lowest 5 pounds. Record these weights on the chart in item 3. Check chapter 7, "Writing a Strength Program," to find a description of each exercise.

Have John do each exercise for as many repetitions as possible. Record the number of repetitions for each exercise on the chart in item 3. John does the following number of repetitions for each exercise: arm curls—15; bench press—12; lat machine pulldown—10 (have someone hold the subject down at the shoulders for the lat machine pulldown); quad lift—21; leg curl—9 (while doing the leg curl, the legs should be brought to a 90-degree angle); curl-up—7 (for the curl-up, hold the weight behind the neck, keep the legs flexed at a 100 degree angle, and have someone hold the feet).

Step 3: Interpreting the strength test correctly

Item 4. Using the Fitness Category Chart in item 4, check the number of repetitions performed for each exercise and determine the number of points John will receive for each exercise and what his fitness category is for each exercise. For example, he will receive 15 points and a fitness category of Excellent for 15 arm curls. Record all of John's ratings on the chart listed in item 3. This information can be used now to indicate to John what his strength fitness is for specific parts of the body. By referring to the weight-training exercises described in chapter 7, "Writing a Strength Program," you can see what exercise tests each area of the body. For example, the bench press tests the shoulders, chest, and the back of the upper arms.

Item 5. Total all of John's points received in the selected exercises listed in item 3 (76 points) and record your answer in the blank next to item 5. This is his Overall Strength Score.

Item 6. Check the rating scale listed in item 6 to determine the Overall Strength Fitness Category. Since John has 76 points he would receive a rating of IV—Good. Record this score in the blank.

Knowing John's strength category will help you write a strength development program for him.

After completing John's Strength Appraisal Work Sheet check your copy with the completed work sheet in figure 2.17.

Strength Appraisal Work Sheet

1. Name _John Jefferson_   Sex _Male_

2. Body Weight _150_

3. Test Administration

Determine the recommended percentage of total body weight for each exercise. Perform as many repetitions as you can, up to the listed maximum, through a full range of motion. See chapter 7 for a description of the exercises.

Exercise	Fraction of Body Weight (Male)	(Female)	Weight	Reps.	Points	Fitness Category
Arm Curl	.35	.18	50	15	15	Excellent
Bench Press	.75	.45	110	12	13	Very Good
Lat Machine Pulldown	.70	.45	105	10	11	Good
Quad Lift	.65	.50	95	21	17	Superior
Leg Curl	.32	.25	45	9	11	Good
Curl-Up	.16	.10	20	7	9	Fair

4. Fitness Category Chart

Exercise and Repetitions

Fitness Category	Points	Arm Curl Male	Female	Bench Press Male	Female	Lat Machine Pulldown Male	Female
Very Poor	5	2 or less	2 or less	0	0	3 or less	2 or less
Poor	7	3–4	3–5	1–2	1	4–5	3–5
Fair	9	5–7	6–7	3–6	2–4	6–8	6–8
Good	11	8–9	8–11	7–10	5–9	9–10	9–10
Very Good	13	10–14	12–15	11–15	11–15	11–15	11–15
Excellent	15	15–20	16–20	16–20	16–20	16–24	16–24
Superior	17	21+	21+	21+	21+	25+	25+

		Quad Lift Male	Female	Leg Curl Male	Female	Curl-Up Male	Female
Very Poor	5	3 or less	1 or less	1 or less	0	1 or less	0
Poor	7	4–6	2–4	2–3	1–2	2	1
Fair	9	7–9	5–7	4–7	3–4	3–7	2–3
Good	11	10–12	8–9	8–10	5–6	8–11	4–5
Very Good	13	13–14	10–12	11–14	7–9	12–16	6–13
Excellent	15	15–19	13–19	15–19	10–16	17–25	14–26
Superior	17	20+	20+	20+	17+	26+	27+

5. Overall Strength Score

_76_

(Total all of the points in the selected exercises)

6. Strength Fitness Category (Check one)

Strength score	Category	
Less than 42	_____	I. Very Poor
42–53	_____	II. Poor
54–65	_____	III. Fair
66–77	____X____	IV. Good
78–89	_____	V. Very Good
90–101	_____	VI. Excellent
More than 101	_____	VII. Superior

Figure 2.17. Strength test. *(Adapted from test developed by W. W. K. Hoeger and D. R. Hopkins and used with their permission.)*

Instructions: The following cases contain information concerning strength testing. Read each case carefully, then answer the multiple-choice items. You may use your Strength Appraisal Work Sheet to determine the correct answer.

1. Sam has a body weight of 180 pounds. What will be the weight used for the bench press test?
   a. 60
   b. 80
   c. 100
   d. 135

2. Sue has a body weight of 120 pounds. What will be the weight used by her for the arm curl?
   a. 20
   b. 40
   c. 60
   d. 80

3. Mike completed 10 repetitions of the leg curl. He will receive how many points?
   a. 5
   b. 7
   c. 9
   d. 11

4. Iris completed 17 repetitions of the lat machine pulldown. What is her fitness category for this exercise?
   a. *Good*
   b. *Very Good*
   c. *Excellent*
   d. *Superior*

5. Helen received 64 points for her overall strength score. What is her strength fitness category?
   a. II
   b. III
   c. IV
   d. V

Answers:

1. d
2. a
3. d
4. c
5. b

If you responded correctly to each item, you are ready to proceed with the next unit.

MEASURING FLEXIBILITY

The effectiveness of movement in most physical activities is affected by the degree of body flexibility. **Flexibility** can be defined as the range of movement in a joint. It is concerned with the degree and ease with which the body can bend or twist by means of contraction and relaxation of the muscles. A person with good flexibility spends less energy in physical movement than does an inflexible person. Increased flexibility of the joints and muscles may also make the individual less vulnerable to injury.

Exactly how much flexibility an individual should possess has not been scientifically determined, and it should be noted that flexibility is specific to each individual joint of the body. As was pointed out earlier, lower-back pain is prevalent among men and women and this is generally related to a lack of flexibility in the lower back, hips, and the back of the legs. Another area of the body that also suffers from a lack of flexibility is the upper torso.

The flexibility tests selected to be used in the *Fitness for Life* program measure the flexibility of the lower back, hips, backs of the legs, shoulder muscles, and the shoulder girdle. Be sure to warm up before performing the flexibility tests. Light calisthenics or slow jogging can be used to increase body heat. Then do some gentle stretching of the body parts to be tested.

Using the Flexibility Appraisal Work Sheet in Appendix C, administering and interpreting flexibility is a simple two-step process:

Step 1: Fill out the work sheet.

Step 2: Plan, administer, and correctly interpret the flexibility tests.

In order to help you become familiar with these procedures we will use a sample case and go through the process step-by-step.

CASE
Susan Jones

Step 1: Filling out the work sheet

Item 1. Fill in Susan's name and sex.

Step 2: Planning, administering, and interpreting flexibility tests

Item 2. Sit-and-Reach Test. This test measures the flexibility of the lower back, hips, and the back of the legs. The person who is being tested assumes a sitting position on the floor. The legs are extended straight in front and the backs of the legs are pressed firmly against the floor. The legs are at right angles to a line drawn on the floor, and the heels should touch the near edge of the line and be about 5 inches apart. A yardstick is placed between the legs of the performer so that it rests on the floor, with the 15-inch mark resting on the near edge of the heel line. The yardstick should be taped to the floor to ensure a constant position. A partner's feet are used to brace the subject's feet so that, on the reach, the heels will not slip over the line. The subject should stretch forward three times and then reach, with both hands held together, as far forward as possible on the yardstick and hold.

The score is the farthest point reached on the yard-stick with the fingertips. Measure to the nearest inch. The best score of three trials is recorded as the test score. Record the inches reached on the chart in item 2 on the work sheet. See figure 2.18 for an example of the sit-and-reach test. Susan has a test score of 21 inches.

Item 3. Check the rating scale in item 3 to determine the flexibility fitness category. Since Susan has a sit-and-reach score of 21 inches, she would receive a rating of *V—Very Good*. Check the blank by the correct fitness category in item 3.

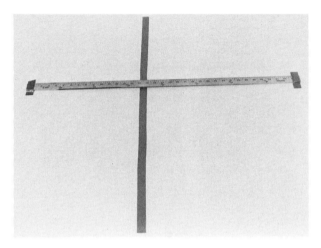

Figure 2.18(a). Sit-and-reach test.

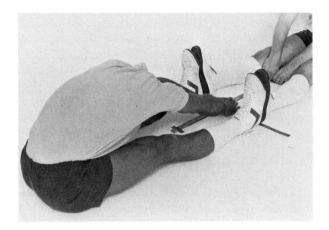

Figure 2.18(b). Sit-and-reach test.

Item 4. Shoulder Lift Test. This test measures the flexibility of the shoulder muscles and the shoulder girdle. The subject lies flat on the floor with the arms extended and a ruler held in both hands. The chin and forehead maintain contact with the floor and a partner stabilizes the buttocks and legs as shown in figure 2.19. The arms are raised as high as possible without the rest of the body losing contact with the floor, and the distance between the floor and the ruler is measured. Three trials are given and the best trial is recorded. Susan has a score of 20 inches for the test and it is recorded next to shoulder lift in item 4.

Item 5. To determine the flexibility fitness category for the shoulder lift, the rating scale in item 5 is used. Susan's score of 20 inches places her in category *IV—Good.* Check the blank by the correct fitness category in item 5.

Now you have an indication of Susan's flexibility and this will help you write a flexibility development program for her.

When you have completed Susan's Flexibility Appraisal Work Sheet, check your copy with the completed work sheet in figure 2.20.

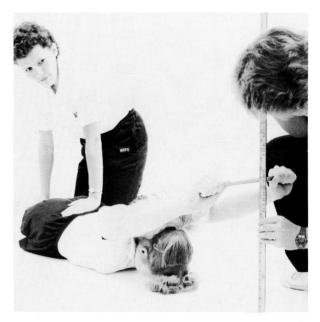

Figure 2.19. Shoulder lift test.

MASTERY CHECK INSTRUCTIONS

Instructions: The following cases contain information concerning flexibility testing. Read each case carefully, then answer the multiple-choice items. You may use your Flexibility Appraisal Work Sheet to determine the correct answer.

1. John had a sit-and-reach score of 16 inches. What is his flexibility fitness category?
   a. III
   b. IV
   c. V
   d. VI

2. Carol had a shoulder lift score of 26 inches. What is her flexibility fitness category?
   a. III
   b. IV
   c. V
   d. VI

Answers:

1. a
2. d

If you responded correctly to each item, you are ready to proceed with the next unit.

Flexibility Appraisal Work Sheet

1. Name _Susan Jones_   Sex _Female_

Test Administration

2. Sit-and-Reach _21_

3. Flexibility Fitness Category

Score		Category
11 or less	_____	I. Very Poor
12–13	_____	II. Poor
14–16	_____	III. Fair
17–19	_____	IV. Good
20–21	__X__	V. Very Good
22–23	_____	VI. Excellent
24 or more	_____	VII. Superior

4. Shoulder Lift _20_
(Inches raised)

5. Flexibility Fitness Category

Score		Category
10 or less	_____	I. Very Poor
11–14	_____	II. Poor
15–18	_____	III. Fair
19–21	__X__	IV. Good
22–24	_____	V. Very Good
25–26	_____	VI. Excellent
27 or more	_____	VII. Superior

Figure 2.20.

MEASURING STRESS AND TENSION

If either the physiological or psychological equilibrium of the body is disturbed, you experience stress. We do not all react the same way to identical stressors. Some people magnify the importance of a given experience and thus view it as a very stressful situation; others may perceive the same experience as having little or no importance.

It is important to point out that not all stress is bad and some is necessary for the body to respond and develop. The type of stress with which the *Fitness for Life* program is concerned is the stress that inhibits the individual from being healthy, happy, and well adjusted.

When measuring physiological variables such as strength and cardiovascular endurance, it is possible to be fairly accurate. The measurement of stress is much more difficult, as we may interpret psychological variables in many different ways; this interpretation is greatly influenced by our different backgrounds and moods.

The following tests selected for the *Fitness for Life* program were developed by the Public Health Service of the former U.S. Department of Health, Education, and Welfare (now the Department of Health and Human Services). A complete explanation can be found in their publication, DHEW Publication No. (PHS) 79–50097, Washington, D.C., 1980.

This is a four-part test. The first three parts are designed to give you an indication of how vulnerable you might be to certain types of stress and to make you aware of how they might affect you. The last part of the test will provide you with information on how to cope with situations that might be of a stressful nature.

Test One

Choose the most appropriate answer for each of the ten questions as it actually pertains to you.

1. When I can't do something "my way," I simply adjust and do it the easiest way.
   (a) Almost always true, (b) Usually true,
   (c) Usually false, (d) Almost always false
2. I get upset when someone in front of me drives slowly.
   (a) Almost always true, (b) Usually true,
   (c) Usually false, (d) Almost always false
3. It bothers me when my plans are dependent upon others.
   (a) Almost always true, (b) Usually true,
   (c) Usually false, (d) Almost always false
4. Whenever possible, I tend to avoid large crowds.
   (a) Almost always true, (b) Usually true,
   (c) Usually false, (d) Almost always false
5. I am uncomfortable when I have to stand in long lines.
   (a) Almost always true, (b) Usually true,
   (c) Usually false, (d) Almost always false
6. Arguments upset me.
   (a) Almost always true, (b) Usually true,
   (c) Usually false, (d) Almost always false
7. When my plans don't flow smoothly, I become anxious.
   (a) Almost always true, (b) Usually true,
   (c) Usually false, (d) Almost always false
8. I require a lot of space in which to live and work.
   (a) Almost always true, (b) Usually true,
   (c) Usually false, (d) Almost always false
9. When I am busy at some task, I hate to be disturbed.
   (a) Almost always true, (b) Usually true,
   (c) Usually false, (d) Almost always false
10. I believe that it is worth waiting for all good things.
    (a) Almost always true, (b) Usually true,
    (c) Usually false, (d) Almost always false

To score: 1 and 10, a = 1 pt., b = 2 pts., c = 3 pts., d = 4 pts. 2 through 9, a = 4 pts., b = 3 pts., c = 2 pts., d = 1 pt.

This test measures your vulnerability to stress from being frustrated or inhibited. Scores in excess of 25 seem to suggest some vulnerability to this source of stress.

Test Two

Circle the letter of the response that best answers the following ten questions. How often do you . . .

1. Find yourself with insufficient time to complete your work?
   (a) Almost always, (b) Very often,
   (c) Seldom, (d) Never
2. Find yourself becoming confused and unable to think clearly because too many things are happening at once?
   (a) Almost always, (b) Very often,
   (c) Seldom, (d) Never

3. Wish you had help to get everything done?
   (a) Almost always, (b) Very often,
   (c) Seldom, (d) Never
4. Feel your boss/professor expects too much from you?
   (a) Almost always, (b) Very often,
   (c) Seldom, (d) Never
5. Feel your family and friends expect too much from you?
   (a) Almost always, (b) Very often,
   (c) Seldom, (d) Never
6. Find your work infringing on your leisure hours?
   (a) Almost always, (b) Very often,
   (c) Seldom, (d) Never
7. Find yourself doing extra work to set an example to those around you?
   (a) Almost always, (b) Very often,
   (c) Seldom, (d) Never
8. Find yourself doing extra work to impress your superiors?
   (a) Almost always, (b) Very often,
   (c) Seldom, (d) Never
9. Have to skip a meal so that you can get work completed?
   (a) Almost always, (b) Very often,
   (c) Seldom, (d) Never
10. Feel that you have too much responsibility?
    (a) Almost always, (b) Very often,
    (c) Seldom, (d) Never

To score: a = 4 pts., b = 3 pts., c = 2 pts., d = 1 pt. Total your score for this exercise.

This test measures your vulnerability to "overload," that is, having too much to do. Scores in excess of 25 seem to indicate vulnerability to this source of stress.

Test Three

Answer each question as it is generally true for you.

1. I hate to wait in lines.
   (a) Almost always true, (b) Usually true,
   (c) Seldom true, (d) Never true
2. I often find myself racing against the clock to save time.
   (a) Almost always true, (b) Usually true,
   (c) Seldom true, (d) Never true
3. I become upset if I think something is taking too long.
   (a) Almost always true, (b) Usually true,
   (c) Seldom true, (d) Never true

4. When under pressure I tend to lose my temper.
   (a) Almost always true, (b) Usually true,
   (c) Seldom true, (d) Never true
5. My friends tell me that I tend to get irritated easily.
   (a) Almost always true, (b) Usually true,
   (c) Seldom true, (d) Never true
6. I seldom like to do anything unless I can make it competitive.
   (a) Almost always true, (b) Usually true,
   (c) Seldom true, (d) Never true
7. When something must be done, I'm the first to begin even though the details may still need to be worked out.
   (a) Almost always true, (b) Usually true,
   (c) Seldom true, (d) Never true
8. When I make a mistake it is usually because I've rushed into something without giving it enough thought and planning.
   (a) Almost always true, (b) Usually true,
   (c) Seldom true, (d) Never true
9. Whenever possible, I try to do two things at once, such as eating while working, or planning while driving or bathing.
   (a) Almost always true, (b) Usually true,
   (c) Seldom true, (d) Never true
10. When I go on a vacation, I usually take along some work to do just in case I get a chance.
    (a) Almost always true, (b) Usually true,
    (c) Seldom true, (d) Never true

To score: a = 4 pts., b = 3 pts., c = 2 pts., d = 1 pt.

This test measures the presence of compulsive, time-urgent, and excessively aggressive behavioral traits. Scores in excess of 25 suggest the presence of one or more of these traits.

Test Four

This scale was created largely on the basis of results compiled by clinicians and researchers who sought to identify how individuals effectively cope with stress. This scale is an educational tool, not a clinical instrument. Its purpose, therefore, is to inform you of ways in which you can effectively and healthfully cope with the stress in your life. At the same time, through a point system, it will give you some indication of the relative desirability of the coping strategies you are currently using. Simply follow the instructions given for each of the 14 items listed. Total your points when you have completed all of the items.

1. Give yourself 10 points if you feel that you have a supportive family.
2. Give yourself 10 points if you actively pursue a hobby.
3. Give yourself 10 points if you belong to some social or activity group that meets at least once a month (other than your family).
4. Give yourself 15 points if you are within 5 pounds of your ideal body weight, considering your height and bone structure.
5. Give yourself 15 points if you practice some form of deep relaxation at least three times a week. Deep relaxation exercises include meditation, imagery, yoga, and so on.
6. Give yourself 5 points for each time you exercise thirty minutes or longer during one average week.
7. Give yourself 5 points for each nutritionally balanced and wholesome meal you consume during one average day.
8. Give yourself 5 points if you do something just for yourself that you really enjoy during an average week.
9. Give yourself 10 points if you have some place in your home that you can go in order to relax and/or be alone.
10. Give yourself 10 points if you practice time management techniques in your daily life.
11. Subtract 10 points for each pack of cigarettes you smoke during one average day.
12. Subtract 5 points for each evening during an average week that you take any form of medication or chemical (including alcohol) to help you sleep.
13. Subtract 10 points for each day during an average week that you consume any form of medication or chemical substance (including alcohol) to reduce your anxiety or just to calm you down.
14. Subtract 5 points for each evening during an average week that you bring work home—work that was meant to be done at your place of employment.

Now calculate your total score. A "perfect" score would be 115 points or more. If you scored in the 50–60 range you probably have an adequate collection of coping strategies for most common sources of stress. You should keep in mind, however, that the higher your score, the greater your ability to cope with stress in an effective and healthful manner.

SUGGESTIONS FOR FURTHER READING

1. Åstrand, P. O., and I. A. Ryhming. "Nomogram for Calculation of Aerobic Capacity from Pulse Rate During Submaximal Work." *Journal of Applied Physiology* 7 (1954):218.
2. Baun, W. B., N. R. Baun, and P. B. Raven. "A Nomogram for the Estimate of Percent Body Fat from Generalized Equations." *Research Quarterly for Exercise and Sport* 52(1981) p. 380.
3. Blanchard, Everard B. "The Blanchard Obesity and Nutritional Index." *Journal of Sports Medicine and Physical Fitness* 14 (1974):132.
4. *Body Composition Assessments in Youth and Adults—Report of Sixth Ross Conference on Medical Research.* Columbus, Ohio: Ross Laboratories, 1985.
5. Bruce, Robert A. "Methods of Exercise Testing." *The American Journal of Cardiology* 33 May (1974):715.
6. Bugyi, Balazs. "Lean Body Weight Estimation in 6–16-Year-Old Children Based on Wrist Breadth and Body Height." *Journal of Sports Medicine and Physical Fitness* 12 (1972):171.
7. Burke, Edmund J. "Validity of Selected Laboratory and Field Tests of Physical Working Capacity." *Research Quarterly* 47 (1976):95.
8. Coates, T. J. "Eating—Psychological Dilemma." *Journal of Nutritional Education* 13 March (1981):49.
9. Cooper, Kenneth H. *The Aerobics Way.* New York: M. Evans & Co., Inc., 1977.
10. Cooper, Kenneth H. "A Means of Assessing Maximal Oxygen Uptake." *Journal of American Medical Association* 203 (1958):135.
11. Crowley, J. A. "Worries of Elementary School Students." *Elementary School Guidance and Counseling* 16 December (1981):98.
12. Cureton, Thomas K. "Are You Fit To Win?" *Aquatic World Magazine,* September 1974.
13. Davis, P. O., and C. O. Datson. "Job Performance Testing: An Alternative to Age Discrimination." *Medicine and Science in Sports and Exercise* 19 April (1987): no. 2, p. 179.
14. Hage, P. "Perceived Exertion: One Measure of Exercise Intensity." *The Physician and Sports Medicine* 9 September (1981): no. 9, p. 136.
15. "How Fit Are You?" *Mademoiselle* 81 (1975):94.
16. Hoeger, W. W. K. *Lifetime Physical Fitness and Wellness—A Personalized Program.* Englewood, Colorado: Morton Publishing Company, 1986.
17. Hutinger, Paul. "How Flexible Are You?" *Aquatic World Magazine,* January 1974.
18. Kline, G. M., J. P. Porcari, R. Hintermeister, P. S. Freedson, A. Ward, R. F. McCarron, J. Ross, and J. M. Rippe. "Estimation Maximum Oxygen Uptake from a One-Mile Track Walk, Gender, Age, and Body Weight." *Medicine and Science in Sports and Exercise* 19 June (1987): no. 3, p. 253.

19. Klein, Karl K. "Stress Mechanisms: Postural and Muscular Imbalance and Mechanical Faults." *Track and Field Quarterly Review* 74 (1974):226.

20. Krahenbuhl, G. S., R. P. Pangrazi, G. W. Petersen, L. N. Burkett, and M. J. Schreider. "Field Testing of Cardiorespiratory Fitness in Primary Children." *Medicine and Science in Sports* 3 (1978).

21. Kraus, Hans. "Evaluation of Muscular and Cardiovascular Fitness." *Preventive Medicine* 1 (1972):178.

22. Kuntzleman, Charles T. "Can You Pass This Fitness Test?" *Fitness For Living* 6 January-February (1972):1.

23. Legwold, G. "Does Lifting Weights Harm a Prepubescent Athlete?" *The Physician and Sports Medicine* 10 July (1982): no. 7, p. 141.

24. Lomaeu, O., and J. G. Allen. "Prediction of Adult Aerobic Capacity from Childhood Tests." *Ergonomics* 16 (1973): no. 6, p. 783.

25. McGavack, T. H. "Optimal Weight Determination—Experiences with the Method of Willoughby as a Guide to Reduction." *Metabolism* 14 (1965):150.

26. Montage, H. J., M. E. Frontz, and A. J. Kozar. "The Value of Age, Height and Weight in Establishing Standards of Fitness for Children." *Journal of Sports Medicine and Physical Fitness* 12 (1972):174.

27. Montoye, H. J., F. H. Epstein, and M. O. Kjelsberg. "The Measurement of Body Fatness." *The American Journal of Clinical Nutrition* 16 (1965):417.

28. National Strength and Conditioning Association Journal. "Body Composition—Round Table." Volume 9, Numbers 3 and 4, 1987.

29. Shepherd, Roy J. "Do Risks of Exercise Justify Costly Caution?" *The Physician and Sports Medicine* 5 (1977):58.

30. Smith, Charles D. "Fitness Testing: Questions About How, Why and with What." *Journal of Health, Physical Education and Recreation* 43 (1972):37.

31. Wells, Katherine F., and Evelyn K. Dillon. "The Sit and Reach Test—A Test of Back and Leg Flexibility." *Research Quarterly* 23 (1952):118.

32. "What Do Stress Tests Show?" *The Physician and Sports Medicine* 8 September (1980): no. 9, p. 44.

33. Wilmore, J. H. *Sensible Fitness*. Champaign, Illinois, 1986.

34. *Youth Fitness Test Manual*. AAHPERD Publications, Washington, D.C., 1981.

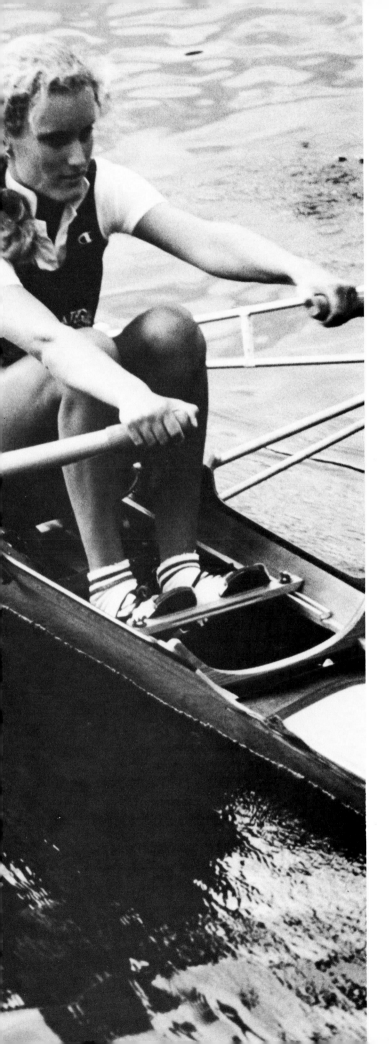

3

WRITING A CARDIOVASCULAR ENDURANCE PROGRAM

Objectives

After study of this chapter you should be able to

1. write a cardiovascular endurance program, tailor-made to age, weight, fitness category, and exercise preference;
2. pass a multiple-choice mastery self-check involving the selection of appropriate cardiovascular endurance programs for individuals varying in age, weight, fitness category, and exercise preference.

Cardiovascular endurance refers to the body's ability to provide oxygen continuously to the cells while they perform work for extended periods of time. It is necessary to have a basic understanding of the circulatory system in order to understand how to train for cardiovascular endurance.

The purpose of the circulatory system is to deliver oxygen and nutrients to body cells and to remove carbon dioxide and other waste products of cell metabolism. Transportation of these substances is accomplished by the movement of blood around the body through a series of arteries, capillaries, and veins. Blood is composed primarily of plasma, which is about 90 percent water. Red blood cells carried within the plasma contain a chemical unit known as **hemoglobin,** which is used to pick up and transport nearly all of the oxygen used by the cells. At the cellular level, oxygen is utilized in chemical reactions to produce the energy necessary to carry on the living processes of the body.

As the blood flows through the lungs the exchange of oxygen and carbon dioxide takes place through a network of tiny air sacs called **alveoli,** which are surrounded by **capillaries.** The efficient exchange of these gases contributes to cardiovascular endurance.

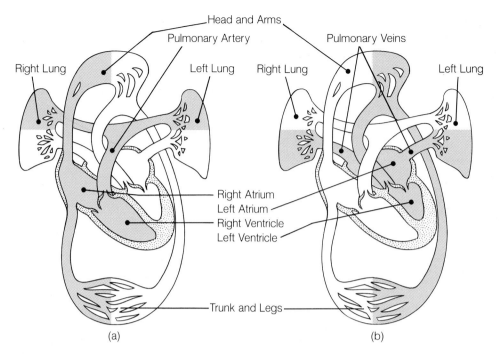

Right Lung
Head and Arms
Pulmonary Artery
Left Lung
Pulmonary Veins
Right Lung
Left Lung

Right Atrium
Left Atrium
Right Ventricle
Left Ventricle

Trunk and Legs

(a)   (b)

Figure 3.1. Blood flow associated with the right heart and left heart. Blood flow associated with the right heart (a). Note that the major purpose of the right heart is to pump blood to the lungs, where oxygen is picked up and carbon dioxide is eliminated. Blood flow associated with the left heart (b). Note that the left heart is responsible for pumping the blood out of the left ventricle via the aorta to all parts of the body. *(Drawn from Robert V. Hockey, Physical Fitness 2d ed., St. Louis: The C.V. Mosby Co., 1973. Drawings by Eugene Sinervo.)*

Figure 3.1 contains a diagram of the blood flow through the body.

In order to keep the blood flowing through the circulatory system and the lungs, a pump is needed to provide the force to keep the fluid in motion. The heart is the pump used for this purpose. The heart is a muscle about the size of your fist. The average heart beats approximately seventy-two times each minute, or one hundred thousand times per day. The amount of blood circulated in a twenty-four hour period is more than two thousand gallons. At rest, the heart ejects about five to six quarts of blood each minute, but during strenuous exercise this will increase to twenty to twenty-five quarts, as a result of the increased capability of the heart to pump blood.

Since the maintenance of life depends upon the chemical reactions taking place within the cell, it is easy to see why the transport and utilization of oxygen are of great importance.

It is possible to bring about some important changes in the circulatory and respiratory systems of the body through a proper training program.

EFFECTS OF TRAINING

Some of the changes due to a proper training program are:

1. The resting heart rate is decreased. By decreasing the resting heart rate by ten beats per minute, you can save approximately five million heart beats a year.

2. Blood volume is slightly increased and the red-blood cell count is increased. This brings about a greater increase in hemoglobin, which increases the capability of the blood to transport oxygen.

3. The amount of time required to recover from a bout of exercise is decreased.

4. The number of capillaries in the body is increased, which increases the efficiency of the exchange of oxygen, carbon dioxide, and nutrients between the blood and the body cells.

5. The body is more able to remove from the cells waste products that are produced as the result of prolonged exercise. The body can keep going longer without a feeling of fatigue.

6. There is a decrease in the respiratory rate (number of breaths per minute), which will decrease the amount of energy used by the respiratory muscles to move air into and out of the lungs.

7. The heart muscle becomes stronger, and this allows the heart to eject more blood (**stroke volume**) with each beat of the heart. The heart can now rest longer between beats and, therefore, is a much more efficient pump.

CORONARY HEART DISEASE

Today when you hear someone speak about "heart problems" it is probably a reference to coronary **heart disease.** This disease is the most common problem that besets American society today. More than one million Americans suffer a heart attack each year. More than half a million people die from coronary heart disease each year, which makes it the principal cause of death in the United States. The American Heart Association indicates that as many as 4.6 million Americans suffer from some type of coronary heart disease.

A **heart attack** is not primarily a disease of the heart muscle. The disease is brought about by the result of a condition in the coronary arteries that supply the heart muscle with blood. Some people believe that the heart receives its blood supply directly from the blood located in the various chambers of the heart that is being pumped throughout the circulatory system, but this is not true.

The heart, like other tissues of the body, receives its blood via arteries and other blood vessels that surround the heart muscle. As shown in figure 3.2, a complex network of arteries grows out of two main trunks, the right and left coronary arteries. These main coronary arteries branch much like a tree, with each branch smaller than the main trunk. Every part of the heart, no matter how small, is now supplied with blood that provides the oxygen and nutrients necessary for life. If anything should interfere with the flow of blood to the cells of the heart, then normal activity would cease for these cells and the result might be a heart attack.

In order to understand coronary heart disease, it is necessary to know the definitions of some commonly used terms.

Arteriosclerosis A general term for various types of arterial problems. It is associated with an increase in rigidity of the arterial wall and is sometimes defined as "hardening of the arteries."

Atherosclerosis A disease of the coronary arteries that develops over time due to a deposit of fat, cholesterol, and other substances on the inner lining of the artery. These deposits, known as **plaque,** narrow the arterial opening and thus restrict the flow of blood to vital tissues of the body. Sometimes a blood clot can result from the formulation of plaque and is known as a thrombus. Atherosclerosis in the blood vessels of the heart is a major cause of coronary heart disease.

Coronary occlusion A narrowing of a coronary blood vessel that restricts the flow of blood.

Coronary thrombosis A coronary occlusion caused by a blood clot (thrombus) that blocks the flow of blood to some part of the heart muscle.

Myocardial infarct A heart attack brought about by an occlusion of blood to the heart muscle. The result is death of the muscle cells of the heart.

Angina pectoris An uncomfortable sensation of pressure or pain in the center of the chest caused by the heart not getting enough oxygen through its blood supply. The pain or discomfort may spread to the left shoulder and arm as a feeling of numbness.

Since coronary heart disease is the leading cause of death in most industrialized nations, a great amount of money and effort is being spent to determine the causes of atherosclerosis and coronary heart disease. Although the actual cause has not been completely discovered, certain **risk factors** have been identified that may contribute to the disease. If a person can either eliminate or modify these risk factors, it might be possible to reduce the risk of developing coronary heart disease.

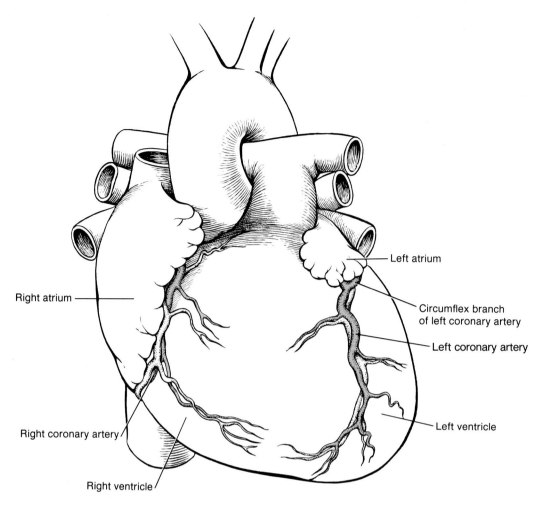

Figure 3.2. The coronary arteries. The heart muscle itself receives its blood supply from the coronary arteries. The main coronary arteries are the left coronary artery, one of its branches named the *circumflex,* and the right coronary artery. Atherosclerosis of these arteries leads to coronary heart disease. *(From Stuart Ira Fox,* Human Physiology. *© 1984 Wm. C. Brown Publishers, Dubuque, Iowa. All Rights Reserved. Reprinted by permission.)*

Table 3.1 Risk Factors Associated with Coronary Heart Disease

Risk Factors	Nonmedication Methods to Improve
Hypertension (high blood pressure)	Proper nutrition, exercise
High blood lipids	Proper nutrition, exercise
Smoking	Stop smoking
EKG abnormalities	Exercise
Over-fatness	Proper nutrition, body fat reduction, exercise
Diabetes	Proper nutrition, body fat reduction, exercise
Stressful life-style	Stress-reduction exercise
Dietary intake	Proper nutrition
Sedentary life-style	Exercise
Family history of heart disease	Not modifiable
Sex	Not modifiable
Age	Not modifiable

RISK FACTORS FOR CORONARY HEART DISEASE

Table 3.1 lists the factors associated with a high incidence of coronary heart disease. Only three of the factors, family history, sex, and age, cannot be affected by a change in life-style. All of the other factors can be modified by engaging in proper nutrition, stress reduction, exercise programs, and smoking cessation. The information concerning nutrition and stress reduction will be completely explained in the following chapters. This chapter will deal with the writing of a proper exercise program.

Exercise and Heart Disease

Physical exercise is not a cure-all for coronary heart disease and regardless of the amount of exercise, neither prevention nor recovery from heart disease can be guaranteed. But it is known that the proper exercise program can have beneficial effects and that there is a strong relationship between physical fitness and a decrease in heart disease.

Following are some of the ways that exercise can help reduce the risk of coronary heart disease.

1. Exercise reduces the incidence of heart disease. Extensive population studies reveal that people who exercise have less heart disease than nonexercisers. The research does not prove that exercise alone is the direct cause of the reduction and it may be a combination of factors that bring about the results. Many times when people begin to exercise, they also stop smoking, their diet improves, body fat decreases, and there is a reduction in stress and tension. The important point is not how exercise decreases heart disease, so long as it works in bringing about positive effects.

2. Exercise helps reduce the amount of fat in the blood. Proper exercise can remove fatty substances from the blood. This helps prevent the buildup of fatty plaques on the walls of the arteries that can narrow the openings of the arteries.

3. Exercise causes the heart muscle to become stronger. Just as the legs and arms become stronger when exercised, so does the heart muscle. The result is a stronger heart that needs fewer beats per minute to get the same job done. A stronger heart muscle will allow you to enjoy physical activity and also help the heart to better resist heart disease.

4. Exercise stimulates the development of **collateral circulation.** This opening of new branches in the coronary circulatory system may offset the effect of atherosclerosis. If a vessel becomes blocked, the new vessels can provide the blood with a pathway to service the heart tissue. This increase in collateral circulation helps to explain why some people who have narrower arteries do not have a heart attack and may also account for the excellent recovery of other individuals who have suffered from a heart attack.

5. Exercise helps reduce emotional stress. Research indicates that a favorable effect of exercise is reducing the tension of stress. In some cases, the training effects of exercise might even produce a protection against

stress. Exercise might help the various systems of the body resist the stresses of daily life that contribute to a breakdown of tissues.

The American Heart Association states, "Exercise training can increase cardiovascular function capacity and decrease myocardial oxygen demand for any given level of physical activity in normal persons as well as most cardiac patients. Regular physical activity is required to maintain the training effects. The potential risk of vigorous physical activity can be reduced by appropriate medical clearance, education, and guidance. Exercise may aid efforts to control cigarette smoking, hypertension, lipid abnormalities, diabetes, obesity, and emotional stress. Evidence suggests that regular, moderate, or vigorous occupational or leisure time physical activity may protect against coronary heart disease and may improve the likelihood of survival from a heart attack."

Dr. Paul O. Thompson, a cardiologist of the Miriam Hospital in Providence, Rhode Island, summed it up very well when he said, "If the only thing you're concerned about is surviving the next sixty minutes of your life, the smartest thing you can do is crawl into bed—alone. But if you're interested in living a long, active, productive life, then one of the smartest things you can do during the next hour is to exercise."

CARDIOVASCULAR ENDURANCE ACTIVITIES

Activities that develop increased oxygen transportation and utilization are sometimes referred to as **aerobic** exercises.

The word *aerobic* means "with oxygen," and indicates that the energy produced to do the work utilizes an oxygen system. By increasing the capacity of our aerobic system, we can become much more efficient organisms.

Aerobic exercises produce a positive training effect on many of the systems of the body such as the heart, lungs, muscles, and the circulatory and endocrine systems. The body increases its capacity to bring in oxygen, transport the oxygen to the necessary areas of the body, and then use the oxygen to produce energy to do work. Aerobic exercise is also the type of activity that helps to prevent cardiovascular disease. Even if a person should suffer a heart attack, this type of exercise helps him or her recover and once again live a normal, healthy life.

Examples of aerobic activities are aerobic dance, bicycling, walking, swimming, jogging, handball, and basketball. As the body is stimulated by participation in these activities, changes occur and an improved fitness level is obtained. The end result is a healthier, more efficient individual.

An all-out effort of short duration, such as the 100-yard dash or weight-training, does not develop the cardiovascular system to any great extent. Exercise of this type is known as *anaerobic activity* and does not utilize oxygen to produce energy. Anaerobic activities can be carried on for only a short period of time. Activities requiring speed rather than endurance impose anaerobic demands and may be exhausting and painful, both physiologically and psychologically.

Anaerobic exercises are necessary for the training of athletes, but have a lesser contribution in a personal physical fitness program. In cases where an individual has been sedentary for a long time, or if the person has damage to the heart, anaerobic exercises may be harmful.

In order to overcome the effects of sedentary living and the risks that accompany our effortless life-style, people can benefit most by engaging in a program of aerobic activities.

INTENSITY, DURATION, FREQUENCY, AND MODE OF ACTIVITY

Before you begin your cardiovascular endurance program you must become acquainted with four variables that affect the attainment of cardiovascular endurance. These are **intensity, duration, frequency,** and **mode** of activity. Intensity refers to how stressful the exercise is; duration has to do with the amount of time each exercise bout requires; frequency is the number of times you exercise each week; and mode is the type of activity selected, such as walking, jogging, aerobic dance, etc. The American College of Sports Medicine has issued a position statement, "The Recommended Quantity and Quality of Exercise for Developing and Maintaining Fitness in Healthy Adults." It provides information that can prove beneficial to anyone interested in a cardiovascular endurance program. The four major guidelines of this statement follow. A complete copy of the position statement, together with a list of references that provide a scientific rationale and research background for the statement, can be found in Appendix A.

Increasing numbers of people are becoming involved in endurance training activities and, thus, the need for exercise prescription guidelines is apparent.

Based on the existing evidence concerning exercise prescribed for healthy adults and the need for guidelines, the American College of Sports Medicine makes the following recommendations for the quantity and quality of training to develop and maintain cardiorespiratory fitness and body composition in the healthy adult:

1. Frequency of training: three to five days per week.

2. Intensity of training: 60 percent to 90 percent of maximum heart rate reserve, or 50 percent to 85 percent of maximum oxygen uptake (Vo_2 max).

3. Duration of training: fifteen to sixty minutes of continuous aerobic activity. Duration is dependent on the intensity of the activity: therefore, lower intensity activity should be conducted over a longer period of time. Because of the importance of the "total fitness" effect and the fact that it is more readily attained in longer duration programs, and because of the potential hazards and compliance problems associated with high-intensity activity, lower-to-moderate-intensity activity of longer duration is recommended for the nonathletic adult.

4. Mode of activity: Any activity that uses large muscle groups, that can be maintained continuously, and is rhythmical and aerobic in nature. For example, activities include running, jogging, walking, hiking, swimming, skating, bicycling, rowing, cross-country skiing, rope skipping, aerobic dance, and various endurance game activities.

The level of training intensity that is sufficient to bring about changes in cardiovascular endurance seems to be a specific target zone in which the activity is difficult enough to achieve fitness, but not of such a high intensity to be above safe limits. In the *Fitness for Life* program we use two methods to monitor intensity—heart rate and caloric expenditure.

RECOMMENDED EXERCISE HEART RATE

A fairly valid and reliable indicator of intensity can be obtained by measuring the heart rate obtained during participation in activity. In order to determine the recommended heart rate necessary to achieve a training effect, you must know your **maximal heart rate.**

To determine your heart rate you must be able to count your pulse. The pulse can be counted by placing the middle fingers over the carotid artery alongside the esophagus in the neck or over the radial artery on the thumb-side of the wrist. Check figure 3.3 for a description of how to perform these two procedures. If you use the carotid artery, be certain you do not apply too much pressure. Excessive pressure may cause the heart rate to slow down by reflex action. After you have determined the heart rate rhythm, start counting, with the first count of zero.

In order to determine maximal heart rate you could measure the pulse after an all-out endurance run. This type of procedure is not recommended, however, for people who are just beginning to exercise or for anyone who may have health problems, such as those associated with cardiovascular disease. It is possible to approximate your maximal heart rate by subtracting your age from 220. For example, a person twenty years of age would have an estimated maximal heart rate of two hundred beats per minute ($220 - 20 = 200$).

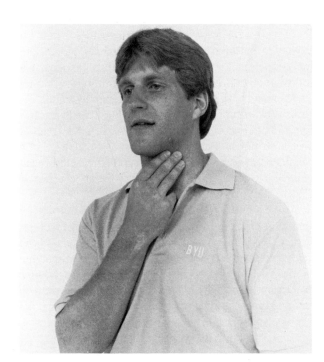

Figure 3.3(a). Carotid pulse.

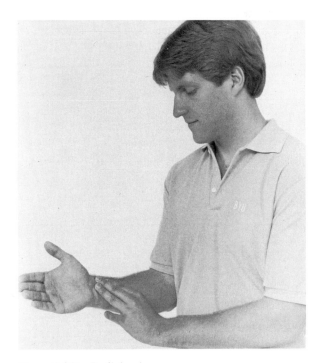

Figure 3.3(b). Radial pulse.

Average Maximal Heart Rates and Target Training Zones

Age	Maximal Heart Rate	Target Training Zones			
		70%	75%	80%	85%
10	210	147	158	168	179
15	205	144	154	164	174
20	200	140	150	160	170
25	195	137	146	156	166
30	190	133	143	152	162
35	185	130	139	148	157
40	180	126	135	144	153
45	175	123	131	140	149
50	170	119	128	136	145
55	165	116	124	132	140
60	160	112	120	128	136
65	155	109	116	124	132
70	150	105	113	120	128
75	145	102	109	116	123

Figure 3.4.

The heart rate necessary to bring about a training effect is between 70 and 85 percent of your maximal heart rate. To determine the heart rate you must achieve to ensure cardiovascular endurance training changes is a very simple matter. Take 70 percent of your maximal heart rate to find the lowest pulse you should have when training, and 85 percent of your maximal heart rate to estimate the highest pulse rate during an aerobic training bout.

Figure 3.4 contains the average maximal heart rates and target zones for training effects for selected age groups. If your age is not listed, compute the **heart rate training zone** as previously explained.

It is important to count the pulse immediately upon stopping the exercise in order to determine the exercise heart rate, because it begins to decrease quite rapidly once the exercise is slowed or stopped. Find your pulse within five seconds and count the number of heart beats for ten seconds; then multiply by six to determine your estimated exercise heart rate for one minute. Remember to start counting at zero.

CALORIC EXPENDITURE

Another factor you must consider is the **caloric expenditure** of the activity. Research by Dr. Thomas K. Cureton, former Director of the University of Illinois Physical Fitness Research Laboratory, indicates that in order to control blood fats (triglycerides) and cholesterol, which are risk factors in cardiovascular disease, a person should expend 300 or more calories in each workout session.[1] If you are just beginning an exercise program, it may take several weeks to attain this caloric expenditure. Associated with the beneficial effects of fat metabolism is the effect of caloric expenditure on weight control. One pound of body fat is the equivalent of approximately 3,500 calories. In order to utilize exercise as a means of achieving and maintaining a proper body weight, you must be willing to expend enough calories over a long enough period of time to achieve the expected results. Though some suggested exercise programs may help maintain a cardiovascular endurance training effect, they require such a low caloric expenditure that it would take approximately twelve weeks to lose 2 pounds of fat.

Appendix B contains a list of activities that have been measured to determine the average number of calories expended per minute for persons of various body weights.

For example, if you weigh 152 pounds and use half-court basketball as an exercise activity, you would expend 4.9 calories per minute. If your specific body weight is not listed, then go to the nearest weight. For example, if you weigh 163 pounds, you would check the caloric expenditure for a body weight of 161 pounds.

Caloric expenditure is directly related to heart rate. The relationship varies with the level of fitness. Therefore, you can use the information contained in figure 3.5 to determine the number of calories used in any activity if you know your current level of cardiovascular endurance.

To use this figure effectively, you need only to engage in an activity and determine your average exercise heart rate. Then find the line that represents your fitness category and corresponds to your heart rate; by lining up these two variables you can read the number of calories expended per minute at the bottom of the figure. This method enables you to determine caloric expenditure for any activity. It also indicates how a gain in fitness corresponds with a gain in caloric expenditure.

Knowing this type of information makes it possible for a person to combine a cardiovascular endurance program with a proper diet in order to engage in a weight-control program. This program will be explained in detail in chapter 5, "Writing a Weight-Control Program."

An effective way to rate the value of exercise and its contribution to cardiovascular endurance is to determine the amount of continuous exertion it requires. The key word in this concept is *continuous*. If we use activities such as weight training, bowling, or golf, which are examples of intermittent activities broken up with extended rest periods, the cardiovascular system is not stressed and, thus, the training effects are not achieved.

1. Thomas K. Cureton, *The Physiological Effects of Exercise Programs Upon Adults* (Springfield, IL.: Charles C. Thomas, Publisher, 1971), pp. 52–55.

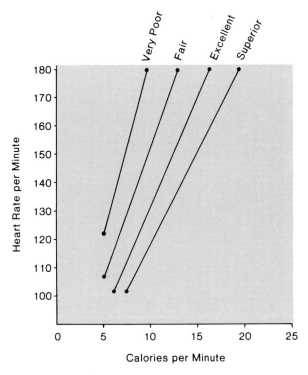

Figure 3.5. Predicting calories burned during physical activity from heart rate. *(Adapted from research of Dr. Brian Sharkey of the University of Northern Colorado. Reprinted by permission of the researcher.)*

Cardiovascular endurance activities should be maintained continuously for fifteen minutes or longer.

Three to five days a week is the recommended frequency of training to obtain cardiovascular endurance benefits. In the *Fitness for Life* program it is recommended that you exercise a minimum of four days per week. This type of exercise schedule ensures that you will not only obtain gains in cardiovascular endurance, but that you also will be better able to obtain and maintain a proper weight as a result of the caloric expenditure of the exercise.

By combining intensity, duration, and frequency you can provide yourself with a training stimulus that will allow you to obtain the many benefits, both physiological and psychological, that have been discussed in previous sections.

EXERCISE PROGRAM

When a person begins to engage in an exercise program the questions he or she usually asks are, "How much exercise do I need?" and "What activity is the best to develop endurance?" The cardiovascular endurance program developed in this chapter makes the answers relatively easy.

The program takes into consideration your present level of cardiovascular endurance (i.e., fitness category). In chapter 2, "Fitness Appraisal," you learned how to test yourself in order to determine your own cardiovascular endurance fitness category.

Following is a list of the categories:

0—Beginner	*IV*—Good
I—Very Poor	*V*—Excellent
II—Poor	*VI*—Superior
III—Fair	

If you haven't engaged in an exercise program for an extended period of time, you should begin on *Fitness Category 0, Beginner.* You should exercise at this level for approximately five weeks before taking the 1.5-mile run or the 3-mile walk.

Because it takes time for the body systems to adjust to increased activity, people initiating a program at a low level of fitness should begin by expending only 75 to 100 calories each workout session, at an intensity of approximately 5 calories per minute. Many individuals forget that they have been sedentary for many years and that it will take longer than a few weeks to get back into good physical condition.

It is recommended, therefore, that people in *Fitness Categories 0* and *I* have a minimum of three to five exercise sessions per week, with an expenditure of 75 to 100 calories per session and an intensity of 5 calories per minute.

For those individuals in *Fitness Categories II* and *III*, activity programs requiring 150 to 200 calories per session are recommended, at an intensity ranging from 5 to 10 calories per minute. A minimum of three to five days per week is recommended. As fitness improves, the intensity and duration can be increased.

Those in *Fitness Categories IV, V,* and *VI* can engage in almost any activity they desire. Caloric expenditures of 300 calories or more can be utilized in each exercise period to obtain the maximum training effects. Expenditures of above 10 calories per minute can be maintained without fear of injury or excessive fatigue.

The simplest way to determine whether you are progressing in your cardiovascular endurance program is to retake the 1.5-mile run or the 3-mile walk periodically. This will give you an assessment of your current status and show whether you have progressed from one fitness category to the next. In most instances, it is recommended that you take the test after the first five weeks of your program.

By being aware of the concepts concerning intensity, duration, frequency, and mode of activity, you can provide yourself with a sound cardiovascular endurance program that will enable you to travel toward the goal of increased physical fitness.

The use of the Cardiovascular Endurance Program Work Sheet located in Appendix C will make writing a fitness program fairly easy. It consists of four steps:

Step 1. Fill in items 1 through 4 of the work sheet.

Step 2. Choose an activity from the list of appropriate cardiovascular endurance exercises contained in Appendix B.

Step 3. Determine how long you or your subject will engage in the selected activity and determine the recommended exercise heart rate.

Step 4. With the information provided, write a cardiovascular endurance program for yourself or for the person who is exercising.

To help you become familiar with these steps we will practice writing a program based on a sample case.

CASE
Paul Reynolds

A businessperson by the name of Paul Reynolds wants to start a cardiovascular endurance program. He is thirty-five years old and prefers to play handball on Tuesdays and Thursdays. He wants to run four other days of the week at a 7-mile-per-hour pace. He weighs 170 pounds and is in *Fitness Category V.* He had a medical examination with a resting EKG two months ago, and has been given medical clearance.

Step 1: Filling out the work sheet

Item 1. Fill in Paul's full name and the current date.

Item 2. Fill in Paul's weight (170 pounds) and age (thirty-five).

Item 3. Paul has had proper medical clearance, so check *No Restrictions.*

Step 2: Selecting the cardiovascular endurance activity

Item 4. Place a check by Paul's fitness category *(V)* in item 4. By reading to the right, you see that Paul can expend a minimum of 300 calories per exercise session at an intensity of 10 calories per minute or higher. He should exercise a minimum of three to five days per week. Paul has stated that he wishes to exercise six days each week.

Item 5. Paul wants to play handball twice a week and run four days at a 7-mile-per-hour pace. Record these in the blanks provided.

Item 6. Check the Calorie-Expenditure-per-Minute table in Appendix B to determine how many calories per minute a person weighing 170 pounds expends. Locate the nearest body weight, which is 170, on the top of the chart and read down until you find handball, which is 11.0 calories per minute, and running (7 mph), which is 15.7 calories per minute. Write these figures in the blank next to item 6.

Item 7. Paul determines the recommended caloric expenditure per exercise session by referring to item 4. For *Fitness Category V,* this is 300 calories or more. Record this number in the blank.

Step 3: Determining the duration of the selected activity

Item 8. In order to determine the minimum number of minutes to exercise for each activity, divide the caloric value in item 7 (300) by the calories per minute for handball (11) and then do the same thing for running (15.7). Round off your answer to the nearest whole number and record these figures in item 8. You should have a minimum of twenty-seven minutes for handball and nineteen minutes for running.

It is important to remember that the duration should always be fifteen or more minutes of *continuous* exercise in order to obtain a cardiovascular endurance training effect.

Item 9. In order to determine Paul's recommended heart rate zone while he is exercising to provide him with a training stimulus, you find his age, thirty-five, in the table in item 9. Read to the right of his age to determine the training zone for 70 percent and 85 percent. The zone for a training effect is between 130 and 157 beats per minute. Record these figures in the blanks provided to the right of item 9. By monitoring his heart rate periodically during his exercise program, he will have an added check to make sure his training intensity is of such a nature as to bring about cardiovascular endurance changes.

Step 4: Filling in the cardiovascular endurance program

On the first line of the *Week* column, write a *1* to represent the first week of the program. In the *Days* column, list the days of the week from *Monday* to *Saturday*.

Because you already know that Paul plays handball on Tuesday and Thursday, write *handball* next to these days, then write *running (7 mph)* beside the remaining days of the week.

In the *Duration* column, write in the time he will spend playing handball and running during each exercise session. This can be obtained from item 9, and will be a minimum of nineteen minutes for running and twenty-seven minutes for handball. If Paul wishes to increase his caloric expenditure, he can increase the amount of time he spends in each exercise session.

When you have completed Paul's work sheet, check your copy with the work sheet in figure 3.6.

MASTERY CHECK INSTRUCTIONS

Instructions: Read each of the cases, then answer the multiple-choice items. You may use the Cardiovascular Endurance Program Work Sheet in Appendix C to determine the correct answers.

A. Jack played high school basketball and would like to play half-court basketball as a conditioning activity. He is twenty years of age and weighs 163 pounds. He has received medical clearance and is in *Fitness Category IV.*
  1. Jack should expend how many calories each workout session?
     a. 100
     b. 200
     c. 300
  2. His suggested exercise intensity (cals./min.) will be
     a. 5.
     b. 5–10.
     c. 10+.
  3. Jack will expend approximately how many calories per minute while playing half-court basketball?
     a. 4.7
     b. 5.3
     c. 6.0

  4. Jack's recommended target zone for heart rate to obtain a training effect will be
     a. 137–166.
     b. 140–170.
     c. 144–174.

B. Sandra, who is in *Fitness Category V,* has received medical clearance for an exercise program. She wants to use timed calisthenics as her activity. She is thirty-five years old and weighs 125 pounds.
  1. Sandra should exercise a minimum of how many days per week?
     a. 1–2
     b. 3–5
     c. 6–7
  2. She should spend a minimum of how many minutes of exercise each session?
     a. 20
     b. 25
     c. 30
  3. Sandra's recommended target zone for heart rate to obtain a training effect will be
     a. 123–149.
     b. 126–153.
     c. 130–157.

Cardiovascular Endurance Program Work Sheet

1. Name _Paul Reynolds_ _____ Date _____

2. Weight _170_ _____ Age _35_ _____

3. Medical Clearance: No Restrictions _X_ _____ Restrictions _____

4. **Fitness Category**

Fitness Category	Minimum Caloric Expenditure per Exercise Session	Exercise Intensity Cals./Min.	Minimum Number of Days to Exercise Each Week
___ 0. Beginner	75	5	3–5
___ I. Very Poor	100	5	3–5
___ II. Poor	150	5–10	3–5
___ III. Fair	200	5–10	3–5
___ IV. Good	300+	10+	3–5
_X_ V. Excellent	300+	10+	3–5
___ VI. Superior	300+	10+	3–5

5. Exercise preference _handball, running_ _____ Rate _7 mph_

6. Calories expended per minute (from Appendix B) _handball = 11   running = 15.7_

7. Recommended caloric expenditure per session (from item 4) _300 +_

8. Number of minutes to exercise each day (item 7 ÷ item 6) _handball = 27   running = 19_
   Note: This should always be a minimum of 15 continuous minutes to obtain training effect. (Round off to nearest whole number.)

9. Recommended exercise heart rate training zone: _130_ to _157_

Age	Maximal Heart Rate	Target Zone 70%	Target Zone 85%	Age	Maximal Heart Rate	Target Zone 70%	Target Zone 85%
10	210	147	179	45	175	123	149
15	205	144	174	50	170	119	145
20	200	140	170	55	165	116	140
25	195	137	166	60	160	112	136
30	190	133	162	65	155	109	132
35	185	130	157	70	150	105	128
40	180	126	153	75	145	102	123

Cardiovascular Endurance Program

Week	Days	Exercise	Duration of Activity
1	Monday	running	19
	Tuesday	handball	27
	Wednesday	running	19
	Thursday	handball	27
	Friday	running	19
	Saturday	running	19

Figure 3.6.

Answers:

A. 1. c   B. 1. b
   2. c   2. b
   3. b   3. c
   4. b

If you responded correctly to each item, you are ready to proceed with the next unit.

SUGGESTIONS FOR FURTHER READING

Check the references given for the American College of Sports Medicine's position statement, "The Recommended Quantity and Quality of Exercise for Developing and Maintaining Fitness in Healthy Adults." This is contained in Appendix A. These references contain excellent material concerning cardiovascular endurance programs.

4

APPLYING A CARDIOVASCULAR ENDURANCE PROGRAM

Objective

After study of this chapter you should be able to

• use your own written cardiovascular endurance program and contract to engage in an appropriate cardiovascular endurance program.

Now that you have completed the chapter, "Writing a Cardiovascular Endurance Program," we assume that you are eager to start your exercise program. There are, however, a few important facts we must consider before heading for the gym, tennis courts, swimming pool, or track.

TIPS TO MAKE EXERCISE MORE BENEFICIAL

In our competitive society we are always in a hurry to achieve our goals. This type of plan doesn't always work in exercise, especially if you are in *Fitness Categories 0, I, II,* and *III*. It has taken your body time to get out of condition and, in most cases, it will take more than a few weeks to get it back into condition. Progression is built into your cardiovascular endurance program. It is there for a reason. Progressive increase will give the heart and circulatory system an opportunity to develop, and also allow the muscles and connective tissue to adjust to the stress of a new exercise program.

Following are some important guidelines that will make your exercise program a more enjoyable experience.

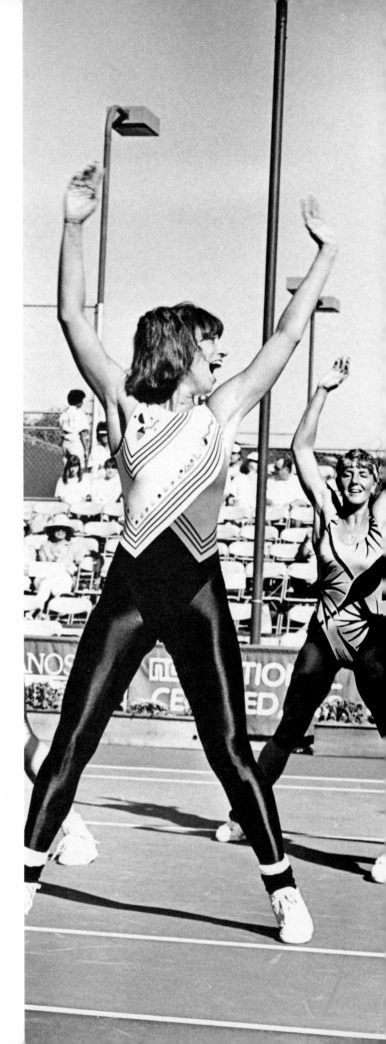

Warm-Up

A person wouldn't start an expensive automobile on a cold morning and immediately attempt to drive it at maximum speed. You are dealing with an expensive machine also—the human body. It is particularly unwise for most people over thirty to start exercising strenuously without first warming up.

A good rule of thumb is to **warm up** with activities related to the sport in which you wish to engage. For example, if you are using swimming in your program, do a few slow laps as warm-up. If you are walking or jogging, start the exercise slowly and then increase the speed. The five or ten minutes spent in warm-up will be time that will reduce muscular aches and pains.

This is also a good time to do your flexibility program, which will be explained in detail in chapter 9, "Writing a Flexibility Program." The stretching exercises will promote development of flexibility as well as help warm up the muscles, joints, tendons, and ligaments for the cardiovascular endurance training session.

Good Judgment

Avoid stress to the point that you are completely fatigued. Signs of overwork are (1) extreme pain in the chest, (2) dizziness, (3) severe breathlessness, (4) lightheadedness, and (5) nausea. These symptoms are the body's way of indicating that you should stop exercising.

Consistency

We wish to emphasize the importance of exercising on a regular time schedule. Research indicates that a person should receive training stimuli at least three to five days a week in order to gain and maintain cardiovascular endurance. Regularity is also a safety precaution. The people who have problems are the "hit-and-miss" exercisers. Their type of program does not develop or maintain fitness.

Although regularity of exercise is important, you should not exercise when you become ill.

Clothing

Wear clothing that is loose and comfortable. Avoid rubberized suits as they can be very dangerous, especially in hot and humid weather. They are **not** an aid in weight reduction.

The shoes you wear while exercising are among the most important items. Purchase a good pair of quality shoes. Good shoes and socks are your best prevention against blisters, sore feet, and aching ankles and knees.

If you desire more information about jogging shoes, *Runner's World,* a monthly magazine for runners of all sexes and ages, has an issue each year that is devoted to a rating of the different brands of running shoes. We suggest that you check this publication for information and a rating of most running shoes in which you might be interested.

Time of Day to Exercise

Almost any time of day, other than an hour or so after a meal, is acceptable for exercise. Exercise during the middle of a hot, humid day should also be avoided. We suggest you set aside a specific time of day for your exercise program. Such a schedule increases the chances that you will adhere to your program.

Motivation

The first five to six weeks of your exercise program will be the most difficult. In many cases you are changing your life-style and taking part in a totally different activity. As you start to experience physiological and psychological changes, however, all your time and effort will be rewarded. You will feel better and, in many cases, look better.

If you find it hard to exercise by yourself, try to work with a group or a friend. Often group effort has provided the stimulus to carry a beginner through the first few weeks.

Following are some tips for maintaining motivation in an exercise program:

1. Keep your workouts moving at a fast, brisk pace.
2. Don't overexercise.
3. Work out in different places.
4. Start your workouts at the same time each day. Use different activities if you wish and, thus, avoid boredom.
5. Set a goal.
6. Keep a progress chart.
7. Concentrate on success.
8. Remember that exercise should be enjoyable.

Cool Down

Cooling down is as important as warming up. A minimum of five minutes should be allowed to give the body the opportunity to recover from the stress of exercise. In order to keep the blood circulating, taper off gradually by walking or jogging slowly.

A series of one-way valves are located in the veins of the circulatory system in order to permit the blood to flow in only one direction. As the muscles contract during the **cool down** they create pressure against the veins, which in turn aid in the return of blood to the heart. Without this cool down period, the blood might pool in the lower body and cause you to experience dizziness or even pass out due to the lack of blood flow to the brain. You also should avoid going into a steam room, sauna, or hot shower immediately after exercise. A general indicator is to cool down until you have stopped sweating profusely and until the heart rate has dropped to one hundred beats or less per minute.

You are now entering a program that should be lifelong. President John F. Kennedy summed up what we hope will be your approach to exercise:

> Physical fitness is not only one of the most important keys to a healthy body, it is the basis of dynamic and creative intellectual activity. The relationship between the soundness of the body and the activities of the mind is subtle and complex. Much is not yet understood. But we do know what the Greeks knew: that intelligence and skill can only function at the peak of their capacity when the body is healthy and strong; that hardy spirits and tough minds usually inhabit sound bodies.[1]

COMMONLY ASKED QUESTIONS

Through the years, we have kept a record of the most common questions that people have asked about exercise.

How can I determine how strenuous an exercise is? An easy method is to count the exercise pulse rate, which is a good indication of exertion. The higher the pulse rate, the greater the intensity of exertion. Another method is to check the caloric expenditure of various activities that you will find listed in Appendix B. The more calories expended per minute, the greater the exertion.

If I am overweight, will running instead of a diet help me? Running, dieting, or both will help. Remember that to lose weight you must decrease the food consumed, or increase exercise, or both. Exercise combined with diet results in a greater reduction of body fat. Caution: dieting alone may result in a loss of muscle tissue along with the fat.

Can I avoid a heart attack if I achieve good cardiovascular endurance? One of the high-risk factors contributing to heart disease is inactivity. Cardiovascular fitness cannot promise immunity from heart disease; however, it decreases your chances of incurring an attack, decreases the severity of most attacks, and increases your chances of survival.

1. John F. Kennedy, "The Soft American," *Sports Illustrated* 13 (26 December 1960):16.

Why do I perspire more after I run than while I am running? The body has a certain amount of blood to send to the various systems. During vigorous exercise there is a great demand for blood by the skeletal muscles. In order to fulfill this demand, blood is shunted from the skin to the muscles, which causes a buildup of heat. At the cessation of exercise, the body can send additional blood to the skin and we begin to perspire more profusely in order to dissipate the excess heat. Also, sweat evaporates more rapidly while we run, thus increasing the efficiency of our cooling mechanism during exercise.

Should I exercise when it is really hot? When a person exercises, only about 30 percent of the energy produced is used for movement. The other 70 percent is converted to heat. If your body can't get rid of this heat, serious consequences can develop. To become acclimated to the heat, work at approximately half your regular caloric output for eight to ten days. Signs of heat distress are a throbbing in your temples and a cold sensation around your sides, chest, and back. Cool off immediately with a cool shower, and drink cool fluids.

The American College of Sports Medicine has given some helpful guidelines for exercise in the heat:

1. Don't run more than ten miles when the temperature on a wet bulb globe thermometer exceeds 82.4° F. To obtain this type of a temperature reading, use an instrument consisting of two thermometers. The bulb of one thermometer will be wet. The wet bulb will be cooled by evaporation and, consequently, will show a temperature lower than that of the dry bulb thermometer. The evaporation is less on a humid day, and so the difference between the thermometer readings is greater when the air is dry. The difference between the two readings constitutes a measure of the dryness of the surrounding air.

2. In hot weather, exercise early in the morning or later in the evening.

3. Drink thirteen to seventeen ounces of fluid ten to fifteen minutes before running, and frequently during long runs.

4. Don't drink fluids with high sugar or electrolyte content. Use only small amounts of sugar (about 2 grams glucose per 100 milliliters of water) and electrolytes (less than 10 mEq sodium and 5 mEq potassium per liter of solution).

5. Make as much of the skin surface as possible available to the circulating air to aid in the evaporation of sweat.

How do you account for the fact that some people will score in the excellent *category in one fitness test, but only in the* fair *or* good *category in another?* The five aspects of physical fitness (cardiovascular endurance, strength, flexibility, weight control, and relaxation) are separate variables. Even though they are interrelated, a person must write and engage in exercise programs for each of the variables to obtain overall physical fitness.

I'm only twenty-five years of age. Should I worry about heart disease? Even though a person may die of heart disease at age fifty-five, it is probable that he or she started to contract the disease at a much earlier age. One study of military personnel (average age twenty-two years) killed in the Korean and Vietnam conflicts showed that approximately 77 percent of them already had evidence of atherosclerosis.

Someone told me that children don't need to exercise since they get plenty of activity. What is your reaction to this statement? The average American child in elementary school spends 90 percent of his or her waking hours in a sitting position, and it is estimated that childhood obesity is increasing each year. The important thing to remember is to make exercise enjoyable and to help children select activities that are fun. The problem with many sports activities is that half of the people are winners and the other half are losers. If we lose all of the time, we tend to avoid the activity. So select an activity in which everyone can win, such as jogging, swimming, hiking, or bicycling.

Do children have to worry about cholesterol and blood fats the way adults do? Heart disease probably starts at a young age, and some children ten or eleven years old have abnormal fatty deposits in the circulatory vessels.

I'm almost seventy years old. Isn't it too late to get any benefits from an exercise program? It may take longer than it would if you were twenty-five and you will want to make sure you have medical clearance, but it is not too late. There is an abundance of research that reports many benefits resulting from exercise programs for older people.

Is it okay to exercise when I have varicose veins? It depends on how bad the veins are. Consult your doctor and ask about wearing support hose that might assist in circulation. You might want to consider walking in waist-high water to obtain hydrostatic support and massage from the water while exercising. You could also use swimming or bicycling as your mode of exercise.

I seem to reach plateaus with my training. I achieve steady progress, and then, for no apparent reason, my performance levels off or decreases. What can I do about this problem? The human body will go through various training stages physiologically as it adapts to the stress placed on it. If you are training for long periods of time, your performance will often be good for six to twelve weeks and then drop off. This is an indication that you should back off on your training and not overwork. This is the cause of the "staleness" that occurs with many athletes.

What are the effects of sleep on exercise? Research seems to indicate that either too much or too little sleep can have a negative effect on performance. Each person has a unique sleep requirement that must be determined by trial and error.

What is second wind? It is not known what causes this phenomenon, but it is usually preceded by intense breathlessness and other distress. This distress leaves as the exercise continues and you are able to continue exercising with ease. It is probably a result of the metabolic processes of the body obtaining a state of equilibrium. An example is a diversion of blood to the working muscles of the body to provide sufficient amounts of oxygen.

If I donate blood, should I reduce my training? Legitimate blood banks will not accept donors who have health problems, so we assume that you are in good health. Follow the guidelines given to you when donating blood and there will not be any problems.

Does smoking affect my ability to exercise? Smoking not only reduces the amount of oxygen carried by the hemoglobin, but it increases the resistance to airflow into and out of the lungs. This, in turn, reduces your ability to do endurance-type activities.

What is interval training? Regardless of the type of activity, such as running, swimming, cycling, and the like, **interval training** is simply repeated periods of physical training interspersed with recovery periods. During recovery periods, activity of reduced intensity, such as walking, is performed. This procedure is repeated a certain number of times, depending on the ability of the individual and the time available. The greatest advantage of interval training over many other forms of endurance training is that a greater amount of work can be performed in a shorter period of time. The total amount of exercise performed by a person can be varied by changing the following factors: speed or intensity of the exercise bout; duration or distance of the effort; number of times the bout of exercise is repeated; the length of the recovery period; and the type of activity utilized during the recovery period.

What are the effects of running during pregnancy? According to Dr. Evalyn Gendel, Director of the Division of Maternal and Child Health for the Kansas State Department of Health, there is no reason why women should not exercise during pregnancy, especially if they were exercising prior to becoming pregnant. In most cases, it is not only permissible but desirable. Consult your personal physician to determine any unique problems you may have, and to decide what form of exercise is best for you.

Are women really different from men in their ability to exercise? There are some basic physiological differences that affect the training potential of women. For instance, women have a slightly lower hemoglobin level and a relatively smaller size heart than men. These two differences can have an effect on the amount of oxygen available to the cells during exercise. Women also have less total muscle mass than men. The quality of their muscle is similar; they just have a smaller quantity and this has an effect on their total body strength compared to that of men. Regardless of the physiological differences, exercise can be enjoyable and fulfilling for both sexes, and the same type of training program can be used to increase physical fitness for both males and females.

I read somewhere that women shouldn't jog because they may displace the uterus or snap ligaments in the breasts, causing them to droop. Are these stories true? There seems to be no research justifying these claims. Most physicians feel positive about the effects of exercise for women. Most women who exercise report an increase in the firmness of the breasts. This increase in firmness is probably due to a loss of body fat, and the action of the arms and chest muscles during exercise may firm up the pectoral muscles, which

are support for the breasts. The uterus has the best shock-absorbing system in the human body and so-called displacement is a fallacy. Dr. Evalyn Gendel reported that women in top physical condition have less menstrual discomfort, fewer backaches, less digestive disorders, fewer colds, and less fatigue than their nonexercising peers.

I am convinced of the positive benefits of exercise, but have a hard time staying with a program. What do you suggest? Try to find a friend with whom to work out and don't make your exercise program a source of great competition. Set some goals and sign a contract, witnessed by a friend, to meet your goals.

At what speed does jogging become running? It is not possible to determine this by a miles-per-hour pace, since everyone has different capabilities. A good test is the "talk test." If you can't talk to someone while exercising, this is probably running, not jogging.

What about exercising in cold weather? Freezing of the lungs does not occur because the air is warmed in the mouth and nasal passages before entering the lungs. The extreme dryness of cold air, however, may cause a cracking and bleeding of the respiratory passages. When exercising in the cold, it is important to protect the hands, head, and feet. You will want to wear several layers of lightweight clothing rather than heavy, bulky garments. Wind velocity is a big factor in cold weather; as the wind increases, it has a tremendous effect on the chill factor.

Should I use salt tablets when exercising? Unless salt tablets are taken with large amounts of water they may upset the gastrointestinal tract and also slow down the absorption process. Liberal salting of your food should provide all the salt you need.

What effect will higher altitudes have on my exercise sessions? As the altitude increases, there is a decrease in the amount of oxygen available for aerobic processes. In time the body will adjust to these changes. It is estimated that you should allow two to three weeks to acclimatize for every 3,000 feet of change in elevation.

Are ten-speed bikes better than three-speed bikes for physical fitness? The important factor is the gear ratio of each bike. Ten-speed bikes have a larger selection of gear ratios than do three-speed bikes. You can adjust the difficulty of exercise by using a three-speed bicycle or a ten-speed bicycle with their different gear ratios, and, therefore, affect the amount of time necessary to obtain a training result.

How should I breathe when I run? Just breathe normally. The demands of the body will determine the number of breaths per minute. Breathe in and out through both the mouth and nose at a rate that feels comfortable. Holding the breath or attempting to regulate breathing does not increase the strength of the respiratory muscles or contribute to cardiovascular fitness.

Is it better to run on a soft surface than on a hard one? What about running in sand on the beach? In most cases it is better to run on a soft surface such as grass in order to reduce the stress on the joints and connective tissue. An important factor is footwear, because proper shoes are a great aid in absorbing the shock of running. Running in sand on the beach is an enjoyable activity, but you will probably find an increase in your running time as a result of the added resistance of the loose sand. Many people enjoy running in the water, which has a cooling effect on the body and is quite refreshing.

What if I get a pain in my side when I exercise? It is not known what causes the pain in the side. One theory is that it is caused by trapped metabolic gases, which create an increase in pressure that brings about pain. Another theory is that it is caused by lack of oxygen to the respiratory

muscles. If you should experience this phenomenon, the best treatment is to stop running and walk until the pain subsides. As you continue your conditioning program and your cardiovascular fitness improves, the problem will be eliminated in most cases.

What if I must interrupt a regular exercise program for a vacation or a business trip or because of illness? Much of the conditioning gained after a four-week training program is lost within two weeks when training is stopped completely. These findings support the recommendation that we exercise at least three to five days a week to maintain cardiovascular fitness. A person can maintain fitness by walking or stair climbing if regular exercise facilities are not available. Exercise should be eliminated, however, when one is ill.

What are shin splints? **Shin splints** are an inflammation of the muscle and/or tendons of the lower leg caused by repetitive running on a hard surface or by running on the toes. Much of the soreness can be eliminated by stretching the legs in a good flexibility program. If this does not help, you may have to discontinue running until the legs heal.

APPLYING A CARDIOVASCULAR ENDURANCE PROGRAM

By using the Cardiovascular Endurance Program Contract in figure 4.1, preparing your own fitness program is a fairly easy six-step process.

Step 1. Prepare your own Cardiovascular Endurance Program Work Sheet.
Step 2. Fill out your Cardiovascular Endurance Program Contract.
Step 3. Get your contract approved.

Step 4. Implement the program and record your progress on the Cardiovascular Endurance Progress Log in figure 4.2.
Step 5. Check progress.
Step 6. Complete contract.

To help you become familiar with these procedures, we will go through them step-by-step.

Step 1: Preparing your own cardiovascular endurance program work sheet

You should have learned how to complete a personal Cardiovascular Endurance Program Work Sheet while you were studying chapter 3. If you have not written out a work sheet for yourself, write one now before going on with this unit.

Step 2: Filling out your Cardiovascular Endurance Program Contract

The work copy of the Cardiovascular Endurance Program Contract in figure 4.1 will help you implement your fitness program. This contract is quite easy to fill out if you have completed a Cardiovascular Endurance Program Work Sheet for yourself, as explained in chapter 3. Using this work sheet, fill out your contract as follows:

Cardiovascular Endurance Program Contract

1. Name _____ Age _____

2. Beginning Fitness Category: ___ 0. Beginner   ___ II. Poor   ___ IV. Good   ___ VI. Superior
                                 ___ I. Very Poor ___ III. Fair ___ V. Excellent

3. Desired cardiovascular exercise(s): _____

4. Recommended exercise heart rate training zone: _____ to _____

Week	Days	Exercise	Rate	Duration
1				
2				
3				
4				
5				
6				
7				
8				
9				
10				

Signature: _____

Contract approval date: _____ Approved by: _____

Progress check date: _____ Approved by: _____

Contract completion date: _____ Approved by: _____

Figure 4.1.

Cardiovascular Endurance Progress Log

Name _____ Age _____

Beginning cardiovascular endurance level _____

Exercise(s): _____ Exercise heart rate training zone: _____ to _____

Week	Date	Day	Exercise	Rate		Duration
				Time	Distance	

Figure 4.2.

Item 1. Fill in your name and age.

Item 2. Place a check by your fitness category. This information can be found in item 4 of the Cardiovascular Endurance Program Work Sheet you filled out while studying chapter 3.

Item 3. Write your desired exercise in the blank. Use the information on your Cardiovascular Endurance Program Work Sheet to fill in the columns on the contract. In the *Week* column are listed the numbers 1 through 10, representing ten weeks of your program. In the *Days* column, write the number of days you will be exercising during each week of your program. In the *Exercise* column, write the aerobic exercises you will be doing every day of every week of your program. In the *Rate* column, write how fast you will walk, run, cycle, swim, and so forth. If your exercise has no measurable rate, ignore this column. In the *Duration* column, write how long you will exercise.

Item 4. Fill in your recommended zone for exercise heart rate. Take this information from item 9 of your Cardiovascular Endurance Program Work Sheet.

Step 3: Getting your contract approved

When you have filled in every week of your contract, it should be approved. If you are a student in a physical education class, it can be signed by your instructor. If you are not enrolled in some organized class, then have it signed by a friend.

The reason for having your contract approved is to reaffirm your commitment to a life-style of personal fitness. It has been found that by involving someone else, people are more likely to continue to engage in their fitness programs.

Step 4: Implementing your program and recording your progress on the cardiovascular endurance progress log

Begin your activity as soon as your contract has been approved. After each exercise period, fill in your Cardiovascular Endurance Progress Log in figure 4.2. This will help you keep an accurate account of your work in the program. After every exercise period, write in the log the number of the week of your program (1–10), the date and the day of your workout, the exercise you engaged in, and the rate and duration of the exercise.

Step 5: Progress check

At the completion of five weeks of your Cardiovascular Endurance Program Contract, it is recommended that you take a progress check by retaking the 1.5-mile test or the 3-mile walking test, as explained in the unit on Administering and Interpreting Cardiovascular Endurance Tests in chapter 2. The progress check will give you some idea of how you are progressing in your fitness program. If you want to make changes in your program after your progress check, you may do so. Make sure you have the progress check approved in order to reaffirm your decision to improve your cardiovascular endurance.

Step 6: Contract completion

When you have completed your exercise program for the selected number of weeks, repeat your fitness appraisal and have your contract approved by the person who originally signed the contract.

This does not mean you will stop exercising; it only indicates you have started a new life-style. You must continue to exercise for the rest of your life either to improve or to maintain your cardiovascular endurance.

SUGGESTIONS FOR FURTHER READING

1. Allen, T. E., P. G. Hatcher, J. B. Lewis, and R. N. Morgan. "Metabolic and Cardiorespiratory Responses of Young Women to Skipping and Jogging." *The Physician and Sports Medicine* 15 May (1987):109.
2. Allsen, Philip E. *Conditioning and Physical Fitness: Current Answers to Relevant Questions.* Dubuque, Iowa: Wm. C. Brown Company Publishers, 1978.
3. Allsen, P. E. "Circulorespiratory Endurance." *Journal of Physical Education, Recreation, and Dance* 52 September (1981):36.
4. American Heart Association. "Subcommittee on External Cardiac Rehabilitation: Statement on Exercise." *Circulation* 64(1981):1302.
5. Barnard, R. James. "The Heart Needs Warm-up Time." *The Physician and Sports Medicine* 4 (1976):40.
6. Barnes, L. "Do Exercise Walkers Need Special Walking Shoes?" *The Physician and Sports Medicine* 15 June (1987):213.
7. Drinkwater, Barbara L. "Aerobic Power in Females." *Journal of Physical Education and Recreation* 46 (1976):36.
8. Duda, M. "The Medical Risks and Benefits of Sauna, Steam Bath, and Whirlpool Use." *The Physician and Sports Medicine* 15 May (1987):170.
9. Feigel, B., and D. Zamzow. "Orthotics." *Runner's World* 17 June (1982): no. 6, p. 40.

10. Fisher, A. Garth, and Philip E. Allsen. *Jogging*. Dubuque, Iowa: Wm. C. Brown Company Publishers, 1987.

11. Fuertges, Don R. "Is There Any Value to Warm-up?" *Coach and Athlete* 38 (1976):14.

12. Holloszy, John O. "Adaptation of Skeletal Muscle to Endurance Exercise." *Medicine and Science in Sports* 7 (1975):155.

13. Krissoff, W. B., and Ben Eiseman. "The Hazards of Exercising at Altitude." *The Physician and Sports Medicine* 3 (1975):26.

14. Martin, B. J., S. Robinson, D. L. Wiegman, and L. H. Aulick. "Effect of Warm-up on Metabolic Responses to Strenuous Exercise." *Medicine and Science in Sports* 7 (1975):146.

15. Massicaffe, Denis R., and Ross B. J. MacNab. "Cardiorespiratory Adaptations to Training at Specified Intensities in Children." *Medicine and Science in Sports* 6 (1974):242.

16. Monahan, T. "Should Women Go Easy On Exercise." *The Physician and Sports Medicine* 14 December (1986):188.

17. Morton, C. "Running Backward May Help Athletes Move Forward." *The Physician and Sports Medicine* 14 December (1986):149.

18. Porcari, J., R. McCarron, G. Hine, P. S. Freedson, A. Ward, J. A. Ross, and J. M. Rippe. "Is Fast Walking an Adequate Training Stimulus for 30-to-69-Year-Old Men and Women?" *The Physician and Sports Medicine* 15 February (1987):119.

19. President's Council on Physical Fitness and Sports. *Conditioning Through Aquatic Activities*. Washington, D.C.

20. President's Council on Physical Fitness and Sports. *Interval Training*. Washington, D.C.

21. President's Council on Physical Fitness and Sports. *Jogging Guidelines*. Washington, D.C.

22. Shephard, Roy J. "What Causes Second Wind?" *The Physician and Sports Medicine* 2 (1974):37.

23. Stockard, J. "Aerobic Dancing May Be Rx for Women's Cardio-Fitness." *Journal of Physical Education and Programs* 78 September (1981):6.

24. "Walking For Fitness—Round Table." *The Physician and Sports Medicine* 14 October (1986):144.

25. Ward, A. "Born To Jog: Exercise Programs for Preschoolers." *The Physician and Sports Medicine* 14 December (1986):163.

26. Williams, M. H. "Blood Doping: An Update." *The Physician and Sports Medicine* 9 July (1981): no. 7, p. 59.

27. Winningham, M. L., M. G. MacVicar, and C. A. Burke. "Exercise for Cancer Patients: Guidelines and Precautions." *The Physician and Sports Medicine* 14 October (1986):125.

28. Work, J. A. "Treating Patients Who Have High Cholesterol Levels: The Role of Screening Tests, Drugs, and Exercise." *The Physician and Sports Medicine* 15 August (1987):113.

29. Zarandona, J. E., A. G. Nelson, R. K. Conlee, and A. G. Fisher. "Physiological Responses to Hand-Carried Weights." *The Physician and Sports Medicine* 14 October (1986):113.

5

WRITING A WEIGHT-CONTROL PROGRAM

Objectives

After study of this chapter you should be able to

1. evaluate your current diet to determine if you are obtaining the recommended daily nutrient requirements;
2. write a weight-control program, tailor-made to age, sex, weight, daily caloric intake, and activity schedule;
3. pass a multiple-choice mastery self-check involving the selection of appropriate weight-control programs for individuals varying in age, sex, weight, daily caloric intake, and activity schedule.

You are what you eat. Even though genetic information dictates the organization of the materials that constitute your body, these materials are all derived from the food, water, and air taken into the body. Although this concept may seem obvious, it has vast implications about your health and well-being. Through better nutrition, you can improve the quality of life. Since you control the types and amounts of food you eat, you alone are ultimately responsible for your body's nutritional state.

Nutrition has a significant effect on health. It affects virtually every function of the body. Nutrients from food are necessary for every heartbeat, nerve sensation, and muscle contraction. Good nutrition not only prevents deficiency diseases such as scurvy and anemia, but also improves resistance to infectious diseases and plays a role in the prevention of chronic disease. Good nutrition is preventive medicine.

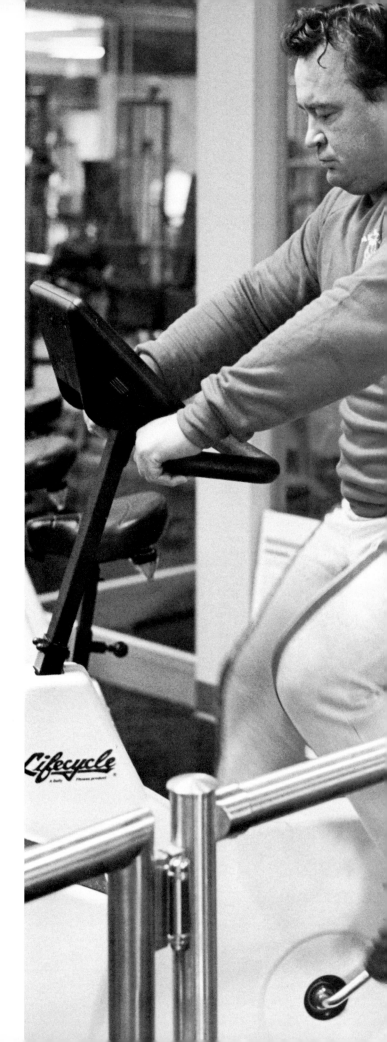

A knowledge of nutrition also is important to you as a consumer. With rising food costs and the accompanying changes in eating patterns, it is important for you to be able to get the best nutrition for your money. Knowing the nutritional value of various foods, you can eat more economically by decreasing or eliminating foods that have little nutritional value. Your pocketbook also may be affected by your ability to differentiate between reliable and unreliable claims about the nutritional properties of foods.

CALORIES

A **calorie** is a measure of heat used to explain the potential energy value of food. One large calorie, which is also known as a kilocalorie (kcal), represents the amount of heat necessary to raise the temperature of a kilogram of water (about a quart) one degree centigrade. In the *Fitness for Life* program, whenever we refer to a calorie, whether in relationship to exercise or food, we will be referring to a large calorie.

To determine how many calories of energy a specific amount of food will yield, a sample of the food is burned in an instrument called a bomb calorimeter. The bomb calorimeter is an insulated metal container that is jacketed by a water chamber containing a measured amount of water. Food is placed in the metal container together with a measured amount of oxygen, allowing it to be ignited by an electric current and burned. The heat of the burning food raises the water temperature and the measurement of this temperature rise can be converted to calories.

The approximate energy values of the three basic energy-yielding food groups are **carbohydrates**—4 calories per gram; **proteins**—4 calories per gram; and **fats**—9 calories per gram. The majority of the energy needed to do work in the human body is obtained from carbohydrates and fats.

The number of calories used by the body each day to maintain a given weight is called the daily caloric need. Of this, part is the minimum caloric need for basal metabolism, or **basal metabolic rate** (BMR). Basal metabolism is the amount of energy needed to maintain the body at rest, while you are awake but reclining and completely relaxed. The remainder of the daily caloric need is utilized by the body in carrying out various work and leisure activities.

If a person takes into the body food that contains a greater caloric potential than is needed by the body to carry on daily requirements, part of the food will be changed to fat, to be stored by the body. It is this metabolic function of storing fat that creates a serious problem in our modern-day society.

Only about one-third of the body's fuel is contributed by carbohydrate under resting conditions, and about two-thirds is contributed by the fat stores. During exercise requiring maximal effort for a short period of time, such as the 100-yard dash, the major fuel is carbohydrate.

During prolonged aerobic exercise lasting five minutes or longer, the major fuels are a combination of carbohydrate and fat, with fat the predominant source of energy.

Using the same caloric measure as a measurement of energy, it is also possible to measure how much energy the body spends to do work. Thus, tables of caloric values of specific activities, such as walking, running, swimming, and other exercises, can be constructed.

These two bodies of information, caloric values of food and activity, can now be combined to write programs of exercise and diet to effect weight control and cardiovascular endurance.

NUTRIENTS

Nutrients are chemical substances obtained from food during digestion. They are needed to build and maintain body cells, regulate body processes, and supply energy.

About fifty nutrients, including water, are needed daily for optimum health. If you obtain the proper amount of the so-called leader nutrients in the daily diet, the other forty or so nutrients will likely be consumed in amounts sufficient to meet the needs of the body. One's diet should include a variety of foods because no single food supplies all fifty nutrients and because many nutrients work together. Figure 5.1 is a chart listing the basic nutrients, important sources from which to obtain the nutrients, the manner in which they are used in energy production, and some of their major physiological functions in the body.

A federal law requires that nutritional labels of foods state the food's nutritional value. This is to help you identify the nutrient content of the foods you buy. All labels with nutrition information must follow the same format. The upper portion of the label shows the number of calories in a serving of the food and lists, in grams, the amount of protein, carbohydrate, and fat.

Nutrient	Sources	Energy Production	Major Physiological Function
Protein	Meat, poultry, fish, dried beans and peas, eggs, cheese, milk	Supplies 4 calories per gram.	Constitutes part of the structure of every cell, such as muscle, blood, and bone; supports growth and maintains healthy body cells; constitutes part of enzymes, some hormones and body fluids, and antibodies that increase resistance to infection.
Carbohydrate	Cereal, potatoes, dried beans, corn, bread, sugar	Supplies 4 calories per gram. Major source of energy for central nervous system.	Supplies energy for movement and for the growth and maintenance of body cells. Unrefined products supply fiber—complex carbohydrates in fruits, vegetables, and whole grains—which aids in regular elimination. Assists in fat utilization.
Fat	Shortening, oil, butter, margarine, salad dressing, fatty meats	Supplies 9 calories per gram.	Constitutes part of the structure of every cell. Stored energy. Supplies essential fatty acids. Provides and carries fat-soluble vitamins A, D, E, and K.
Vitamin A (retinol)	Liver, carrots, sweet potatoes, greens, butter, margarine		Assists formation and maintenance of skin and mucous membranes that line body cavities and tracts, thus increasing resistance to infection. Functions in visual processes and forms visual purple, promoting healthy eye tissues and eye adaptation in dim light.
Vitamin C (ascorbic acid)	Broccoli, orange, grapefruit, papaya, mango, strawberries		Forms cementing substances such as collagen that holds body cells together, thus strengthening blood vessels, hastening healing of wounds and bones, and increasing resistance to infection. Aids utilization of iron.

Figure 5.1. Chart adapted from *Guide to Good Eating: A Recommended Daily Pattern,* developed by the National Dairy Council, Rosemont, Illinois. Reprinted with permission of the publisher.

Nutrient	Sources	Energy Production	Major Physiological Function
Thiamine (B$_1$)	Lean pork, nuts, fortified cereal products	Aids in utilization of energy.	Functions as part of a coenzyme to promote the utilization of carbohydrate. Promotes normal appetite. Contributes to normal functioning of nervous system.
Riboflavin (B$_2$)	Liver, milk, yogurt, cottage cheese	Aids in utilization of energy.	Functions as part of a coenzyme in the production of energy within body cells. Promotes healthy skin, eyes, and clear vision.
Niacin	Liver, meat, poultry, fish, peanuts, fortified cereal products	Aids in utilization of energy.	Functions as part of a coenzyme in fat synthesis, tissue respiration, and utilization of carbohydrate. Promotes healthy skin, nerves, and digestive tract. Aids digestion and fosters normal appetite.
Calcium	Milk, yogurt, cheese, sardines and salmon with bones, collard, kale, mustard and turnip greens		Combines with other minerals within a protein framework to give structure and strength to bones and teeth. Assists in blood clotting. Functions in normal muscle contraction and relaxation and normal nerve transmission.
Iron	Enriched farina, prune juice, liver, dried beans and peas, red meat	Aids in utilization of energy.	Combines with protein to form hemoglobin to carry oxygen and carbon dioxide to and from the cells. Prevents nutritional anemia and its accompanying fatigue. Increases resistance to fatigue. Functions as part of enzymes involved in tissue respiration.

Figure 5.1—*Continued.*

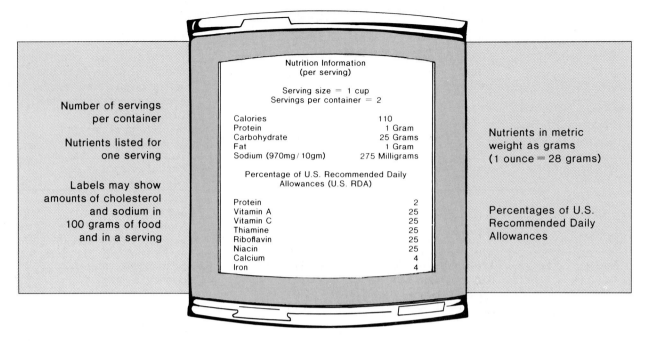

Number of servings
per container

Nutrients listed for
one serving

Labels may show
amounts of cholesterol
and sodium in
100 grams of food
and in a serving

Nutrition Information
(per serving)

Serving size = 1 cup
Servings per container = 2

Calories	110
Protein	1 Gram
Carbohydrate	25 Grams
Fat	1 Gram
Sodium (970mg / 10gm)	275 Milligrams

Percentage of U.S. Recommended Daily
Allowances (U.S. RDA)

Protein	2
Vitamin A	25
Vitamin C	25
Thiamine	25
Riboflavin	25
Niacin	25
Calcium	4
Iron	4

Nutrients in metric
weight as grams
(1 ounce = 28 grams)

Percentages of U.S.
Recommended Daily
Allowances

Figure 5.2. Nutritional label. Adapted from DHEW
Publication No(FDA)76–2049.

The lower portion of the label tells the percentage of the **United States Recommended Daily Allowance (U.S. RDA)** for protein and the seven leader **vitamins** and **minerals** provided in one serving. Figure 5.2 contains a diagram of the nutrition information contained on such a label.

OTHER USES OF NUTRITIONAL LABELS

The Department of Health and Human Services suggests that shoppers can also use nutritional labels for the following purposes:

To Serve Better Meals

1. Compare labels to select foods that round out the nutrients you need daily. For example, if you need more Vitamin A, compare food labels to find the best sources of this vitamin.
2. Use nutrition labels to help count calories.
3. If you are on a special diet recommended by your physician, you can use nutrition labels to help avoid restricted foods.
4. Read labels on new foods to see what nutrients they supply.

To Save Money

1. Use labels to compare the cost per serving of similar foods (see figure 5.3).
2. Read labels to make sure you get the most for your food dollar. For example, compare two frozen pot pies of the same weight. One costs

Yields: 4 (½–cup)*
servings
(31¢ ÷ 4 = cost)
Cost 7.8¢ per serving

Yields: 7 (½–cup)*
servings
(49¢ ÷ 7 = cost)
Cost: 7¢ per serving

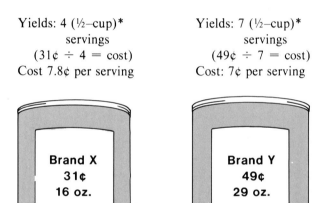

Figure 5.3. Calculating cost per serving.

thirty-nine cents, the other twenty-nine cents. But when you read the nutrition label, you may see the pot pie that costs thirty-nine cents provides a high percentage of the U.S. RDA for protein. So if you are serving the pot pie as a main dish and protein content is important, the one that costs thirty-nine cents may be a better buy from the standpoint of nutrition.
3. Read labels to find less costly substitutes for more expensive foods. For instance, you may be surprised to learn that many canned and packaged foods have high amounts of protein at a reasonable price.

Evaluating your diet is fairly easy if you use the Dietary Evaluation Work Sheet found in figure 5.4. Following are the four steps for evaluating your diet:

Step 1. Fill out the personal information.
Step 2. Determine whether you use iodized salt.

Step 3. Keep a daily record of food intake.
Step 4. Utilize the Evaluation Key to rate your diet.

To help you become familiar with these steps, we'll practice writing an evaluation step-by-step.

Dietary Evaluation Work Sheet

Name _____ Date _____

Do you use iodized salt?   yes _____   no _____

Food Eaten	Amount	Protein	Calcium	Iron	Vitamin A	Thiamin	Riboflavin	Vitamin C (ascorbic acid)
Totals								
Ratings								

Figure 5.4.

Step 1: Filling in personal information

Item 1. Fill in your name and the date on the Dietary Evaluation Work Sheet.

Step 2: Determining the use of iodized salt

Item 2. Look for the word *iodized* on the label of the salt you use. If you are not obtaining iodine from other sources, you should be using iodized salt.

Step 3: Keeping a food record

Item 3. Keep a record for one day of everything you eat and the corresponding amounts or measures. Write these down under the columns *Food Eaten* and *Amount*. Now use the table, Nutritional Values of Common Foods, in figure 5.5 to fill in the values of the nutrients in the foods you have eaten. The specific classes of foods listed in the table of nutritional values were selected because, if you eat adequate amounts of these foods, all other vitamins and minerals will also be included in your diet. If the protein intake is adequate—and corn is not the major source of protein in the diet—then the niacin will generally be adequate. Niacin can be synthesized by the human body if adequate amounts of noncorn protein are also eaten. Carbohydrates and fats are not listed since the average diet is not deficient in those two foods. For example, if you had one cup of milk for breakfast, find milk on the table, and write on the Dietary Evaluation Work Sheet the amount of nutrients listed for one cup: eighteen for protein, twenty-nine for calcium, and so forth. If you had two cups of milk, multiply these values by two, of course. The values given are expressed as a percentage of the United States Recommended Daily Allowances. When you have filled in the nutrient values for the foods you have eaten, each column will ideally add up to one hundred. Total the columns at the bottom of the work sheet for your daily nutrition intake.

Step 4: Rating your diet

Item 4. Use the Evaluation Key in figure 5.5 to rate your diet for each of the nutrients evaluated. Write these ratings below the daily total for each nutrient on the Dietary Evaluation Work Sheet.

How Does Your Diet Rate?

If your ratings weren't all *good* or *excellent,* you should again refer to the table, Nutritional Values of Common Foods, and determine what foods could have been eaten to supply the nutrients you are lacking. With the possible exception of iron for women, you should be able to obtain all the vitamins and minerals you need in the food you eat.

For More Information

The Nutritional Values of Common Foods table was designed for a quick, general dietary evaluation. For more extensive information on the nutrient content of foods, you can write for "Nutritive Value of Foods," *Home and Garden,* bulletin no. 72, for sale by the Superintendent of Documents, U.S. Government Printing Office, Washington, D.C. 20402.

NUTRITION AND HEALTH

The knowledge that you have concerning nutrition will certainly determine how healthy your life will be. This section will discuss some factors concerning food that can have an impact on your daily nutritional plans.

Fats and Cholesterol

Technically called lipids, fats come in solid or liquid form and both are insoluble in water. Fats are a concentrated source of food energy and supply essential fatty acids that the body cannot manufacture and must obtain from food sources. Most fats in foods are **triglycerides,** which consist of three fatty acids attached to a glycerol molecule. These fatty acids vary in degree of saturation by hydrogen atoms. All fats are combinations of saturated and unsaturated fatty acids.

When fatty acid molecules are loaded with all the hydrogen atoms they can carry, they are said to be saturated. Highly **saturated fats** are usually solid at room temperature. Animal sources include butter, milk, and meat fat; and vegetable sources are peanut and palm oils. Unsaturated fatty acid molecules do not have all the hydrogen atoms they can carry, are generally liquid at room temperature, and may become rancid quite quickly. Vegetable, plant, and animal sources of **unsaturated fats** include corn, safflower, and fish. Polyunsaturated fatty acid molecules are the least saturated with hydrogen atoms. These fats and oils are also usually liquid at room temperature. They are found mainly in foods of plant origin.

Kind of Food	Size of Serving (Ready to Eat)	Protein	Calcium	Iron	Vitamin A	Thiamine	Riboflavin	Vitamin C (ascorbic acid)
Milk Group								
Milk	1 cup	18	29	0	7	5	25	3
Cheese	1 slice	15	21	2	7	0	8	0
Cottage cheese	¼ cup	17	5	1	2	1	8	0
Ice cream	½ cup	6	8	0	7	2	7	1
Meat Group								
Liver	1 oz.	14	0	20	149	3	55	10
Oysters	5-8	19	9	3	6	9	10	0
Pork	1 oz.	17	0	5	0	4	5	0
Other meats, fish and poultry	1 oz.	16	0	1	1	2	2	0
Dried beans and peas	½ cup	11	3	10	0	15	5	0
Egg	1	14	3	6	11	3	8	0
Nuts	6-8	2	1	3	0	6	1	0
Peanut butter	1 Tbsp.	4	1	2	0	1	1	0
Fruit and Vegetable Group								
Cabbage, raw	½ cup	1	2	1	1	1	1	23
Dark green vegetables	½ cup	4	8	11	146	4	8	42
Deep yellow vegetables	½ cup	2	3	4	152	4	4	24
Potato	medium, ½ c.	2	1	3	0	6	2	27
Tomato, tomato juice	½ cup	2	1	7	19	4	2	33
Other vegetables	½ cup	3	2	6	5	6	3	13
Apricots	½ cup	2	2	3	54	2	2	27
Cantaloupe	¼ (6″ diam.)	1	1	5	68	3	2	55
Citrus fruit or juice	½ cup	1	1	1	5	7	2	103
Raisins	1 Tbsp.	0	0	2	0	1	1	0
Strawberries	1 cup	2	3	8	2	3	6	146
Other fruits	½ cup	1	1	2	10	3	2	5
Bread and Cereal Group								
Bread, enriched or whole grain	1 slice	3	2	3	0	4	2	0
Cereal, dry, ready to eat	¾ cup	2	0	2	0	5	1	0
Cereal, cooked variety	½ cup	4	1	4	0	4	1	0
Macaroni, enriched	½ cup	5	1	4	0	8	4	0
Rice	½ cup	2	1	3	0	5	1	0
Other Foods								
Butter or margarine	1 tsp.	0	0	0	3	0	0	0
Brewer's yeast	1 Tbsp.	6	2	9	0	98	23	0
Molasses	1 Tbsp.	0	12	13	0	4	3	0
Sugar	1 Tbsp.	0	0	0	0	0	0	0

Evaluation Key

Protein, Vitamin A, Vitamin C, Calcium:		Iron:				Thiamine and Riboflavin:		
		Men	Women			Men	Women	
Above 90%	Excellent	Above 50%	Above 90%	Excellent		Above 90%	Above 65%	Excellent
75-89%	Good	40-49%	75-89%	Good		75-89%	50-64%	Good
45-74%	Fair	30-39%	45-74%	Fair		45-74%	40-49%	Fair
30-44%	Poor	20-29%	30-44%	Poor		30-44%	25-39%	Poor
0-29%	Very poor	0-19%	0-29%	Very poor		0-29%	0-25%	Very poor

Figure 5.5.

Cholesterol and Risk of Heart Disease (Values in mg/dl)

Age	Total Cholesterol		LDL-Cholesterol		HDL-Cholesterol
	Moderate Risk	High Risk	Moderate Risk	High Risk	Increased Risk
Male					
0–14	173	190	106	120	38 or less
15–19	165	183	109	123	30
20–29	194	216	128	148	30
30–39	218	244	149	171	29
40–49	231	254	160	180	29
50+	230	258	166	188	29
Female					
0–14	174	190	113	126	36 or less
15–19	173	195	115	135	35
20–29	184	208	127	148	35
30–39	202	320	143	163	35
40–49	223	246	155	177	34
40+	252	281	170	195	36

Figure 5.6.

Cholesterol is a fatlike substance found in the cells of humans and other animals. Cholesterol is used to form hormones, cell membranes, and other body substances. Cholesterol is especially concentrated in the liver, kidneys, adrenal glands, and the brain. The body produces about 80 percent of the total cholesterol found in the blood and tissues; the other 20 percent is furnished by dietary sources. The amount of saturated fat and cholesterol in the diet determines to a great extent how much cholesterol is located in the bloodstream. Dietary cholesterol is found exclusively in animal products. The American Heart Association recommends that people should limit their daily intake of cholesterol to less than 300 milligrams.

In atherosclerosis, part of the plaque that is developed in the arterial walls is composed of fats and cholesterol. A high level of blood lipids, such as triglycerides and cholesterol, are associated with the increased formation of plaque. Most of the triglycerides and cholesterol are transported in the blood as lipoproteins, which are chemical units composed of triglycerides, cholesterol and another lipid called phospholipids. These are attached to a protein carrier that gives them the name of **lipoproteins.**

There are different forms of lipoprotein in the blood and they are classified by their density. Two of the lipoproteins seem to have a relationship with the onset of coronary heart disease and have different amounts of cholesterol in their molecular makeup. The **low-density lipoprotein-cholesterol (LDL-C)** molecule contains high amounts of cholesterol and the **high-density lipoprotein-cholesterol (HDL-C)** molecule has a high concentration of protein.

Individuals with high levels of HDL-cholesterol seem to experience less coronary heart disease when compared to people who have high levels of LDL-cholesterol. It is not known exactly why this happens, but one theory suggests that the HDL-cholesterol molecule helps prevent the process of atherosclerosis by blocking the movement of LDL-cholesterol into the artificial wall to form plaques and by aiding the transport of cholesterol to the liver for removal by the body.

Total cholesterol in the blood is important, but an analysis of the different types of lipoprotein cholesterol should also be made when blood tests for lipids are conducted. Figure 5.6 contains a presentation of the various cholesterol levels and their relationship to the risk of heart disease.

Another important factor in heart disease is the ratio of total cholesterol to HDL-cholesterol. You can determine this ratio by dividing the total cholesterol level by the value for HDL-cholesterol. The smaller the ratio, the less risk there is for coronary heart disease. Figure 5.7 contains the ratios for both men and women and the risk of heart disease.

Ratio of Total Cholesterol to HDL-Cholesterol and Risk of Heart Disease

T-C/HDL-C Men	T-C/HDL-C Women	Risk
3.43	3.27	One-half average risk
4.97	4.44	Average risk
9.55	7.05	Twice average risk
23.59	11.04	Three times average risk

Figure 5.7.

Levels of Omega-3 Fatty Acids in Fish and Seafood

High in Omega-3 Fatty Acids	Medium to Low in Omega-3 Fatty Acids	
Anchovies	Amberjack	Orange Roughy
Atlantic Herring	Bass	Oysters
Lake Trout	Brill	Pompano
Lake Whitefish	Cod	Red Snapper
Atlantic Mackerel	Crab	Scallops
Sablefish	Flounder	Shrimp
Salmon	Haddock	Sole
Sardines	Halibut	Squid
Sturgeon	Lobster	Swordfish
Tuna	Mahi-Mahi	Thresher Shark
	Mussels	

Figure 5.8.

Studies indicate that people who are lean, non-smokers, exercisers, and eat a diet low in saturated fats have higher levels of HDL-cholesterol and lower levels of total cholesterol. Thus, it appears that a combination of diet and exercise is helpful in combating heart disease.

Omega-3 Fatty Acids

Findings published in the New England Journal of Medicine indicate that fish oils, rich in unsaturated fats called **Omega-3 fatty acids** actually change the chemistry of the blood to lower the likelihood of heart disease. The oil in certain seafood seems to depress low-density lipoprotein-cholesterol and raise the amount of high-density lipoprotein-cholesterol. Not all fish contain the same amount of Omega-3 fatty acids. Figure 5.8 contains a list of fish and seafood and the levels of Omega-3 fatty acids found in them.

It appears that the consumption of as little as two to four fish or seafood dishes per week of about 6 ounces can contribute to the following benefits:

1. lowering of cholesterol levels
2. altering the blood chemistry in such a way that blood clots are less likely to form
3. helping to slow the formation of plaques that bring about atherosclerosis
4. in conjunction with a low-fat, high-fiber diet, Omega-3 fatty acids may help to prevent certain cancers

As a result of the research concerning the effect of Omega-3 fatty acids, there are currently a number of fish oil capsules on the market. Offered as a new approach to warding off heart disease, they contain fat extracted from fish whose tissues are rich in Omega-3 fatty acids. The important question is Do these capsules provide all the benefits that are advertised? The answer may be no. According to the American Heart Association, the American Medical Association, and many researchers studying fish oils, the clinical research does not seem adequate to determine the proper dosage of fish oil capsules that might work. Also, it may not just be the oil from the fish that provides protection, but a combination of components contained in fish that work together to bring about beneficial effects. Thus, the evidence at this time would support the addition of fish and seafood to the diet rather than using fish oil capsules as a supplement.

Fiber

Fiber is found in all plants and is an inert material that does not break down while passing through the digestive tract. Thus, fiber adds bulk to the diet and can contribute some beneficial effects to the body. High-fiber foods include whole-grain breads, cereals, pasta, brown rice, fruits, vegetables, dried beans, nuts, and seeds.

There is research that indicates an adequate amount of fiber in the diet can help prevent many colon problems, reduce the incidence of cancer of the colon, and aid in blood-sugar control in diabetes. Fiber has also been associated with having a lowering effect on cholesterol. Fiber soaks up water in the gastrointestinal tract and can bring about larger, softer bowel movements that tend to move fairly quickly through the system.

Although there are no Recommended Daily Allowances for fiber, an estimate of between 25 and 50 grams of dietary fiber would be a proper goal to achieve per day. The point to remember is if you eat portions of fruits and vegetables each day along with whole-grain products, you will probably have no trouble meeting the recommendation of the National Cancer Institute and many other nutritionists.

Complex Carbohydrates

Carbohydrates are one of the prime sources of energy during exercise and are the basic foodstuffs formed by plants using energy from the sun. Carbohydrates can be divided into either simple or complex carbohydrates. The **simple carbohydrates** are usually known as sugars and the **complex carbohydrates** are commonly known as starches. Most of the carbohydrates in the plant world are in the form of starch.

The human body uses both the sugars and starches for energy to perform bodily functions. The question is Why does it matter if the energy comes from sugars or starches? To answer this question, you must understand the different ways starch and sugars are packaged in food. Many of the foods high in starch are nutrient-dense; that is, in proportion to the number of calories in them, there is also an ample supply of vitamins and minerals and, in some cases, a large amount of protein. Foods high in simple sugars, such as cake, candy, and cookies often have a lot of fat and many times are extremely low in vitamins and minerals.

This can be illustrated by comparing a baked potato to a portion of candy. Both of them may contain about 100 calories. The potato, which is rich in carbohydrates in the form of starch, also provides vitamin C, some protein, the B-complex vitamins, minerals, and fiber. Many of the complex carbohydrates are high in fiber and this has been shown to be beneficial to health. The candy, on the other hand, is composed of sugar and a large amount of fat. Even though the caloric values are the same, the nutritional effects are quite different.

Complex carbohydrates are an aid in weight control since the process of digestion utilizes more energy metabolizing starch than it does metabolizing fat. It has been stated that you don't get fat from overeating complex carbohydrates, but from overeating fat. Complex carbohydrates also seem to be better than fats at informing the body it has taken in enough food and is therefore, a good control of appetite. It should be pointed out that this doesn't mean you can eat all the complex carbohydrates you wish and still not gain weight, but there will be less of a chance than on a diet high in sugar and fats.

Currently people in the United States have a diet that is about 45 percent carbohydrate, but only half of the carbohydrate is complex or starch. Nutritionists usually agree that 50 to 60 percent of the total calories per day should be derived from carbohydrate, and most should be in the form of complex carbohydrates.

Protein and Essential Amino Acids

Proteins are the building blocks of body tissues and also help control chemical reactions in the human body. There are twenty-two or more **amino acids** the body uses in various ways to form the proteins used for various functions. Eight of these amino acids can't be manufactured by the body and must come from outside sources in the diet. These are known as **essential amino acids.** If one or more of these essential amino acids is lacking, then protein construction may be hindered. One of the problems associated with many quick weight-loss programs is a shortage of essential amino acids and, in some cases, death has been the result.

It is estimated that a person needs about 1–2 grams of protein for every 2–3 pounds of body weight. This can usually be achieved by having 12 percent or more of the daily caloric intake come from protein. Milk, cheese, meat, and eggs are excellent sources of the essential amino acids. You must be aware that these products are also high in fat and thus it is a good idea to balance your protein intake between both animal and plant protein.

Vitamin and Mineral Supplements

Vitamins and minerals are involved in regulating many of the body processes. Since many of these functions are critical during exercise, a deficiency of key vitamins or minerals might prove detrimental to optimal physical performance. Many people believe the vitamin and mineral supplementation industry has attempted to convince the public that the foods we eat are lacking in vitamins and minerals and, thus, our health is being threatened. Current research and the recommendation of qualified nutritionists indicate there is no need for a supplement if a person eats a balanced diet.

If you decide to take a supplement because you want a margin of safety in your diet, the sensible guide is to select a combination multi-vitamin and mineral supplement that contains a variety of vitamins and minerals in no greater than 100 percent of the United States Recommended Daily Allowances (U.S. RDA). The U.S. RDA values appear on the labels of food products and represent the percentage of the Recommended Daily Allowances developed by the Food and Nutrition Board of the National Academy of Sciences. These are generous allowances based on research to more than meet the nutritional needs of most Americans. By examining the label, it becomes easy to determine the dietary value of the supplement. Since the body probably does not need more than these recommended values, megadoses or the use of so-called high-potency supplements are of little use.

OBESITY

In contrast with the problem of undernutrition in many parts of the world, overnutrition in the form of excess fat affects the health of many Americans. Obesity has become a national health problem in the United States. It has also become a national obsession. Newspapers, magazines, radio, and television all indicate that eating and reducing are increasingly prominent topics of concern to Americans. This concern of the general population is shared by health professionals who associate excess body fat with increasing incidence of disease and

mortality. The prevalence of obesity among Americans may be due in part to increased mechanization of our society, resulting in decreased activity and increased leisure time for many people. Insufficient knowledge and/or lack of motivation in regard to weight control might also be reasons for the prevalence of this condition.

What Is Obesity?

It is important to differentiate between the terms **obese** and **overweight.** An obese person is one who has an excess accumulation of body fat. As you read in chapter 2, the amount of fat in the body is commonly expressed as a percentage of total body weight and is called percent body fat. A desirable percent body fat for the average person is estimated to be from 10 to 15 for men and from 15 to 22 for women. It may be noted that some highly trained male athletes have a percent body fat as low as 4.

Most health authorities indicate that obesity for men is a percent body fat above 20 percent, and for women when the percent body fat is above 28 percent. An overweight person is generally defined as someone who weighs more than 10 percent above the desired weight. By these definitions a person could be obese without being overweight, or could be overweight without being obese. It may not be how heavy a person is but how much excess body fat the person possesses that is important in regard to health problems associated with obesity.

The body's energy balance determines whether or not a person gains body fat. Ideally, the energy (expressed in calories) expended for body functions and activities equals the food energy consumed, and the body has some fat reserve to call on for energy in times of emergency or stress. When more food energy is consumed than is used for activity, this energy is put into storage in the form of fatty tissue. This extra fat can be lost by tipping the balance the other way, so that the energy expenditure for activity is greater than the food energy consumed. In this way the body is forced to use its stored fuel to meet part of its energy needs.

OBESITY AND DISEASE

Statistics show a significant association between obesity and early mortality from a number of diseases. Obesity may increase the risk of developing some diseases or may aggravate diseases caused by other factors.

Diseases of the heart and circulatory system are frequently associated with obesity. Both high blood pressure and atherosclerosis (a type of hardening of the arteries) appear to be related to obesity. Because extra fatty tissue requires extra blood and capillaries, there is an increased burden on the heart to pump blood to that tissue. Thus, obesity can contribute to the development of cardiovascular disease and decrease the chance of recovery from a myocardial infarction (heart attack). Obesity may also contribute to the development of varicose veins and intermittent claudication, a vascular disease of the limbs.

The burden of excess fatty tissue may aggravate many types of bone and joint disease, such as osteoarthritis and the rupture of intervertebral discs. Extra weight and pressure may be more than the bones and joints can easily bear, and may make diseases like osteoarthritis extremely painful.

Obesity also increases the risk of death from diabetes and cerebral hemorrhage. Life insurance figures have shown that mortality in overweight males from all causes is 150 percent that of the normal mortality rate. Thus we can conclude that obesity does create a health hazard!

ANOREXIA NERVOSA

Much attention is given to the disorder of excessive body fat, but there are also problems that can be associated with individuals who become desperate to achieve extreme leanness. This disorder is also dangerous and can become a serious threat to health.

Anorexia nervosa is defined by the American Anorexia Nervosa Association as a serious illness of deliberate self-starvation with profound psychiatric and physical components. Because of a terror of body fat and a desire to obtain extreme thinness, the individual may refuse to eat or may engage in bizarre eating behaviors. Anorexics seem to lose a sense of reality when it comes to food and the feeling of hunger or fullness. As the problem persists, they believe they have conquered the need to take in food, which leads to metabolic disturbances within the body and may result in death.

A review of the research reveals that about 90 percent of the anorexics are young women, with about 5 to 10 percent being men.

Another problem associated with about 50 percent of all anorexics is the development of **bulimia**. This disorder is characterized by periods of voracious eating binges, followed by a purging of the offending food in order to prevent a weight gain. In order to purge the food from the body, individuals may use diuretics, laxatives, and/or self-induced vomiting.

According to the American Medical Association, the following diagnostic criteria are used in identifying a victim of anorexia nervosa:

1. An intense fear of becoming obese that does not diminish with weight loss. Regardless of how much weight is lost, the victim is still terrified of becoming grossly overweight.

2. A disturbed body image; the anorexic claims there is still excessive fat when the body is skeletal in appearance.

3. A loss of at least 25 percent of the original body weight has occurred. If the anorexic is under the age of eighteen, there may be a loss of at least 25 percent of the original body weight plus the projected weight that should have been gained as an adolescent.

4. A refusal to maintain the minimal normal weight for age and height.

5. The presence of no known physical illness that could explain the weight loss.

Other symptoms of this problem are dry, brittle fingernails and hair, absence or irregularity of menstruation, dry mouth, sore and burning tongue, and irregular heartbeat.

It is not known what the definite causes of anorexia are and it may be a combination of many factors that make it difficult for a person to accept his or her body and make a correct interpretation of body image.

The treatment of this illness is beyond the scope of this textbook and there is a need for professional help and advice to combat the danger of anorexia nervosa. Following is a questionnaire that can reveal your feelings about eating, dieting, and your body.

FACTS VERSUS FALLACIES CONCERNING WEIGHT CONTROL

Even though the communications media have deluged the public with information concerning weight control, much of the information is inaccurate. Seymour K. Fineburg, M.D., states,

Regrettably, scientific half-truths, unproven and unsubstantiated conclusions, and just plain bunk about obesity and its treatment are still being welcomed by many as the ultimate truth and are often enthusiastically espoused. The trouble with most popular books about obesity and reducing diets is that only half of what they say is accurate, but the reader does not know which half![1]

1. Seymour K. Fineburg, "The Realities of Obesity and Fad Diets," *Nutrition Today* 7 July/August (1972):26.

ANOREXIA NERVOSA: ARE YOU AT RISK?

How do you think about eating, dieting and your body? To find out, see if these statements are true for you:

True	False	
☐	☐	1. A day rarely passes that I don't worry about how much I eat.
☐	☐	2. I am embarrassed to be seen in a bathing suit.
☐	☐	3. There are many foods I always feel guilty about eating.
☐	☐	4. Most attractive people I see are thinner than I am.
☐	☐	5. I usually begin the day with a vow to diet.
☐	☐	6. My thighs are too fat.
☐	☐	7. I feel uncomfortable eating anything fattening in front of people.
☐	☐	8. It makes me nervous if people can watch me from behind.
☐	☐	9. After I eat a lot, I think about ways of getting rid of or burning up calories.
☐	☐	10. I hate seeing myself in a mirror.
☐	☐	11. I feel terrible about myself if I don't do a lot of exercise every day.
☐	☐	12. I find my naked body repulsive.
☐	☐	13. If I eat too much, I sometimes vomit or take laxatives.
☐	☐	14. My worst problem is the appearance of my body.

Answers

The odd-numbered questions tell whether your eating and exercise patterns have gone awry. The even ones tell if you're overly critical of your body. Add up the number of "true" answers. If your score is:

2–4, You're typical, and probably not at risk.

5–8, You're overly concerned with your weight. Watch your attitudes and behavior carefully.

9–14, You may well be developing an eating disorder. Consider professional psychological help.

—American Health Magazine copyright 1986

It is human nature to want a quick and easy way to affect body weight. This accounts for the popularity of every new fad diet that comes along. Fad dieting invariably leads to failure because these methods of reducing are based on the supposition that losing weight is only a temporary, short-term problem. It is relatively easy to lose pounds on any low-calorie diet, but after weight loss the dieter goes back to his or her regular way of eating and regains the weight lost and perhaps more. Fad diets don't teach one how to eat in order to maintain weight loss permanently. It is important that a person have some knowledge of nutrition in order to choose a proper reducing plan.

SET POINT THEORY OF WEIGHT CONTROL

Current research indicates that located in the brain is a regulatory center that may very closely control body weight. This mechanism appears to be set at a particular level much the same way you set the thermostat in your home to control temperature at a certain degree. This mechanism keeps body weight at a given **set point** by controlling food intake; it gives you a feeling of hunger, thus triggering the desire to eat, or a feeling of fullness that reduces the desire. It is also hypothesized that this center affects how much energy the body may use in normal daily activities. This may be one of the reasons that some people can eat large amounts of food and stay thin and others seem to stay fat even when they restrict their food intake. This metabolic mechanism that conserves energy to protect fat may be a defense to protect a person against starvation. The human body has no way of determining the difference between starvation and a low-food intake diet. Both seem to stimulate the body to move the set point of the regulatory center in the brain to a higher level, and thus the person may attempt to store more fat as a protective device. This is a possible answer to what happens to people who have a quick weight loss but then return to the same weight or, in some cases, even an increase in body fat when they go off the low-calorie diet.

Permanent success in fat control requires a program that will lower the set point and thus allow the body to lose weight, but not view the fat loss as a threat to its well-being.

Two major factors that aid in lowering the set point are the increase of exercise and the decrease of the intake of refined carbohydrates. Exercise increases the muscle mass, decreases appetite, increases the fat-burning enzymes, and increases energy levels. Aerobic activities that use large muscle groups, such as jogging, cycling, swimming, and aerobic dance, for over fifteen continuous minutes and at a heart rate of 70 percent of maximum heart rate or higher, are the best type of exercise in which to engage. A decrease in refined carbohydrates with a high sugar content seems to lower the set point and helps control insulin levels that affect the feeling of hunger.

It is also important that you don't eat too little during the course of the day. When a person misses meals or seriously restricts food intake, various sensors throughout the body send signals to the regulatory center in the brain that conditions similar to starvation are taking place. A number of changes then start to occur in the body to conserve energy and protect fat. The end results of these changes, which might raise the set point, would actually defeat the attempt to reduce body fat.

EXERCISE AND WEIGHT CONTROL

The key to effective weight control is keeping energy intake (food) and energy output (physical activity) in balance. The person who has a proper body weight and wants to keep it should exercise regularly and eat a balanced diet that provides enough calories to make up for the energy expended. The thin individual who wishes to gain weight should exercise regularly and increase the number of calories consumed until the desired body weight is attained. The overly fat person should decrease food intake and increase the amount of physical activity. Figure 5.9 points out the importance of physical activity combined with diet in bringing about positive results in both a weight-gain and a weight-loss program.

A large proportion of the population is overly fat, and it is this group that needs help in combining a diet and exercise program. Lack of exercise has been cited as the most important cause of "creeping obesity" found in modern mechanized societies. As figure 5.10 shows, it doesn't take many calories to affect fat changes. For example, if you eat one extra slice of bread and butter (approximately 106 calories) each day and you don't expend the energy in activity, in one year you will have consumed enough calories to be 11 pounds fatter and, in five years, you could have an excess of 55 pounds of fat. It should be pointed out that there is a positive side to this information. If you reduce your caloric intake by a slice of bread and butter and expend an extra 106 calories in exercise (an example would be to walk approximately 1.5 miles at a 4 mph pace), you could lose approximately 22 pounds of fat in one year!

Some desirable characteristics that should be a part of any reducing program are:

1. The diet must produce a negative caloric balance. In other words, the energy expended in calories will be more than the energy consumed as food, so some of the excess fatty tissue will be used.

2. The diet must contain a balance of required nutrients. To meet the body's need for protein, carbohydrates, fat, vitamins, and minerals, food should be selected from a variety of sources—dairy products; fruits and vegetables; breads and cereals; and meat, fish, and poultry.

3. The reducing program should promote a gradual weight loss. The suggested rate is no more than 2 or 3 pounds per week. Diets that promise more than this likely have so few calories that the body's nutritional needs are not met. Much of the weight lost on a semi-starvation diet is quickly regained because it is not fatty tissue that is lost, but lean muscle tissue and water.

4. An exercise program should be a part of the reducing plan. Exercise helps build muscle at the expense of excess body fat. Dieting alone will cause loss of fatty tissue as well as some

Body Composition Changes

Cause of Weight Gain	Composition of Weight Change		
	Fat	Other Cells	Extracellular Fluid
Gluttony	66%	20%	14%
Gluttony and indolence	109%	−20%	11%
Physical activity and diet	−38%	120%	18%

Method of Weight Loss	Composition of Weight Change		
	Fat	Other Cells	Extracellular Fluid
Obese — Dieting alone	75%	10%	15%
Obese — Dieting and exercise	98%	−10%	12%
Starvation	50%	50%	0%

Figure 5.9. Adapted from *Alive Man: The Physiology of Physical Activity* by Roy J. Shephard, pp. 484, 488. Copyright 1972 by Charles C. Thomas. Reprinted by permission of the publisher.

Caloric Imbalance

Pounds Gained per Year	Excess Calories per Day	Pounds Gained per Year	Excess Calories per Day
1	9.6	13	124.8
2	19.2	14	134.4
3	28.8	15	144.0
4	38.4	16	153.6
5	48.0	17	163.2
6	57.6	18	172.8
7	67.2	19	182.4
8	76.8	20	192.0
9	86.4	21	201.6
10	96.0	22	211.2
11	105.6	23	220.8
12	115.2	24	230.4

Yearly Weight Gain

Year	1 lb./yr.	3 lb./yr.	5 lb./yr.	7 lb./yr.	10 lb./yr.
1988	150	150	150	150	150
1989	151	153	155	157	160
1990	152	156	160	164	170
1991	153	159	165	171	180
1992	154	162	170	178	190
1993	155	165	175	185	200
1994	156	168	180	192	210
1995	157	171	185	199	220

Figure 5.10.

muscle tissue. By combining dieting with exercise, more of the weight lost will be from fatty tissue. A weight-control program should be a fat-control program.

5. A good reducing program should be adaptable to lifetime use. Assuming that a person is obese, at least in part because of faulty eating habits, a reducing plan should teach desirable eating habits. Unfortunately for many persons who are obese, control of this problem is not short lived, but lifelong. These individuals must have a diet that is acceptable to them and not detrimental to health.

The American College of Sports Medicine has developed a position stand regarding proper and improper weight-loss programs. The complete reference can be found in Appendix A.

GAINING BODY WEIGHT

Although many people have a problem with excess body fat, there are some individuals who may have a desire to increase their body weight. The important point to remember in a weight-gain program is to make sure the majority of the increased weight comes from a gain in lean body tissue, such as muscle, and not from an increase in body fat.

A person should first make sure there are no medical problems that might be the cause of the reduced body weight. Once it has been determined that reduction in body weight is due to expending more calories than are being consumed, then a program that manipulates input of calories and the output of calories can be undertaken.

As indicated in figure 5.9, by combining physical activity with diet, it is possible to bring about the most beneficial changes in the composition of weight gain.

Dr. Melvin Williams, the director of the Human Performance Laboratory at Old Dominion University, has some excellent guidelines to help maximize gains in muscle tissue and keep body fat increases relatively low.

1. Set a reasonable goal within a certain time period. In general, about 1 to 2 pounds per week is a sound approach.

2. An individual on a weight-gain program should follow the same dietary principles advocated for those who are maintaining or even trying to lose body weight. The dietary intake should be selected using the Food Exchange Guide in figure 5.11, as explained in the weight-control program. The only major difference will be that greater amounts of foods will be consumed in order to gain weight.

3. Increase your caloric intake. It is not known exactly how many additional calories are necessary to form one pound of muscle tissue in human beings, nor is it known in what form

Food Exchange Guide for Various Daily Calorie Intakes

Number of Calories per Day

Food Exchange	1,200	1,300	1,400	1,500	1,600	1,700	1,800	1,900	2,000	2,100	2,200	2,300	2,400	2,500
Vegetables	2	2	3	3	5	4	6	6	7	8	8	9	9	9
Breads	5	5	6	6	7	8	8	8	8	8	8	9	10	10
Meats	4	5	3	5	4	5	5	4	6	6	6	6	6	6
Milk	2	2	3	3	3	3	3	4	4	4	4	4	4	4½
Fruits	4	5	4	4	4	4	4	5	6	6	7	7	8	8
Fats	2	2	2	2	2	2	3	2	2	2	3	3	3	3

Note: If your diet requires more than 2,500 calories, you can still use the food selection guide. For example, if you wish to write a diet for 3,000 calories, all you need to do is double the diet suggested in the 1,500-calorie list. For 3,200 calories you would double the 1,600-calorie list.

Figure 5.11.

these calories have to be consumed. However, the general recommendation is to increase your caloric intake approximately 1,000 calories above your daily energy needs. The 7,000 extra calories per week should be sufficient to help produce 2 pounds of muscle.

4. Start a strength-training exercise program in addition to a cardiovascular endurance training program. A strength-training program will serve as a stimulus to build muscle tissue. A complete explanation of how to write a strength program can be found in chapter 7, "Writing a Strength Program."

5. Use a tape to take body measurements. Be sure to take them at the same place every one to two weeks. Those body parts measured should include the neck, upper and lower arm, chest, abdomen, thigh, and calf. This is to ensure that body weight gains are proportionately distributed. You should look for good gains in the chest and limbs, but the abdominal girth increase should be kept low because that is where fat usually increases the most.

By following the preceding suggestions, you can plan a program that will be very effective in gaining the proper kind of body weight.

WRITING A WEIGHT-CONTROL PROGRAM

Writing a weight-control program is fairly easy if you use the Weight-Control Work Sheet in Appendix C. Here are the steps to follow.

Step 1. Fill in the general information on the work sheet.

Step 2. Determine the exercise program and average daily caloric expenditure for exercise.

Step 3. Determine the estimated daily caloric intake.

Step 4. Determine the diet and daily food plan to be followed.

Step 5. Follow the diet-exercise program.

Step 6. Maintain body weight.

CASE
Ann Hathaway

Ann Hathaway is twenty-one years old and weighs 145 pounds. One month ago, she had a medical checkup and the doctor gave her a clean bill of health, but he also suggested that she lose some weight. After a body weight appraisal, as explained in chapter 2, her estimated target weight was found to be 125 pounds. She is in *Fitness Category III* and prefers running at 5.5 miles per hour for her exercise for five days a week. Her exercise heart rate training zone is 137 to 168 beats per minute.

With this information, we will write a complete weight-control program for Ann.

Step 1: Filling in the general information on the work sheet

Item 1. Write in Ann's name, age, sex, and the current date.

Item 2. Write in Ann's weight (145 pounds) and her estimated target weight. Her target weight can be determined by utilizing the appraisal

procedure for determining body weight that was explained in chapter 2. This weight is 125 pounds. Also write in her exercise heart rate training zone of 137 to 168.

Item 3. Since Ann has met the medical requirements and her doctor recommended she lose weight, check *No Restrictions*.

Item 4. Place a check by Ann's fitness category *(III)* in item 4.

Step 2: Determining the exercise program and average daily caloric expenditure for exercise

Item 5. In selecting an exercise program, Ann consults item 4 to determine the suggested exercise intensity for her fitness category. It is 5–10 calories per minute. By working at this intensity, Ann will not only lose weight but also will gain in cardiovascular endurance. She has asked to run at 5.5 miles per hour. By checking Appendix B, Calorie Expenditure Per Minute for Various Exercises, she finds that this activity requires 10.2 calories per minute for her body weight (145 pounds). This is within the suggested intensity for her fitness category. Write in "running" for exercise preference and "5.5 mph" for rate next to item 5.

Item 6. Ann finds that she expends 10.2 calories per minute for running and records this figure in the blank.

Item 7. By checking item 4, she finds that she should expend a minimum of 200 calories each exercise session. Record this number next to item 7.

Item 8. To determine the minimum number of minutes to exercise each session, Ann divides item 7 by item 6 (200 ÷ 10.2) and records her answer (20). Remember to round your answer to the nearest whole number. Note: It is important to remember that in order to obtain a cardiovascular endurance training effect, the minimum duration is fifteen minutes of *continuous* activity.

Item 9. By checking item 4, Ann finds she should exercise a minimum of three to five days each week. She wants to run five days each week as she knows that exercise combined with diet will allow her to lose a greater amount of fat from her body. She also wants to increase her cardiovascular endurance as she loses weight. Record the number 5 in the blank.

Item 10. To determine the recommended number of calories expended in exercise each week, multiply item 7 by item 9 (200 × 5). Record the answer (1,000) in the blank.

Item 11. Divide item 10 by the number 7, the number of days in one week, (1,000 ÷ 7) to determine the average daily caloric expenditure Ann will use in exercise. Even though Ann exercises only five days each week, it is necessary to divide by seven days, as this number will be used in determining the daily caloric intake when Ann plans her diet. Round off the answer to the nearest whole number (143).

Step 3: Determining the estimated daily caloric intake

Item 12. To decide how much you should eat to lose weight, you should know how much you are now eating to maintain a constant weight. Since there is so much individual variance, the best way to determine how much food you require is to keep a record of what you eat for a week in which you neither gain nor lose weight. Then use a calorie counter to calculate the number of calories this represents and divide by seven to get your average daily caloric intake.

If a person is unsure of the accuracy of this seven-day intake record, he or she can compare it to the following estimate. A moderately active adult who maintains a specific body weight will usually require 15 calories per pound of body weight to maintain this weight. The daily caloric intake, therefore, can be estimated to be 15 calories times the current weight in pounds. Multiply item 2, Ann's current weight, by 15 (145 × 15 = 2175) to obtain an estimate of the daily caloric intake. Record the number in the blank by item 12.

Item 13. The loss of a pound of fatty tissue represents a reduction in food intake of about 3,500 calories. It is not recommended that a person lose more than 2 pounds per week without medical supervision. The program developed in this text is planned for a 2 pound per week weight loss. In order to lose 2 pounds per week, you must eliminate from the diet about 7,000 calories per week, or 1,000 calories per day. The number 1,000 has already been provided in the blank.

Item 14. Subtract item 13 from item 12 to determine Ann's daily caloric intake if she is using a diet alone to lose 2 pounds per week. The answer is 1175.

Item 15. Since Ann is combining her diet with an exercise program, she can add these calories to her weight-control program. It is important to note that a greater percentage of fat is lost by combining exercise and diet than by just using a diet to lose weight. Also, she will be gaining in cardiovascular endurance. Add items 11 and 14 to obtain this figure. Always round this number to the lowest 100 calories. In this case the number of calories will be 1,300. Write your answer in the blank. IMPORTANT: This number must be at least 1,500 calories for men and 1,200 calories for women in order to meet the body's need for protein, vitamins, and minerals. If your calculation is ever less than this, it should be adjusted upward to those amounts.

Step 4: Determining the diet and daily food plan to be followed

Now that you have completed Ann's Weight-Control Work Sheet, you can advise her on the diet to follow in order to provide her with a well-balanced eating program.

The Food Exchange Guide For Various Daily Calorie Intakes in figure 5.11 gives food plans for several different levels of caloric intake. Locate the column heading corresponding to the number of calories in Ann's diet (this is obtained from item 15, and in Ann's case is 1,300 calories). By running your finger down this column you can determine how many servings of a given food group Ann should eat in her diet. You will notice that this food plan is divided into six food groups. These groups are called **food exchange groups,** because any food on one of the six lists can be freely exchanged for any other food on the *same* list. The advantage of this diet is that it enables you to select your own foods rather than following a specific menu that may not suit your tastes or economic situation. It enables you to choose what to eat and still to know that you have a nutritionally balanced diet that does not exceed your daily caloric allotment.

The average American diet is approximately 43 percent fat, with a high amount of saturated fat; 45 percent carbohydrate that consists of sugar rather than complex carbohydrates; and 12 percent protein. It is this type of diet that has contributed to the nutritional problems of many Americans. The food exchange groups have been organized in the *Fitness for Life* program to be approximately 50 percent carbohydrate, 30 percent fat, and 20 percent protein, regardless of the number of calories eaten. Thus, you can be assured of taking in a balanced diet that will provide you with the necessary nutrients you require. Each food-group list contains foods that are approximately the same in calorie, carbohydrate, protein, and fat content. A few foods therefore may

appear in unexpected places. For example, you may think of potatoes and corn as vegetables, but since their composition is more like that of the foods in the breads and cereals group, they appear on that list. Measurements are given for each food to make certain that the caloric content of the foods on a list will be the same. To use another example from the bread and cereals group, one slice of white bread has the same number of calories as ½ cup of macaroni or ⅓ cup of corn. These foods, *in these amounts,* therefore, are interchangeable. The same applies to each of the other lists: vegetables, fruits, meats, and fats. Remember that you should not exchange between groups (i.e., a fruit exchange for a meat exchange) but only within a group (i.e., a fruit exchange for a different fruit exchange).

You may also note that as the number of calories per day increases, there will be an increase in the number of food exchanges for vegetables, breads, and fruits. This is to increase the amount of complex carbohydrates in the diet. If the diet recommends ten vegetable exchanges, this does not mean you must select ten different exchanges. You can double or triple the portions of any vegetable so that the total intake equals the given amount of exchanges.

In addition to the six food-group lists, there is a list of free choices of foods that contain few or no calories and a list to help you apply the exchange groups to commercially prepared mixtures.

Almost any food you desire to eat will appear on these lists. The exceptions are foods high in sugar content. You have decreased your caloric intake to go on a reducing diet. The foods that you do eat, therefore, must be chosen carefully so that you can still get all the nutrients you need, such as protein, vitamins, and minerals. Sugar contains essentially no other nutrient except carbohydrates, so it and the desserts that contain it should be eliminated from a reducing diet. A glass of skim milk and the same amount of a soft drink, for example, will have about the same number of calories. The skim milk, however, provides a bonus of protein, calcium, riboflavin, and other essential nutrients. (By substituting a fresh apple for a piece of apple pie, you can save 250 calories—without a substantial sacrifice of nutrients!)

To illustrate how you might use the 1,300 calorie daily food plan for Ann, a plan for two possible menus follows.

Breakfast

1 bread exchange
1 meat exchange
1 milk exchange
1 fruit exchange
1 fat exchange

Menu I

½ cup hashbrowns
1 fried egg
1 cup skim milk
½ cup orange juice
1 tsp. margarine*

Menu II

1 slice bread
1 oz. cheese
1 cup skim milk
½ grapefruit
1 tsp. butter on bread

Lunch

2 bread exchanges
2 meat exchanges
1 milk exchange
2 fruit exchanges
1 fat exchange

Menu I

1 cup mashed potatoes
2 oz. halibut
1 cup skim milk
4 fresh apricots
1 tsp. butter on potatoes

Menu II

½ cup sweet potatoes
1 oz. turkey
1 cup skim milk
1 small banana
1 tsp. butter on potatoes

Dinner

2 vegetable exchanges
2 bread exchanges
2 meat exchanges
2 fruit exchanges

Menu I

1 cup green beans
2 small rolls
2 oz. beef
2 cups strawberries

Menu II

1 cup carrots
⅓ cup cooked corn
2 oz. ham
1 cup canned (unsweetened) peaches

*for preparation of egg and hashbrowns

There are an infinite number of possibilities for a day's menus. Furthermore, you should be able to select from the regular foods your family uses, with the exception of sweets like sugar, syrups, candy, pies, cakes and cookies, jams, and regular soft drinks (diet soft drinks are allowed). You will want to have plenty of vegetables and fruits available.

You may make slight alterations in your food plan as long as you do not change the total number of exchanges allowed in each food group per day. For example, you may want to save a fruit exchange from lunch to have as an afternoon snack. Or perhaps you would like to move a bread exchange up to the next meal. Do not combine your daily total into just one or two meals, however. Eat at least three meals a day to avoid getting too hungry and thus eating more than you should. For the same reason, do not "borrow" food from the next day's food plan.

The exchange lists, with a little care and creativity, can be applied to mixed dishes. For example, a spaghetti dish might include hamburger (from the meat exchange), spaghetti (from the bread and cereal exchange), and tomato sauce (¼ cup counts as one vegetable and one fat). See exchange values for commercially prepared foods later in this chapter. Mushrooms and spices are free!

To be sure you are eating neither more nor less than is allowed, you will initially need to measure your foods. It may be impossible for you to measure your food in all situations, so you will want to have a mental picture of what some of the common measures look like (do the actual measurements often to check yourself). You will probably rely on the exchange lists heavily at first, but soon you will find that you remember the measurements for the exchanges you use most, and you may refer to the lists only occasionally (remember to check yourself periodically).

Step 5: Following the diet-exercise program

To check your progress, weigh yourself at least once a week on the same scales at about the same time of day, and wear no clothing. You will lose approximately 2 pounds per week, but this should be considered an average over one to two month's time. Individual metabolism and activity can cause the rate of weight loss to vary. Ann may have a rapid weight loss for the first week, followed by one to three weeks of no weight change. Weight loss will resume and she will be able to *average* a loss of approximately 2 pounds per week.

Step 6: Maintaining body weight

When Ann reaches her target weight it is possible to make a final check to see if that is the weight she desires. She will measure her percent body fat as explained in chapter 2, "Fitness Appraisal." By using this information she will be able to obtain another indication of what her body weight should be.

Item 16. Ann will now have to readjust her diet in order to determine what her caloric intake should be to maintain her target weight. An estimate of her caloric intake can be made by multiplying the target weight by 15 calories (125 × 15 = 1,875). She can continue to use the exchange lists as a guide in menu planning to ensure that she has a balanced diet. She should keep weighing herself at least once a week to make certain that she is maintaining her desired weight. Her weight should not fluctuate more than 2 pounds over or under her desired weight. If she starts either to gain or lose, she can control it by manipulating her diet and exercise program to effect such changes.

Exercise will help Ann keep extra fat and body weight from creeping up on her. A plan for continual exercise should be part of everyone's life.

Check your Weight-Control Work Sheet with the example in figure 5.12 to determine whether you have made any mistakes in writing a weight-control program.

MASTERY CHECK INSTRUCTIONS

Instructions: Circle the letter that corresponds to the best answer in the following situations. There is only one correct answer for each. Assume proper medical clearance for all cases. Use a blank copy of the Weight-Control Work Sheet in Appendix C to answer questions A and B.

A. Your brother, age twenty-three, weighs 193 pounds. His estimated target weight is 170 pounds. He is in Fitness Category II and wants to exercise five days per week.
   1. Your brother will expend an *average* of _____ calories per day in exercise.
      a. 75
      b. 107
      c. 150
   2. His estimated typical daily caloric intake is
      a. 2,795.
      b. 2,895.
      c. 3,095.
   3. His recommended daily caloric intake to lose 2 pounds per week, *including exercise* is
      a. 1,800.
      b. 1,900.
      c. 2,000.
   4. When he reaches his target weight, his caloric intake to maintain this weight (without exercise) will be
      a. 2,895.
      b. 2,550.
      c. 1,895.

B. Susan, age twenty-one, weighs 150 pounds and needs to reduce to 128 pounds. She is in Fitness Category III and prefers to exercise five days per week, using bicycling at 13.0 mph as her activity.
   1. The number of calories expended per minute for her selected activity is
      a. 10.8.
      b. 11.5.
      c. 12.1.
   2. The recommended number of minutes to exercise each day is
      a. 17.
      b. 18.
      c. 19.
   3. Her total daily caloric intake, without exercise, to lose 2 pounds per week is
      a. 1,200.
      b. 1,250.
      c. 1,300.
   4. When Susan reaches her target weight, her caloric intake to maintain her weight (without exercise) will be
      a. 2,250.
      b. 2,130.
      c. 1,920.

C. If you followed a food exchange diet of 1,300 calories per day, you would eat _____ fruits.

D. A typical medium fat meat exchange contains _____ grams of protein.

Weight-Control Work Sheet

1. Name _Ann Hathaway_ Age _21_ Sex _Female_ Date _____

2. Weight _145_ Target Weight _125_ Exercise Heart Rate Training Zone: _137_ to _168_

3. Medical Clearance: No Restrictions _X_ Restrictions _____

4. **Fitness Category**

Fitness Category	Minimum Caloric Expenditure per Exercise Session	Suggested Exercise Intensity (Cals./Min.)	Minimum Number of Days of Exercise Each Week
___ 0. Beginner	75	5	3–5
___ I. Very Poor	100	5	3–5
___ II. Poor	150	5–10	3–5
_X_ III. Fair	200	5–10	3–5
___ IV. Good	300+	10+	3–5
___ V. Excellent	300+	10+	3–5
___ VI. Superior	300+	10+	3–5

5. Exercise preference _Running_ Rate _5.5 mph_

6. Calories expended per minute (from Appendix B) _10.2_

7. Recommended caloric expenditure per session (from item 4) _200_

8. Number of minutes to exercise each day (item 7 ÷ item 6) _20_
Note: This should always be a minimum of 15 continuous minutes to obtain training effect. (Round off to nearest whole number.)

9. Number of days to exercise each week _5_

10. Number of calories expended in exercise each week (line 7 × line 9) _1,000_

11. Average number of calories expended daily in exercise (line 10 ÷ 7 days) _143_
(Round off answer to nearest whole number.)

Determining Caloric Intake

12. Typical daily caloric intake (Current weight × 15 cals.) _2,175_

13. Caloric reduction per day to lose two pounds per week _−1,000_

14. Total daily caloric intake, without exercise, to lose two pounds per week _1,175_
(line 12 − line 13)

15. Daily caloric intake to lose two pounds per week, including exercise (line 14 + line 11). This figure should not be below 1,200 for women or 1,500 for men. (Always round answer to the *lowest* 100 calories.) _1,300_

16. Maintaining body weight (target weight × 15 cals.) _1,875_

Figure 5.12.

If you responded correctly to each item, you are ready to proceed with the next unit.

VEGETABLE EXCHANGE LIST

$$\text{Each exchange} = \begin{cases} 30 \text{ calories} \\ 5 \text{ g carbohydrate} \\ 2 \text{ g protein} \end{cases}$$

$$\text{One exchange} = \tfrac{1}{2} \text{ cup}$$

If fat is added in the cooking or preparation of the vegetables, remember to count this when determining your fat exchanges.

Artichoke (½ medium)	Eggplant	*Peppers
Asparagus	†Escarole	Pimento
Bean sprouts	†Greens	Radishes
Beans, green or wax	Beet greens	Romaine
	Chard	Rhubarb
Beets	Collards	Rutabagas
*†Broccoli	Dandelion	Sauerkraut
*Brussels sprouts	Kale	Squash, summer (zucchini, gooseneck)
*Cabbage	Mustard	
†Carrots	Poke	
*Cauliflower	Spinach	*Tomatoes
Celery	Endive	Tomato juice
†Chicory	Turnip greens	Turnips
Cucumbers	Lettuce	Vegetable juice
	Mushrooms	†Watercress
	Okra	
	Onions	
	Parsley	

*These vegetables are good sources of vitamin C. At least one good source of vitamin C should be eaten each day.

†These vegetables are good sources of vitamin A. A good source of vitamin A should be eaten at least every other day.

BREADS AND CEREALS EXCHANGE LIST

$$\text{Each exchange} = \begin{cases} 70 \text{ calories} \\ 15 \text{ g carbohydrate} \\ 2 \text{ g protein} \end{cases}$$

Bread

White (including French and Italian)	1 slice
Whole wheat	1 slice
Rye or pumpernickel	1 slice
Raisin	1 slice
Bagel, small	½
English muffin, small	½
Plain roll, bread	1
Frankfurter roll	½
Hamburger bun	½
Dried bread crumbs	3 tbsp.
Tortilla, 6″	1

Cereal

Bran flakes	½ cup
Other ready-to-eat unsweetened cereal	¾ cup
Puffed cereal (unfrosted)	1 cup
Cereal (cooked)	½ cup
Grits (cooked)	½ cup
Rice or barley (cooked)	½ cup
Pasta (cooked), spaghetti, noodles, macaroni	½ cup
Popcorn (popped, no fat added)	3 cups
Cornmeal (dry)	2 tbsp.
Flour	2½ tbsp.
Wheat germ	¼ cup

Crackers

Arrowroot	3
Graham, 2½″ sq.	2
Matzoh, 4″ × 6″	½

Oyster	20
Pretzels, 3⅛″ long × ⅛″ dia.	25
Rye wafers, 2″ × 3½″	3
Saltines	6
Soda, 2½″ sq.	4

Dried Beans, Peas and Lentils

Beans, peas, lentils (dried and cooked)	½ cup
Baked beans, no pork (canned)	¼ cup

Starchy Vegetables

Corn	⅓ cup
Corn on cob	1 small
Lima beans	½ cup
Parsnips	⅔ cup
Peas, green (canned or frozen)	½ cup
Potato, white	1 small
Potato (mashed)	½ cup
Pumpkin	¾ cup
Winter squash, acorn or butternut	½ cup
Yam or Sweet Potato	¼ cup

Prepared Foods

Biscuit, 2″ dia. (omit 1 Fat Exchange)	1
Corn bread, 2″ × 2″ × 1″ (omit 1 Fat Exchange)	1
Corn muffin, 2″ dia. (omit 1 Fat Exchange)	1
Crackers, round butter type (omit 1 Fat Exchange)	5
Muffin, plain small (omit 1 Fat Exchange)	1
Potatoes, french fried, length 2″ to 3½″ (omit 1 Fat Exchange)	8
Potato or corn chips (omit 2 Fat Exchanges)	15
Pancake, 5″ × ½″ (omit 1 Fat Exchange)	1
Waffle, 5″ × ½″ (omit 1 Fat Exchange)	1

MEAT EXCHANGE LIST

Lean Meat

One Exchange of Lean Meat (1 oz.) contains 7 grams of protein, 3 grams of fat and 55 calories.

Beef: Baby beef (very lean), chipped beef, chuck, flank steak, tenderloin, plate ribs, plate skirt steak, round (bottom, top), all cuts rump, spare ribs, tripe	1 oz.
Lamb: Leg, rib, sirloin, loin (roast and chops), shank, shoulder	1 oz.
Pork: Leg (whole rump, center shank), ham, smoked (center slices)	1 oz.
Veal: Leg, loin, rib, shank, shoulder, cutlets	1 oz.
Poultry: Meat (without skin) of chicken, turkey, cornish hen, guinea hen, pheasant	1 oz.
Fish: Any fresh or frozen	1 oz.
Canned salmon, tuna, mackerel, crab and lobster,	¼ cup
Clams, oysters, scallops, shrimp,	5 or 1 oz.
Sardines, drained	3
Cheeses containing less than 5% butterfat	1 oz.
Cottage cheese, dry and 2% butterfat	¼ cup
Dried beans and peas (omit 1 Bread Exchange)	½ cup

Medium-Fat Meat

For each Exchange of Medium-Fat Meat omit ½ Fat Exchange. One Exchange = 7 g protein, 5.5 g fat, 77 calories

Beef: Ground (15% fat), corned beef (canned), rib eye, round (ground commercial)	1 oz.
Pork: Loin (all cuts tenderloin), shoulder arm (picnic), shoulder blade, boston butt, canadian bacon, boiled ham	1 oz.
Liver, heart, kidney and sweetbreads (these are high in cholesterol)	1 oz.
Cottage cheese, creamed	¼ cup
Cheese: mozzarella, ricotta, farmer's cheese, neufchatel,	1 oz.
Parmesan	3 tbsp.
Egg (high in cholesterol)	1
Peanut butter (omit 2 additional Fat Exchanges)	2 tbsp.

High-Fat Meat

For each Exchange of High-Fat Meat omit 1 Fat Exchange. One Exchange = 7 g protein, 8 g fat, 100 calories

Beef: Brisket, corned beef (brisket), ground beef (more than 20% fat), hamburger (commercial), chuck (ground commercial), roasts (rib), steaks (club and rib)	1 oz.
Lamb: Breast	1 oz.
Pork: Spare ribs, loin (back ribs), pork (ground), country style ham, deviled ham	1 oz.
Veal: Breast	1 oz.
Poultry: Capon, duck (domestic), goose	1 oz.
Cheese: Cheddar types	1 oz.
Cold Cuts	4½″ × ⅛″ slice
Frankfurter	1 small

MILK EXCHANGE LIST

This list shows the kinds and amounts of milk or milk products to use for one Milk Exchange. Since certain milk products contain fat, you must omit Fat Exchanges from your diet when they are used in your menu planning.

$$\text{Each exchange} = \left\{ \begin{array}{l} 170 \text{ calories} \\ 12 \text{ g carbohydrate} \\ 8 \text{ g protein} \\ 10 \text{ g fat} \end{array} \right.$$

Non-Fat Products

Skim or non-fat milk	1 cup
Powdered (non-fat dry before adding liquid)	⅓ cup
Canned, evaporated-skim milk	½ cup
Buttermilk made from skim milk	1 cup
Yogurt made from skim milk (plain, unflavored)	1 cup

Low-Fat Products

1% fat fortified milk (omit ½ Fat Exchange)	1 cup
2% fat fortified milk (omit 1 Fat Exchange)	1 cup
Yogurt made from 2% fortified milk, plain and unflavored (omit 1 Fat Exchange)	1 cup

Whole Milk Products (omit 2 Fat Exchanges)

Whole milk	1 cup
Canned, evaporated whole milk	½ cup
Buttermilk made from whole milk	1 cup
Yogurt made from whole milk (plain, unflavored)	1 cup

FRUIT EXCHANGE LIST

$$\text{Each exchange} = \left\{ \begin{array}{l} 40 \text{ calories} \\ 10 \text{ g carbohydrate} \end{array} \right.$$

Apple/1 small (2″ diameter)
Apple juice/⅓ cup
Applesauce/½ cup
Apricots, fresh/2 medium
Apricots, dried/4 halves
Apricots, canned (unsweetened)/½ cup
Apricot nectar/⅓ cup
Banana/½ small
Berries (blackberries, raspberries,

Grape juice/¼ cup
Honeydew melon/⅛ (7″ diameter)
Mango/½ small
Nectarine/1 medium
Orange/1 small
Orange juice/½ cup
Papaya/⅓ medium
Peach/1 medium
Peach, canned (unsweetened)/½ cup or 2 halves
Pear/1 small

strawberries)/1 cup
Blueberries/⅔ cup
Cantaloupe/¼ (6″ diameter)
Cherries, fresh/10 large
Cherries, canned (unsweetened)/½ cup
Cranberry juice cocktail, canned/¼ cup
Dates/2
Figs, fresh or dried/1
Fruit cocktail/1 cup
Grapefruit/½ small
Grapefruit juice/½ cup
Grapes/12 large, 30 small

Pear, canned (unsweetened)/½ cup or 2 halves
Pineapple, canned (unsweetened)/½ cup or 2 small slices
Pineapple juice (unsweetened)/½ cup
Plums/2 medium
Pomegranates/1 small
Prunes, dried/2
Prune juice/¼ cup
Raisins/2 tbsp.
Tangerine/1 large
Watermelon/1 cup or ½ slice, ¾″ thick

FAT EXCHANGE LIST

Each exchange = { 45 calories
                 { 5 g fat

To plan a diet low in saturated fat, select only those exchanges that appear in **bold type.** They are **polyunsaturated.**

Margarine, soft, tub or stick	**1 tsp.**
Avocado (4″ in diameter)	**⅛**
Oil, corn, cottonseed, safflower, soy, sunflower	**1 tsp.**
Oil, olive	**1 tsp.**
Oil, peanut	**1 tsp.**
Olives	**5 small**
Almonds	**10 whole**
Pecans	**2 large whole**

Peanuts	
Spanish	**20 whole**
Virginia	**10 whole**
Walnuts	**6 small**
Nuts, other	**6 small**
Butter	1 tsp.
Bacon fat	1 tsp.
Bacon, crisp	1 strip
Cream, light	2 tbsp.
Cream, sour	2 tbsp.
Cream, heavy	1 tbsp.
Cream cheese	1 tbsp.
French dressing	1 tbsp.
Italian dressing	1 tbsp.
Lard	1 tsp.
Mayonnaise	1 tsp.
Salad dressing, mayonnaise type	2 tsp.
Salt pork	¾″ cube

FREE LIST

The following foods are low in caloric content and may be eaten as desired.

Broth, fat-free	Horseradish	Salad dressings, low-calorie/less than 5 calories per tbsp.	Soy sauce
Bouillon	Hot sauce		Steak sauce
Carbonated beverages, low-calorie/less than 5 calories per bottle	Jams, jellies, and syrups—that are artificially sweetened, low calorie	Seasonings and spices (cinnamon, basil, celery salt, garlic, mint, mustard, nutmeg, oregano, parsley, pepper, etc.)	Sweeteners, low-calorie (saccharin, Sugar Twin, etc.)
Consommé	Lemon juice		Taco sauce
Cranberries, unsweetened	Mustard, prepared		Vanilla
Gelatin, unflavored or artificially sweetened	Pickles, sour or dill		Vinegar
	Rennet tablets		

This list may be used in applying some commercially prepared products to the exchange lists.

Exchange Values for Fast Foods

Exchange Equivalent

	Bread	Meat	Fat	Calories
Arthur Treacher's (fish, chips, cole slaw)				
3-piece dinner	6	4	9	1100
2-piece dinner	3½	2½	8	905
Burger Chef				
Hamburger	1½	1	1½	250
Double hamburger	2	2½	1	325
Super Chef	2½	3½	2	530
Big Chef	3	3	3	535
French fries	2	—	2	240
Chocolate shake	3	½	1	310
Burger King				
Hamburger	1½	1½	½	230
Double hamburger	2	3	—	325
Whopper	3	3	4	630
Whopper, Junior	1½	2	1	285
French fries	2	—	2½	220
Chocolate shake	4½	—	1½	365
Kentucky Fried Chicken (fried chicken, mashed potato, coleslaw, roll)				
3-piece dinner, original	4	6	2½	830
3-piece dinner, crispy	5	6	6½	1070
2-piece dinner, original	3½	2	1½	595
2-piece dinner, crispy	3	4½	3½	665
Long John Silver's (fish, chips, cole slaw)				
3-piece dinner	7	6	7	1190
2-piece dinner	6	4	6	955
McDonald's				
Hamburger	1½	1	1½	260
Double hamburger	2	2	1	350
Quarter Pounder	2½	3	1	420
Big Mac	3	2	4	550
French fries	1½	—	2	180
Chocolate shake	3½	—	1½	315
Pizza Hut (cheese pizza)				
Individual—thick crust	9½	7½	—	1030
Individual—thin crust	8½	6	—	1005
½ of 13"—thick crust	7½	7	—	900
½ of 13"—thin crust	7	5	—	850
½ of 15"—thick crust	10	9	—	1200
½ of 15"—thin crust	9½	7	—	1150

Supplementary Exchange List

Description	Serving Size	Exchange Equivalents	Calories
Tomato catsup	2 tbsp.	1 Vegetable	25
Tomato paste	2 tbsp.	1 Vegetable	25
Gooseberries	⅔ cup	1 Fruit	40
Loganberries	½ cup	1 Fruit	40
Mulberries	½ cup	1 Fruit	40
Fruit cocktail, unsweetened	½ cup	1 Fruit	40
Mixed fresh fruit, unsweetened	½ cup	1 Fruit	40
Unsweetened fruit nectars	⅓ cup	1 Fruit	40
Pineapple, canned in pineapple juice	2 slices, drained or 1 slice & 2 tbsp. juice	1 Fruit	40
Bread cubes or plain croutons	1 cup	1 Bread	70
Bread sticks (8″ long, ½″ diameter)	2	1 Bread	70
Bread sticks (4″ long, ½″ diameter)	6	1 Bread	70
Thin sliced bread (diet type)	1½ slices	1 Bread	70
Shredded wheat biscuit	1	1 Bread	70
Grapenuts	3 tbsp.	1 Bread	70
Cornstarch	2½ tbsp.	1 Bread	70
Cornflake crumbs	3 tbsp.	1 Bread	70
Melba toast rectangles	5 each	1 Bread	70
Graham cracker crumbs	¼ cup	1 Bread	70
Dutch pretzels	1	1 Bread	70
3-Ring pretzels	6	1 Bread	70
Zwieback toast	3 pieces	1 Bread	70
Chick peas or garbanzo beans, cooked	¼ cup	1 Bread	70
Lima beans, dried & cooked	⅓ cup	1 Bread	70
Ice milk	½ cup	1 Bread	70
Taco shell (ready to eat)	1	1 Bread + 1 Fat	115
Hash brown potatoes	¼ cup	1 Bread + 1 Fat	115
Instant mashed potatoes, made from flakes with fat as desired	½ cup	1 Bread + 1 Fat	115
Chow mein noodles	½ cup	1 Bread + 1 Fat	115
Ice cream, high fat	½ cup	1 Bread + 2 Fat	160
Shoestring potatoes	¾ cup	1 Bread + 2 Fat	160
Tater Tots, potato puffs	½ cup	1 Bread + 2 Fat	160
Onion rings, frozen	10 medium	1 Bread + 2 Fat	160
Vienna sausages	3	1 Meat	68
Parmesan cheese	4 tbsp.	1 Meat	68
Link sausage	2 links	1 Meat + 2 Fat	158
Blue cheese or Roquefort dressing	2 tsp.	1 Fat	45
Whipped butter, unsweetened	2 tbsp.	1 Fat	45
Whipped cream, unsweetened	2 tbsp.	1 Fat	45
Thousand Island or Russian dressing	2 tsp.	1 Fat	45
Brazil nuts	2 whole	1 Fat	45
Cashews	5	1 Fat	45
Chocolate, unsweetened, melted	2 tsp.	1 Fat	45
Salad dressings, mayonnaise type	2 tsp.	1 Fat	45
Powdered coffee cream substitute	3 tsp.	1 Fat	45

Description	Serving Size	Exchange Equivalents	Calories
Unsweetened coconut, grated or shredded	3 tbsp.	1 Fat	45
Macadamia nuts, whole	3 medium	1 Fat	45
Pine nuts	1 tbsp.	1 Fat	45
Sunflower seed kernels	2 tbsp.	1 Fat	45
White sauce, medium	2 tbsp.	1 Fat	45
Gravy, brown (limit to one exchange)	2 tbsp.	1 Fat	45
Liquid frozen coffee cream substitute	2 tbsp.	1 Fat	45

Combination Choices

Description	Serving Size	Exchange Equivalents	Calories
Meat pies (commercial frozen) chicken, turkey or meat pot pie (1 crust)	1	2 Bread + 1 Meat + 1 Fat	253
Chicken, turkey, or meat pot pie (2 crust)	1	3 Bread + 1 Meat + 1 Fat	323
Chili con carne with beans	⅔ cup	1 Bread + 1 Meat + 1 Fat	183
Enchiladas (cheese)	1 medium	1 Bread + 1 Meat + 1 Fat	183
Pork & beans	½ cup	1 Bread + 1 Meat	138
Taco (as purchased)	1 medium	1 Bread + 1 Meat + 1 Fat	183
Pizza with meat	¼ of 12″	2 Bread + 2 Meat + 2 Fat	366
Tamales with sauce	2 medium	1 Bread + 1 Meat + 1 Fat	183
Spanish rice without meat	½ cup	1 Bread	70
Macaroni & cheese	½ cup	1 Bread + 1 Meat + 1 Fat	183
Chop suey with meat	½ cup	½ Bread + ½ Meat	69
Chow mein with meat	½ cup	½ Bread + ½ Meat	69
Tuna casserole	½ cup	1 Bread + 1 Meat + 1 Fat	183

Betty Crocker

Description	Serving Size	Exchange Equivalents	Calories
Cheeseburger Macaroni Hamburger Helper Mix	⅓ package	2 Bread + 1 Fat	185
Chili-Tomato Hamburger Helper Mix	⅓ package	2 Bread + ½ Fat	165
Creamy Noodles 'N Tuna Hamburger Helper Mix	⅓ package	2 Bread + 2 Fat	230
Creamy Rice 'N Tuna Hamburger Helper Mix	⅓ package	2 Bread + 1 Fat	185
Dry Hash Brown Potato Mix	⅛ package	1½ Bread	105
Dry Scalloped Potato Mix	⅛ package	1½ Bread	105
Hamburger Stew Hamburger Helper Mix	⅓ package	1½ Bread	105
Instant Mashed Potato Buds	⅓ cup	1 Bread	70
Lasagna Hamburger Helper Mix	⅓ package	2 Bread	140
Packaged Noodles Almondine Mix (Prepared)	¼ package	2 Bread + 2 Fat	230
Packaged Noodles Romanoff Mix (Prepared)	¼ package	1 Bread + ½ Milk + 2 Fat	240
Spaghetti Hamburger Helper Mix	⅓ package	2 Bread	140

Birds Eye

Description	Serving Size	Exchange Equivalents	Calories
Frozen Bavarian-Style Beans with Spaetzle	3.3 oz.	2 Vegetable	70
Frozen Chinese-Style Vegetables	3.3 oz.	1 Vegetable	35
Frozen Corn and Peas with Tomatoes	3.3 oz.	1 Bread	70

Description	Serving Size	Exchange Equivalents	Calories
Frozen Danish-Style Vegetable	3.3 oz.	1 Vegetable	35
Frozen French-Style Green Beans with Mushrooms	3 oz.	1 Vegetable	35
Frozen Green Peas & Onions	3.3 oz.	2 Vegetable	70
Frozen Italian-Style Vegetables	3.3 oz.	½ Bread	35
Frozen Japanese-Style Vegetables	3.3 oz.	1 Vegetable	35
Frozen Mexican-Style Vegetables	3.3 oz.	1 Bread	70
Frozen Mixed Vegetables with Onion Sauce	2.6 oz.	2 Vegetable + 1 Fat	80
Frozen Rice and Peas with Mushrooms	2.3 oz.	1½ Bread	105

Campbell's Condensed Soups

Description	Serving Size	Exchange Equivalents	Calories
Asparagus, Cream of	10 oz.	1 Bread + 1 Fat	100
Bean with Bacon	11 oz.	2 Bread + 1 Meat + ½ Fat	200
Beef	11 oz.	1 Bread + 1 Meat	110
Beef Broth (Bouillon)	10 oz.	1 Vegetable	35
Beef Noodle	10 oz.	1 Bread	90
Black Bean	11 oz.	1½ Bread	150
Celery, Cream of	10 oz.	½ Bread + 1½ Fat	110
Cheddar Cheese	11 oz.	1 Milk + 3 Fat	200
Chicken Alphabet	10 oz.	1 Bread + 1 Fat	110
Chicken Broth	10 oz.	1 Lean Meat	50
Chicken, Cream of	10 oz.	½ Bread + 2 Fat	140
Chicken 'N Dumplings	10 oz.	½ Bread + 1 Meat + 1 Fat	120
Chicken Gumbo	10 oz.	1 Bread	70
Chicken Noodle	10 oz.	1 Bread	90
Chicken Noodle O's	10 oz.	1 Bread	90
Chicken with Rice	10 oz.	1 Bread	80
Chicken and Stars	10 oz.	1 Bread	80
Chicken Vegetable	10 oz.	1 Bread	90
Chili Beef	11 oz.	2 Bread + 1 Meat + ½ Fat	210
Clam Chowder (Manhattan)	10 oz.	1 Bread + ½ Fat	100
Clam Chowder (N.E. made with milk)*	10 oz.	½ Milk + 1 Bread + 1 Meat + 1 Fat	200
Consommé (Beef)	10 oz.	1 Meat	45
Curly Noodle with Chicken	10 oz.	1 Bread + ½ Fat	100
Golden Vegetable Noodle O's	10 oz.	1 Bread	90
Green Pea	11 oz.	2 Bread + 1 Meat	190
Hot Dog Bean	11 oz.	2 Bread + 1 Meat + 1 Fat	230
Meatball Alphabet	10 oz.	1 Bread + 1 Meat + ½ Fat	140
Minestrone	10 oz.	1 Bread + ½ Fat	110
Mushroom, Cream of	10 oz.	1 Bread + 2 Fat	150
Mushroom, Golden	10 oz.	1 Bread + 1 Fat	110
Noodles & Ground Beef	10 oz.	1 Bread + 1 Fat	110
Onion	10 oz.	1 Bread	80
Onion, Cream of (made with water & milk)*	10 oz.	½ Milk + 1 Bread + 1½ Fat	180
Oyster Stew (made with milk)*	10 oz.	½ Milk + ½ Bread + 2 Fat	170
Pepper Pot	10 oz.	1 Bread + 1 Meat + ½ Fat	130
Potato, Cream of (made with water & milk)*	10 oz.	½ Milk + 1 Bread + 1 Fat	140

*Exchanges based on addition of whole milk.

Description	Serving Size	Exchange Equivalents	Calories
Scotch Broth	10 oz.	1 Bread + 1 Fat	100
Shrimp, Cream of (made with milk)*	10 oz.	½ Milk + 1 Bread + 2 Fat	210
Split Pea with Ham & Bacon	11 oz.	2 Bread + 1 Meat + ½ Fat	230
Stockpot	11 oz.	1 Bread + 1 Meat	130
Tomato	10 oz.	1 Vegetable + 1 Bread	110
Tomato (made with milk)*	10 oz.	½ Milk + 1 Veg. + 1 Bread + 1½ Fat	210
Tomato-Beef Noodle O's	10 oz.	1½ Bread + 1 Fat	160
Tomato Bisque	11 oz.	2 Bread + ½ Fat	160
Tomato Rice-Old Fashioned	11 oz.	2 Bread	150
Turkey Noodle	10 oz.	1 Bread	80
Turkey Vegetable	10 oz.	1 Bread	90
Vegetable	10 oz.	1 Vegetable + 1 Bread	100
Vegetable Beef	10 oz.	½ Bread + 1 Meat	90
Vegetable, Old Fashioned	10 oz.	1 Bread	90
Vegetarian Vegetable	10 oz.	1 Bread	90
Campbell's Soup for One			
Bean, Old Fashioned	11⅝ oz.	2 Bread + 1 Fat	210
Clam Chowder, New England (made with milk)*	11⅝ oz.	1 Fat + ½ Milk + 1 Bread + 1 Meat	200
Golden Chicken & Noodles	11⅝ oz.	1 Bread + 1 Fat	120
Mushroom, Cream of, with wine	11¼ oz.	1 Bread + 2 Fat	160
Tomato Royale	11⅝ oz.	2 Bread + 1 Fat	180
Vegetable, Old World	11⅝ oz.	1 Bread + 1 Fat	125
Campbell's Chunky Soups			
Chunky Beef	9½ oz.	1 Bread + 2 Meat	190
Chunky Chicken	9½ oz.	1 Vegetable + 1 Meat + 1 Bread	200
Chunky Chicken with Rice	9½ oz.	1 Bread + 2 Meat	160
Chunky Chicken Vegetable	9½ oz.	1½ Bread + 1 Meat + 1 Fat	190
Chunky Chili Beef	9½ oz.	2 Bread + 2 Meat	260
Chunky Clam Chowder (Manhattan Style)	9½ oz.	1½ Bread + 1 Meat	160
Chunky Minestrone	9½ oz.	1½ Bread + 1 Meat	160
Chunky Old Fashioned Bean with Ham	9½ oz.	1 Veg. + 2 Bread + 1 Meat + 1 Fat	260
Chunky Old Fashioned Vegetable Beef	9½ oz.	1 Veg. + 1 Bread + 1 Meat + 1 Fat	160
Chunky Sirloin Burger	9½ oz.	1 Veg. + 1 Bread + 1 Meat + 1 Fat	210
Chunky Split Pea w/Ham	9½ oz.	2 Bread + 1 Meat + ½ Fat	220
Chunky Steak & Potato	9½ oz.	1 Bread + 2 Meat	190
Chunky Turkey	9½ oz.	1 Veg. + 1 Bread + 1 Fat	160
Chunky Vegetable	9½ oz.	1 Veg. + 1 Bread + 1 Fat	140
Campbell's Low Sodium Products			
Chunky Beef, Low Sodium	7½ oz.	1 Vegetable + 1 Bread + 1 Meat + 1 Fat	170
Chunky Chicken, Low Sodium	7½ oz.	1 Bread + 1 Meat + 1 Fat	170
Green Pea, Low Sodium	7¼ oz.	1 Veg. + 1 Bread + 1 Meat	150

*Exchanges based on addition of whole milk.

Description	Serving Size	Exchange Equivalents	Calories
Mushroom, Cream of, Low Sodium	7¼ oz.	½ Bread + 2 Fat	140
Tomato, Low Sodium	7¼ oz.	1 Veg. + 1 Bread + 1 Fat	130
Turkey Noodle, Low Sodium	7¼ oz.	1 Bread	60
Vegetable, Low Sodium	7¼ oz.	1 Bread	90
Vegetable Beef, Low Sodium	7¼ oz.	1 Vegetable + 1 Meat	80
"V-8" Cocktail Vegetable Juice, Low Sodium	6 oz.	1 Vegetable	35
Chili Con Carne with Beans, Low Sodium	7¾ oz.	2 Bread + 2 Meat + 1½ Fat	310

Other Campbell's Canned Products

Barbecue Beans	4 oz.	2 Bread	140
Beans and Franks	4 oz.	1 Bread + 1 Meat + 1 Fat	185
Home Style Beans	4 oz.	2 Bread	150
Old Fashioned Beans	4 oz.	2 Bread	145
Pork & Beans	4 oz.	2 Bread	130
Tomato Juice	6 oz.	1 Vegetable	35
"V-8" Cocktail Vegetable Juice	6 oz.	1 Vegetable	35
"V-8" Spicy Hot Cocktail Vegetable Juice	6 oz.	1 Vegetable	35

Chef Boy-Ar-Dee Mixed Dishes

Spaghetti Sauce/Meat	4 oz., ½ can	1 Bread + ½ Meat + 1 Fat	151
Spaghetti Sauce/Mushroom	4 oz., ½ can	1 Bread + ½ Meat + 1 Fat	151
Pizza Sauce	2 oz., ¼ can	1 Fat	45
Mushrooms in Brown Gravy	5 oz., ½ can	1 Vegetable + 1 Fat	70
Beefaroni	5 oz., ⅓ can	1 Bread + 1 Meat	138
Cheese Ravioli	5 oz., ⅓ can	1½ Bread + ½ Meat + 1 Fat	186
Chili Con Carne w/Beans	5 oz., ⅓ can	1½ Bread + 1 Fat	150
Marinara Sauce	4 oz., ½ cup	1 Bread	70
Meatballs w/Gravy	5 oz., ⅓ can	½ Bread + 2 Meat + 1 Fat	216
Spaghetti Sauce/Meat	5 oz., ⅓ can	1 Bread + 1 Fat	115
Ravioli w/Beef	5 oz., ⅓ can	1½ Bread + 1 Fat	150
Spaghetti & Meat Balls	5 oz., ⅓ can	1 Bread + 1 Meat	142
Spaghetti Sauce w/Meat Balls	5 oz., ⅓ can	1½ Bread + 1 Meat + 1 Fat	218
Spaghetti Sauce w/Mushrooms	5 oz., ⅓ can	1 Bread + ½ Fat	92
Meat Ball Stew	7 oz., ¼ can	1 Bread + 1 Meat + 1 Fat	188
Lasagna	8 oz., ⅕ can	2 Bread + 1 Meat + 2 Fat	298
Ravioli w/Beef	8 oz., ⅕ can	2½ Bread + 1 Fat	220
Spaghetti & Meat Balls	8 oz., ⅕ can	2 Bread + 1 Meat + ½ Fat	231
Pizza Pie Mix (made w/water)	¼	2 Bread + 1 Fat	185
Spaghetti & Meatball Dinner	1/6	3 Bread + 1 Meat	278
Spaghetti w/Meat Dinner	1/6	2½ Bread + 1 Meat	243
Spaghetti w/Mushroom Dinner	1/6	2½ Bread	175
Pizza w/Sausage	1/6	1½ Bread + ½ Meat + 1 Fat	184
Frozen Beef Ravioli	8 oz., ½ can	2½ Bread + 1 Meat + 1 Fat	290
Frozen Cheese Ravioli	8 oz., ½ can	2 Bread + 1 Meat + 1 Fat	253
Frozen Lasagna	8 oz., ½ can	2 Bread + 2 Meat + 1 Fat	321
Frozen Manicotti	8 oz., ½ can	2 Bread + 2 Meat + 3 Fat	411

Chun King Corporation

Chicken Divider Pak Chow Mein	¼ total mix	2 Bread + 2 Meat	276
Beef Divider Pak Chow Mein	¼ total mix	2 Bread + 2 Meat + 1 Fat	321

Description	Serving Size	Exchange Equivalents	Calories
Mushroom Divider Pak Chow Mein	¼ total mix	2 Bread	140
Meatless Chow Mein	½ can	1 Bread	70
Subgum Chicken Chow Mein	½ can	1 Bread	70
Beef Chop Suey	½ can	1 Bread	70
Chinese Vegetables	½ can	1 Bread	70
Chop Suey Vegetables	½ can	1 Vegetable	35
Bean Sprouts	½ can	1 Vegetable	35
Chow Mein Noodles	½ can	1½ Bread + 2 Fat	195
Chicken Chow Mein (Frozen)	8 oz., ½ pkg.	1 Bread + 1 Meat	138

Contadina
Seasoned Bread Crumbs	3 tbsp.	1 Bread	70

Del Monte
Pudding Cups
Chocolate	5 oz.	2½ Bread + 1 Fat	197
Vanilla	5 oz.	2 Bread + 1 Fat	186
Tapioca	5 oz.	2 Bread + 1 Fat	172
Butterscotch	5 oz.	2 Bread + 1 Fat	180
Banana	5 oz.	2 Bread + 1 Fat	179
Strawberry	5 oz.	2 Bread + 1 Fat	165

Dinty Moore
Beef Stew	7½ oz.	½ Bread + 1½ Meat + 1 Fat + 1 Vegetable	180
Vegetable Stew	7½ oz.	1 Bread + 1 Vegetable + 2 Fat	160
Noodles 'N Chicken	7½ oz.	1 Bread + 1 Meat + 2 Fat	215

Durkee
Spaghetti Sauce Mix (made with tomato paste)	¼ package	1 Bread	70
Hollandaise Sauce Mix	¼ package	½ Bread + ½ Fat	55
Cheese Sauce Mix	¼ package	½ Bread + 1 Meat	105
Sour Cream Sauce Mix (made with whole milk)	¼ package	½ Bread + ½ Fat	55
Teriyaki Sauce Mix	½ package	½ Bread	35
Taco Seasoning Mix	½ package	½ Bread	35
Brown Gravy Mix	½ package	½ Bread	35
Chicken Gravy Mix	½ package	½ Bread	35

Franco-American
Beef Ravioli in Meat Sauce	7½ oz.	1 Veg. + 2 Bread + 1 Meat	220
Beef RavioliO's in Meat Sauce	7½ oz.	1 Veg. + 2 Bread + 1 Meat	220
Beefy Mac-Macaroni 'N Beef in Tomato Sauce	7½ oz.	1 Fat + 1 Veg. + 1½ Bread + 1 Meat	220
Elbow Macaroni & Cheese	7¼ oz.	2 Bread + 1 Fat	180
Macaroni & Cheese	7¼ oz.	2 Bread + 1 Fat	180
Meatball Mac-Macaroni & Meatballs in Tomato Sauce	7½ oz.	1 Meat + 1 Fat + 1 Vegetable + 1½ Bread	220
Rotini in Tomato Sauce	7½ oz.	1 Veg. + 2 Bread + 1 Fat	200
Rotini & Meatballs in Tomato Sauce	7¼ oz.	1 Meat + 1 Fat + 1 Vegetable + 1½ Bread	230

Description	Serving Size	Exchange Equivalents	Calories
Spaghetti in Meat Sauce	7¾ oz.	1 Vegetable + 1 Bread + 1 Meat + 1½ Fat	220
Spaghetti in Tomato Sauce with Cheese	7½ oz.	1 Vegetable + 2 Bread	170
Spaghetti with Meatballs in Tomato Sauce	7¼ oz.	1 Meat + 1 Fat + 1 Vegetable + 1 Bread	210
"SpaghettiO's" in Tomato and Cheese Sauce	7½ oz.	2 Bread	160
"SpaghettiO's" with Little Meatballs in Tomato Sauce	7½ oz.	1 Meat + 1 Fat + 1 Vegetable + 1 Bread	210
"SpaghettiO's" with Sliced Franks in Tomato Sauce	7½ oz.	1 Veg. + 1½ Bread + 2 Fat	210
Beef Gravy	2 oz.	1 Fat	30
Brown Gravy with Onions	2 oz.	1 Fat	25
Chicken Gravy	2 oz.	1 Fat	50
Chicken Giblet Gravy	2 oz.	1 Fat	35
Mushroom Gravy	2 oz.	1 Fat	35

General Foods

Description	Serving Size	Exchange Equivalents	Calories
Fruit-Flavored Gelatin (prepared)	½ cup	1 Bread	70
Cheesecake Mix (prepared)	⅛ of 8″ cake	2½ Bread + 2 Fat	265
Egg Custard Mix (prepared with milk)	½ cup	½ Milk + 1 Bread + 1 Fat	195
Low-Calorie Pudding (prepared with skim milk)	½ cup	½ Milk + ½ Bread	65

Green Giant

Description	Serving Size	Exchange Equivalents	Calories
Frozen Broccoli in Cheese Sauce	3½ oz.	½ Meat	35
Frozen Cauliflower in Cheese Sauce	3½ oz.	1 Vegetable + 1 Fat	80
Frozen Creamed Peas	3½ oz.	1 Bread + 1 Fat	115

Heinz

Description	Serving Size	Exchange Equivalents	Calories
Spaghetti with Meat Sauce	7½ oz.	1 Veg. + 1 Bread + ½ Meat + 1 Fat	170

Heinz
Soups, Condensed, Diluted

Description	Serving Size	Exchange Equivalents	Calories
Alphabet with Vegetables	1 cup	½ Bread + 1 Fat	80
Bean, with Smoked Pork	1 cup	1½ Bread + 1 Meat	175
Beef Noodle	1 cup	½ Bread + ½ Fat	60
Beef, Vegetable and Barley	1 cup	½ Bread + ½ Meat	70
Celery, Cream of	1 cup	½ Bread + 1 Fat	80
Chicken, Cream of	1 cup	½ Bread + 1 Fat	80
Chicken Gumbo	1 cup	½ Bread + ½ Fat	60
Chicken Noodle	1 cup	½ Bread + ½ Fat	60
Chicken Vegetable	1 cup	½ Bread + ½ Meat	70
Chicken with Rice	1 cup	½ Bread + ½ Fat	60
Chili with Beef	1 cup	1 Bread + 1 Meat + ½ Fat	165
Clam Chowder (Manhattan Style)	1 cup	½ Bread + ½ Fat	60
Consommé (Chicken)	1 cup	Free	
Green Pea, Cream of	1 cup	1½ Bread + ½ Fat	130
Minestrone	1 cup	1 Bread + ½ Fat	95
Mushroom, Cream of	1 cup	2 Fat + ½ Bread	125
Split Pea	1 cup	1½ Bread + 1 Meat	175
Tomato	1 cup	1 Bread + ½ Fat	95

Description	Serving Size	Exchange Equivalents	Calories
Tomato with Rice	1 cup	1 Bread + 1 Fat	115
Turkey Noodle	1 cup	½ Bread + ½ Fat	60
Turtle, Genuine	1 cup	½ Bread	105
Vegetable Beef	1 cup	1 Bread + ½ Fat	95
Vegetable with Beef Broth	1 cup	1 Bread + ½ Fat	95
Vegetable without Meat	1 cup	1 Bread + ½ Fat	95

Heinz
Minute Meals

Beef Stew	1 cup	1 Bread + 2 Meat	210
Chicken Noodle Dinner	1 cup	1 Bread + 1 Meat	140
Chicken Stew with Dumplings	1 cup	1 Bread + 2 Fat	160
Macaroni with Cheese Sauce	1 cup	1½ Bread + 1 Meat + 1 Fat	200
Macaroni Creole	¾ cup	1½ Bread + ½ Fat	130

Heinz Beans

With Pork & Molasses Sauce	½ cup	1 Meat + 2 Bread	210
With Pork & Tomato Sauce	½ cup	1 Meat + 1½ Bread	175
Beans in Tomato Sauce (Vegetarian)	½ cup	1 Meat + 2½ Fruit + 1 Fat	140

Heinz Condiments & Pickles

Tomato Ketchup	1 tbsp.	½ Fruit	20
Chili Sauce	1 tbsp.	½ Fruit	20
Barbecue Sauce with Savory Bits of Onion	1 tbsp.	½ Fruit	20
57 Sauce	1 tbsp.	½ Fruit	20
Savory Sauce	1 tbsp.	Free	
Worcestershire Sauce	1 tbsp.	Free	
French Dressing	1 tbsp.	1 Fat	45
Salad Dressing	1 tbsp.	1 Fat	45
Dill Pickle	1–4″ long	½ Vegetable	20
Dill Pickle (Processed)	1–3″ long	Free	
Dill Hamburger Pickles	3 slices	Free	
Fresh Cucumber Pickles	3 slices	½ Vegetable	20
Sour Pickles	1–2″ long	Free	
Sweet Gherkins	1–2″ long	1 Vegetable	35
Sweet Mixed Pickles	3 slices	½ Fruit	20
Sweet Mustard Pickles	1 tbsp.	1 Vegetable	35
Barbecue Relish	1 tbsp.	1 Vegetable	35
Hot Dog Relish	1 tbsp.	½ Fruit	20
Hamburger Relish	1 tbsp.	½ Vegetable	20
India Relish	1 tbsp.	½ Fruit	20
Piccalilli	1 tbsp.	½ Fruit	20
Sweet Relish	1 tbsp.	½ Fruit	20
Mustard	1 tsp.	Free	
Horseradish, Dehydrated	1 tsp.	Free	

Heinz Great American Soup

Savory Bean with Smoked Ham	1 cup	1 Meat + 1 Bread + 1 Fruit	180
Bountiful Chicken Noodle with Dumplings	1 cup	½ Meat + 1 Fruit	75
Tempting Chicken Rice with Mushrooms	1 cup	½ Meat + 1 Fruit + ½ Fat	100

Description	Serving Size	Exchange Equivalents	Calories
Golden Cream of Chicken	1 cup	1 Meat + 1 Fruit	110
Velvety Cream of Mushroom	1 cup	½ Milk + 1 Vegetable	115
Luscious Split Pea with Smoked Ham	1 cup	1 Meat + 1 Bread + ½ Fruit	160
Buttered Tomato with Vegetables	1 cup	1 Bread + 1 Fat	115
Hefty Vegetable with Ground Beef	1 cup	1 Meat + 1½ Vegetable	120
Hearty Vegetable Beef	1 cup	1 Meat + 1 Bread + ½ Fat	160
Full Bodied Vegetable with Beef Broth	1 cup	1 Meat + 1 Bread + ½ Fat	160
Tasty Turkey Noodle	1 cup	½ Meat + 1½ Vegetable	85
Delicious Beef Noodle with Dumplings	1 cup	½ Meat + 2 Vegetable	105
Abundant Vegetarian Vegetable	1 cup	½ Meat + 1 Bread + ½ Veg.	140

Hormel

Description	Serving Size	Exchange Equivalents	Calories
Noodles 'N Beef	7½ oz.	1 Bread + 1 Meat + 2 Fat	240
Spaghetti & Meatballs	7½ oz.	1½ Bread + ½ Meat + 1 Fat	170
Beef Goulash	7½ oz.	1 Bread + 1½ Meat + 2 Fat + ½ Vegetable	240

Hunt's

Description	Serving Size	Exchange Equivalents	Calories
Canned Pizza Sauce	1 cup	1½ Bread + 1 Fat	150
Canned Tomato Sauce	1 cup	1 Bread	70
Canned Tomato Paste	¾ cup	2 Bread	140

Hunt's
Snack puddings

Description	Serving Size	Exchange Equivalents	Calories
Chocolate, Banana	5 oz.	1½ Bread + 2 Fat	180
Vanilla, Butterscotch	5 oz.	1½ Bread + 2 Fat	190
Tapioca	5 oz.	1½ Bread + 2 Fat	180

Jell-O
Pudding mixes, prepared with nonfat milk

Description	Serving Size	Exchange Equivalents	Calories
Butterscotch	½ cup	½ Milk + 1½ Bread	140
Chocolate	½ cup	½ Milk + 1½ Bread	130
Vanilla	½ cup	½ Milk + 1½ Bread	120
Vanilla Tapioca	½ cup	½ Milk + 1½ Bread	130

Kraft

Description	Serving Size	Exchange Equivalents	Calories
Macaroni & Cheese Dinner Mix (prepared)	¾ cup	2 Bread + ½ Meat + 2 Fat	270
American-Style Spaghetti Dinner Mix (prepared)	1 cup	3 Bread + 1 Fat	255
Cheese Pizza Mix	¼ box	2½ Bread + 1 Meat	245
Sausage Pizza Mix	¼ box	2½ Bread + 1 Meat + 2 Fat	270

Lipton
Cup-A-Soup,
all one serving size

Description	Serving Size	Exchange Equivalents	Calories
Dry Cream-Style Chicken Soup Mix (prepared)	6 oz.	1 Bread + 1 Fat	105
Dry Bean Soup Mix (prepared)	6 oz.	1 Bread + ½ Meat	105
Dry Vegetable Beef Soup Mix (prepared)	6 oz.	1 Vegetable	35

Description	Serving Size	Exchange Equivalents	Calories
Cream of Mushroom Soup Mix (prepared)	6 oz.	1 Bread + 1 Fat	105
Beef Flavored Noodle Soup Mix (prepared)	6 oz.	½ Bread	35
Chicken Noodle with Meat Soup Mix (prepared)	6 oz.	½ Bread	35
Green Pea Soup Mix (prepared)	6 oz.	1½ Bread + ½ Meat	140
Cream of Tomato Soup Mix (prepared)	6 oz.	1 Bread + ½ Fat	95
Spring Vegetable Soup Mix (prepared)	6 oz.	2 Vegetable	70

Minute

Description	Serving Size	Exchange Equivalents	Calories
Packaged Precooked Rice Mixes (Beef-Flavored, Spanish, Chicken-Flavored, Fried)	½ cup	2 Bread + 1 Fat	185

Mrs. Paul's

Description	Serving Size	Exchange Equivalents	Calories
Frozen Deviled Crab Cakes	1 cake	1 Meat + 1 Bread	140
Frozen Fish Sticks	4 sticks	1 Meat + 1 Bread	140

Morningstar Farms

Description	Serving Size	Exchange Equivalents	Calories
Breakfast Patties	2 patties	2½ Meat + 1½ Fat + ⅓ Bread	221
Breakfast Strips	3 strips	½ Meat + 1¾ Fat	114
Breakfast Links	3 links	2 Meat + 1½ Fat	186
Luncheon Slices	2 slices	1 Meat + ⅓ Bread	87

Nabisco

Description	Serving Size	Exchange Equivalents	Calories
Shredded Wheat Wafers	5 crackers	1 Bread + ½ Fat	95
Thin Wheat Crackers	12 crackers	1 Bread + 1 Fat	115
Zwieback Toast	3 pieces	1 Bread + ½ Fat	95
Animal Crackers	8 crackers	1 Bread + ½ Fat	95
Oyster Crackers	25 crackers	1 Bread + ½ Fat	95
Plain Chocolate Wafers	3 wafers	1 Bread + ½ Fat	95
Graham Crackers	4 crackers	1½ Bread + ½ Fat	130
Thin Pretzel Sticks	67 sticks	1 Bread	70
Arrowroot Biscuits	4 biscuits	1 Bread + ½ Fat	95
Plain Vanilla Wafers	5 wafers	1 Bread + ½ Fat	95
Saltine Crackers	7 crackers	1 Bread + ½ Fat	95
American Harvest	7 crackers	1 Bread + 1 Fat	115
Cheese Tid-Bit	28 crackers	1 Bread + 1 Fat	115
Chicken in a Biskit	12 crackers	1 Bread + 1 Fat	115
Corn Diggers	26 pieces	1 Bread + 1 Fat	115
French Onion	9 crackers	1 Bread + 1 Fat	115
Ritz	7 crackers	1 Bread + 1 Fat	115
Sociables	12 crackers	1 Bread + 1 Fat	115
Bacon Flavored Thins	12 crackers	1 Bread + 1½ Fat	140
Buttery Flavored Sesames	9 crackers	1 Bread + 1½ Fat	140
Cheese Flavored Flings Curls	22 crackers	1 Bread + 3½ Fat	230
Korkers Corn Chips	18 crackers	1 Bread + 1½ Fat	140
Cheese Ritz	8 crackers	1 Bread + 2 Fat	160
Shapies Cheese Flavored (Either Dip Delights or Shells)	15 crackers	1 Bread + 1½ Fat	140
Swiss in Ham Flavored Fling Curls	18 crackers	1 Bread + 2½ Fat	185

Description	Serving Size	Exchange Equivalents	Calories
Nestlé			
Souptime,			
one serving size			
Chicken Noodle Soup Mix (prepared)	6 oz.	½ Bread	35
Beef Noodle Soup Mix (prepared)	6 oz.	½ Bread	35
Cream of Chicken Soup Mix (prepared)	6 oz.	1 Bread + 1 Fat	105
Tomato Soup Mix (prepared)	6 oz.	1 Bread	70
French Onion Soup Mix (prepared)	6 oz.	1 Vegetable	35
Green Pea Soup Mix (prepared)	6 oz.	1 Bread + ½ Meat	105
Mushroom Soup Mix (prepared)	6 oz.	1 Bread + 1 Fat	115
Cream of Vegetable Soup Mix (prepared)	6 oz.	1½ Vegetable + 1 Fat	150
Ore-Ida			
Frozen French Fries	3 oz.	1½ Bread + 1 Fat	150
Frozen Cottage Fries	3 oz.	1½ Bread + 1½ Fat	175
Frozen Southern-Style Hash Brown Potatoes	3 oz.	1 Bread	70
Frozen Shredded Hash Brown Potatoes	3 oz.	1 Bread	70
Frozen Plain Tater Tots	3 oz.	1½ Bread + 2 Fat	195
Frozen Onion Rings	2½ oz.	1 Bread + 2 Fat	160
Pepperidge Farm			
German Chocolate Cake	⅒ cake	1½ Bread + 1 Fat	160
Pound Cake—Butter or Chocolate	⅒ cake	1 Bread + 1½ Fat	130
Goldfish Crackers—Cheddar Cheese, Parmesan Cheese, Lightly Salted, Pizza, Sesame-Garlic, or Taco	45–50 crackers	1 Bread + 1½ Fat	140
Goldfish Thins—Cheddar Cheese, Rye, or Lightly Salted	6 crackers	1 Bread + 1 Fat	105
Croutons—Cheddar Cheese	½ cup	1½ Bread + 1 Fat	130
Croutons—Plain, Seasoned, or Onion-Garlic	½ cup	1½ Bread + 1 Fat	140
Pet			
Canned Imitation Sour Cream	1 tbsp.	½ Fat	22
Dry Nondairy Coffee Creamer	1 tbsp.	½ Fat	22
Pillsbury			
Apple, Blueberry, or Cherry Turnovers	1 turnover	1½ Bread + 1½ Fat	175
Brownie Mix (prepared)	2 1½″ squares	1 Bread + 1 Fat	115
Gingerbread Mix (prepared)	3″ square	2 Bread + 1 Fat	185
Date Bread Mix (prepared)	⅒ loaf	1½ Bread + ½ Fat	130
Cranberry Bread Mix (prepared)	⅒ loaf	1½ Bread + ½ Fat	130
Nut Bread Mix (prepared)	⅒ loaf	1½ Bread + ½ Fat	130
Oatmeal-Raisin Bread (prepared)	⅒ loaf	1½ Bread + ½ Fat	130
Hot Roll Mix (prepared)	2 rolls	2 Bread + 1 Fat	185
Refrigerated Hot Loaf	1 slice	1 Bread + ½ Fat	95
Refrigerated Apple-Cinnamon Muffins	1 muffin	1 Bread + 1 Fat	95
Refrigerated Corn Muffins	1 muffin	1½ Bread + 1 Fat	150
Refrigerated Plain Buttermilk Biscuits	2 biscuits	1½ Bread	105

Refrigerated Butterflake Dinner Rolls	1 roll	1 Bread + ½ Fat	95
Refrigerated Crescent Rolls	1 roll	1 Bread + 1 Fat	115
Applesauce Bread Mix (prepared)	⅒ loaf	1½ Bread + ½ Fat	130
Apricot-Nut Bread Mix (prepared)	⅒ loaf	1½ Bread + ½ Fat	130
Banana Bread Mix (prepared)	⅒ loaf	1½ Bread + ½ Fat	130
Blueberry-Nut Bread Mix (prepared)	⅒ loaf	1½ Bread + ½ Fat	130
Cherry-Nut Bread Mix (prepared)	⅒ loaf	1½ Bread + 1 Fat	150

Royal Regular Pudding Mixes
prepared with nonfat milk

Vanilla, Vanilla Tapioca, Banana, and Butterscotch	½ cup	½ Milk + 1½ Bread	120
Chocolate, Chocolate Tapioca, and Dark 'n Sweet	½ cup	1 Milk + 1½ Bread	160

Sara Lee

Cinnamon Rolls	1 roll	1 Bread + 1 Fat	105
Caramel Sticky Buns	1 roll	1 Bread + 1 Fat	118
Croissant Rolls	1 roll	1 Bread + 1 Fat	109
Parker House Rolls	1 roll	1 Bread + ½ Fat	73
Poppy Seed Rolls	1 roll	½ Bread + ½ Fat	55
Pound Cake	⅒ cake	1 Bread + 1 Fat	124
Golden Cake	⅛ cake	2 Bread + 1½ Fat	188
Chocolate Cake	⅛ cake	1½ Bread + 2 Fat	185
Strawberry French Cream Cheesecake	⅛ cake	2 Bread + 3 Fat	258
Chocolate Brownies	⅛ package	1½ Bread + 2 Fat	200

Stove Top

Packaged Stuffing Mix (prepared with butter)	½ cup	1½ Bread + 2 Fat	195

Swanson
Canned Products

Boned Chicken	2½ oz.	2 Meat	110
Boned Turkey	2½ oz.	2 Meat	110
Chicken Spread	1 oz.	1 Meat	70
Beef Broth	6¾ oz.	Free*	
Chunk White Chicken	2½ oz.	2 Meat	110
Chicken Broth	6¾ oz.	Free**	
Beef Stew	7½ oz.	1 Vegetable + 1 Bread + 1 Meat + 1 Fat	190
Chicken Stew	7½ oz.	1 Vegetable + 1 Bread + 1 Meat + 1 Fat	180
Chicken a la King	5¼ oz.	½ Bread + 2 Meat + 1 Fat	190
Chicken & Dumplings	7½ oz.	1 Bread + 2 Meat + 1 Fat	230
Chili Con Carne with Beans	7¾ oz.	2 Bread + 2 Meat + 1½ Fat	310

Frozen Products

Beef Meat Pie	8 oz.	3 Bread + 1 Meat + 4 Fat	430
Chicken Meat Pie	8 oz.	3 Bread + 1 Meat + 4 Fat	450
Turkey Meat Pie	8 oz.	3 Bread + 1 Meat + 4 Fat	450
Macaroni & Cheese	7 oz.	2 Bread + 1 Meat + 1 Fat	230

*Contains 20 calories per serving.
**Contains 25 calories per serving.

Hungry-Man Meat Pies

Beef	16 oz.	1 Vegetable + 4 Bread + 3 Meat + 7 Fat	770
Chicken	16 oz.	1 Vegetable + 4 Bread + 3 Meat + 7 Fat	780
Sirloin Burger	16 oz.	1 Vegetable + 4 Bread + 3 Meat + 7 Fat	800
Turkey	16 oz.	1 Vegetable + 4 Bread + 3 Meat + 7 Fat	790

Entrees

Chicken Nibbles w/French Fries	6 oz.	2 Bread + 2 Meat + 3 Fat	370
English Style (Fish 'n Chips)	5 oz.	1½ Bread + 2 Meat + 2 Fat	290
French Toast w/Sausages	4½ oz.	2 Bread + 2 Meat + 1 Fat	300
Fried Chicken w/Whipped Potatoes	7 oz.	2 Bread + 2 Meat + 2 Fat	360
Gravy & Sliced Beef w/Whipped Potatoes	8 oz.	1½ Bread + 1 Meat + 1 Fat	190
Meatballs w/Brown Gravy & Whipped Potatoes	9¼ oz.	2 Bread + 2 Meat + 2 Fat	330
Meatloaf w/Tomato Sauce & Whipped Potatoes	9 oz.	2 Bread + 2 Meat + 2 Fat	330
Pancakes and Sausages	6 oz.	3 Bread + 1 Meat + 5 Fat	500
Salisbury Steak w/Crinkle-Cut Potatoes	5½ oz.	2 Bread + 2 Meat + 3 Fat	370
Spaghetti w/Breaded Veal	8¼ oz.	2 Bread + 1 Meat + 2 Fat	290
Turkey/Gravy/Dressing w/Whipped Potatoes	8¾ oz.	2 Bread + 2 Meat	260

Swanson

Hungry-Man Entrees

Barbecue Flavored Fried Chicken w/Whipped Potatoes	12 oz.	3 Bread + 4 Meat + 3 Fat	550
Fried Chicken w/Whipped Potatoes	12 oz.	2 Bread + 5 Meat + 4 Fat	620
Lasagna and Garlic Roll	12¾ oz.	3 Bread + 2 Meat + 5 Fat	540
Salisbury Steak w/Crinkle-Cut Potatoes	12½ oz.	2½ Bread + 4 Meat + 5 Fat	640
Sliced Beef w/Whipped Potatoes	12¼ oz.	1½ Bread + 4 Meat	330
Turkey/Gravy/Dressing w/Whipped Potatoes	13¼ oz.	2 Bread + 4 Meat	380

Swift

Sizzlean	2 strips	1 Meat	101

Van Camp's

Canned Spanish Rice	1 cup	2 Bread + 1 Fat	185

Source: The information contained in the food exchange lists was adapted from research and work done by the following:

American Diabetes Association, Inc.

University of Iowa Medical Center, Iowa City, Iowa, *Recent Advances in Therapeutic Diets.*

Long Beach Veterans Administration Hospital.

Peter Bent Brigham Hospital.

Barbara M. Prater; Nancy J. Benton; and Kathleen Fisher, *Food and You.* Published by the authors, 1970, and research completed by Department of Food Science and Nutrition, Brigham Young University, Provo, Utah.

WARF Institute, Madison, Wisconsin, nutritional analysis of McDonald's foods. This information was converted to food exchanges by the American Diabetes Association, based on the values listed in the publication *Exchange Lists for Meal Planning* (1976). Persons wishing the nutrient values of McDonald's foods or additional copies of this list may write to McDonald's Corporation, Corporate Social Policy, Oak Brook, Illinois 60521.

Jill Paxman, Dietitian, Cottonwood Hospital, Salt Lake City, Utah, *Convenience Food Exchange List—A Guide To Enjoyable Eating.*

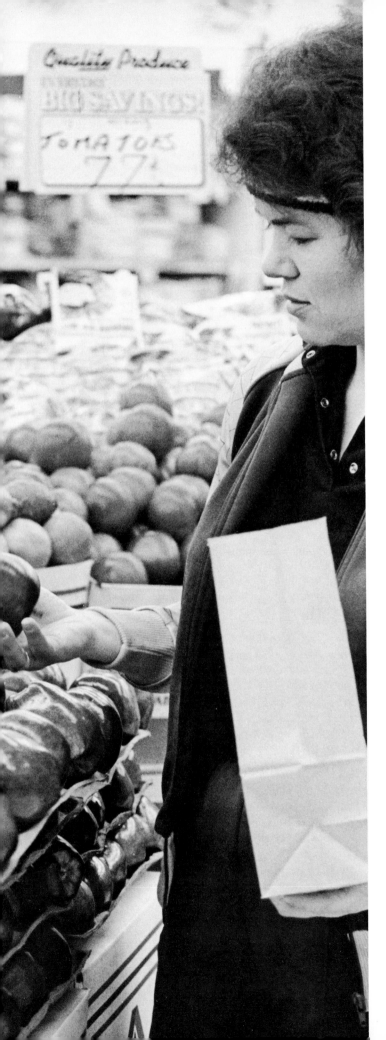

6

APPLYING A WEIGHT-CONTROL PROGRAM

Objective

After study of this chapter you should be able to

- use your own written weight-control program and contract to engage in an appropriate weight-control program.

For many years, two widely held misconceptions have discouraged the coupling of exercise with weight-control programs. It has been falsely asserted that (1) exercise requires little caloric expenditure and does not significantly affect caloric balance, and (2) an increase in physical activity is always followed by an increase in appetite that impairs the effectiveness of the diet. Scientific research has found that these statements are false.

Many Americans rely solely on some form of diet to control excessive fat. Most of these are fad diets that may be damaging to the dieter's health, and evidence is available to show that diets are successful with only a small percentage of persons. One study indicated that of every one hundred people who were concerned enough about weight control to see their doctor, only 7 percent actually attained their desired weight and only 2 percent were able to maintain it for a period of one year.

Jean Mayer, M.D., states:

Inactivity is the most important reason behind the problem of overweight in modern Western societies. The regulation of food intake was never designed for the highly mechanized, sedentary conditions of modern life. If a person is to live a sedentary life without getting fat, he will have to step up his activity or be hungry all his life.

Studies indicate that fat children often eat less and are much less active than children of normal weight. The same conclusions have been derived from controlled animal studies.[1]

Research shows that it is possible to bring about a significant fat loss with increased activity and, more important, the loss resulting from exercise is likely to be a lasting condition. Together with the loss in body fat, increased activity brings about an improvement in strength and endurance.

Remember that diet alone is a much slower method of reducing than a combination of diet and exercise. It should be emphasized that a daily program of activity is much better than a hit-or-miss, once-a-week program. Once a person starts a regular exercise plan, he or she must be as strict in following it as in following the diet.

The authors believe the concepts concerning diet and exercise can be summed up by a poem given to them by one of their students by the name of J. K. Liechty, who combined diet and exercise to overcome his problem.

Whose Fat is It?
(A parody of an Edgar A. Guest poem)

I am the person
Who has to decide
Whether to eat it,
Or push it aside,

Whether to walk for
An hour each day,
Or just be content
With how much I weigh.

I am the person,
The 'porker', the 'sow'
Who didn't like jogging,
But ate all the chow.

I tried 'Ipso-Fatso',
A new diet pill,
To dampen my hunger
Without needing will.

But after the loss,
And one dizzy spell,
I got my fat back.
(With interest, as well!)

I am responsible!
I gained this weight!
It wasn't my genes,
Or metabolic rate!

I have allowed it,
Through choices each day,
And I can't ignore it.
It won't go away,

Unless I address it,
And watch what I eat,
With regular exercise,
Walking my feet.

The method of diet,
The way to get thin,
Is not through another,
But comes from within.

Nobody else
Can change me, they've tried.
For I am the person
Who has to decide.

—J. K. Liechty

COMMONLY ASKED QUESTIONS

Can I gain weight and lose fat at the same time? Yes. It is possible to lose fat and gain muscle weight at the same time when you combine a diet and exercise program. The important consideration is to notice the loss of fat in the obvious body areas such as the waist, hips, and thighs.

What effect will exercise have on my appetite? Contrary to common belief, exercise is not automatically followed by an increase in the intake of food. This increase takes place only if the individual is normally fairly active and then increases his or her activity level even higher. If the person is sedentary, activity can normally be stepped up without any such increase in appetite.

I gained five pounds after I started the cardiovascular endurance program, but I look great and feel great. What happened? Should I try to lose five pounds? Not necessarily. Check your body weight ratio to determine if you need to lose weight. It may be that you have gained lean body tissue and lost fat. Even though you have gained five pounds, there may be a loss of body circumference as a result of the decrease in body fat. It should also be pointed out that muscle tissue is more dense and, therefore, weighs more than fat tissue.

What is wrong with going on a crash diet for a few days? The main thing wrong with this type of diet is that it simply doesn't work. The number of calories allowed is usually so low that the dieter is miserable and consequently finds it difficult to stay on the diet. A large part of the weight loss on a crash diet is protein from lean muscle tissue and water. This weight is replaced rapidly when eating is resumed.

What about diets that eliminate or greatly reduce carbohydrates? There are currently several widely publicized diets that eliminate or severely restrict carbohydrate-rich foods while allowing unlimited amounts of foods containing protein and fat. The body needs a combination of protein, fat, and carbohydrates to function properly. An imbalance of any of these nutrients may be dangerous.

Do carbohydrates have more calories than protein? No. Equal amounts of carbohydrates and protein have the same energy, or caloric value. Fats have almost two-and-one-half times the calories of carbohydrates or protein. Eating an extra piece of meat instead of a potato won't help you lose weight if you are not cutting down on calories by reducing the amount of food you eat.

1. Jean Mayer, *Overweight: Causes, Cost, and Control* (Englewood Cliffs, NJ: Prentice-Hall, 1968), p. 83.

How does the preparation of foods affect their caloric values? Ordinary preparation (cooking, freezing, cutting, blending) does not appreciably change the amount of calories in a food. To dispel a myth, toasted bread does not have fewer calories than untoasted bread. Frying foods does increase the number of calories to the extent that fat is added. On the other hand, if you drain some fat from browned hamburger, you can reduce the calories.

Do some foods or combinations of foods have special chemical properties? No. This is another myth that was circulating a few years ago as a reducing diet. The grapefruit-and-egg diet was supposed to have a special chemical combination that "burned" your fat off. Unless you get so tired of the one or two foods allowed on these diets that you decrease your caloric intake, you won't lose weight. More important, these diets may actually be dangerous.

What is cholesterol and how is it related to heart disease? Cholesterol is a special type of fat found primarily in fats from animal sources. It is not an abnormal compound; the body synthesizes much of its own cholesterol and uses it in making sex hormones, bile, and other compounds that are necessary for normal body function. The amount of cholesterol in the blood is affected by many factors including diet, exercise, and heredity. High levels of blood cholesterol have been associated with atherosclerosis in some patients. Persons who have high blood cholesterol may be instructed by their doctors to decrease the cholesterol in their diet. For persons with normal blood cholesterol and fat levels, however, a moderate intake of cholesterol and animal fat is not considered harmful.

What is the difference and effect of high-density lipo-proteins (HDL) and low-density lipoproteins (LDL)? Some of the cholesterol in the body is packaged in small fatty-cholesterol particles that have a high density and are labeled high-density lipoproteins. Other types have a less dense particle and are known as low-density lipoproteins. In problems with the circulatory system, the LDL particles are the offenders, as they appear to stick in the walls of the arteries and start the atherosclerotic process. The HDL particles seem to be of help in preventing cholesterol from depositing in the arteries, thus retarding the process of atherosclerosis. There is some research stating that a combination of diet and exercise can reduce the LDL level and increase the amount of HDL, and this would aid in the prevention of circulatory problems.

What is "cellulite" and how do I get rid of it? Certain proponents maintain that **cellulite** is a particular type of fatty deposit that is lumpy and bumpy and causes the overlying skin to have a puckered appearance similar to an orange peel. All creditable nutritionists and medical authorities maintain, however, that there is no such a thing as cellulite, and the lumpy bulges are ordinary fat and thus will respond to a diet and exercise program that affects caloric intake.

What does vitamin E do? There has been considerable controversy about the function and the therapeutic benefits of this vitamin. However, very little of the scientific evidence has been conclusive. Much more research needs to be done to determine the functions of vitamin E. (It is known that vitamin E helps prevent chemical changes in some types of body fat.) A healthy person eating a nutritionally balanced diet should not need a vitamin E supplement.

How do we get vitamin D from the sun? Vitamin D is not a chemical that the sun sends down for us to "soak up" out of the air. Rather, the sun acts on the chemical substance, 7-dehydrocholesterol, which is present in the skin, and changes it to vitamin D. Vitamin D is also added to dairy products.

Is it possible to get too much of a nutrient? Yes! Large amounts of vitamins A and D may be toxic, as are excess amounts of many minerals, such as iron. High amounts of other nutrients, though not toxic, may result in "conditioned deficiencies." In other words, the body may adapt to increased amounts of the nutrient and experience deficiency symptoms when only normal amounts are consumed. Once again, a balanced and varied diet will supply the proper amounts of nutrients without supplements.

Are whole grains superior to refined? Yes. Several nutrients are known to be removed during the refining of grains, particularly some of the B vitamins and trace amounts of minerals. The enrichment of refined grains adds back some of these nutrients (thiamin, riboflavin, niacin, and iron), but not all. It is advisable to consume some whole-grain products, particularly if grain products are a major element of your diet. When purchasing refined grains, make sure they are labeled *enriched*.

What happens if I diet but don't exercise? Part of your weight loss will be lean body mass. On a diet program, approximately 75 percent of the weight loss is fat while the rest is lean body mass and extracellular fluid.

What is the difference between being obese and being overweight? A person is considered overweight when he or she does not meet standards of weight as determined by age, height, and weight (these, by the way, are poor indicators). Obesity refers to the percentage of fat in the body. In men, 20 percent body fat or more is considered obese; in women, over 28 percent body fat is so considered.

Why should I not attempt to lose weight by exercising with a plastic sweat suit or figure-wrapping device? The problem here is in adverse effects on the body's heat-regulating mechanisms. The excessive sweating is a false loss of weight since it represents a loss of body fluids, not fat.

Figure wrapping does not cause a loss of inches from loss of body fat but a change in inches due to the shifting of body fluids resulting from the pressure of the wraps. In time, the fluids will stabilize and the measurements will return to their original diameters.

What happens when I crash diet? The body is without many essential proteins, vitamins, and minerals that are often unavailable in a "crash diet," and much of the weight loss is not fat but lean body tissue.

What about grapefruit diets? Do they really burn the fat off? No. The body fat is lost because the body has to turn to its reserve of fat for fuel to provide energy that is not available in the grapefruit. In a grapefruit diet, a person also runs the risk of upsetting the metabolism of the body because of a shortage of essential nutrients.

I want to lose weight on my thighs only. Is this possible? So-called **spot-reducing** is not possible. A person will lose body fat throughout the entire body, though it should be noted that a greater percentage of fat loss will be from those areas where the greater amount of fat is deposited. If a person has a great deal of fat deposited in the area of the thighs, then a proportional amount will be lost in this area.

Why can't I go on a one-meal-a-day diet or a starvation diet? This type of diet upsets the body's metabolism. Eating all your calories in one meal may act as a stimulus to cause the body to store more of the calories as fat, and thus you defeat your purpose. A one-meal-a-day schedule will also cause a great deal of hunger, which is one of the chief reasons for breaking a diet.

In a starvation diet, an individual deprives the body of essential nutrients such as vitamins, minerals, and some proteins that cannot be stored by the body. In addition, only about 50 percent of the weight loss on a starvation diet is fat; the rest is lean body tissue.

Why do people get too heavy? Inactivity causes the greatest number of people to be overweight because their physical activity has decreased much more rapidly than their food intake.

PUTTING A WEIGHT-CONTROL PROGRAM TO USE

Through the use of the Weight-Control Program Contract in figure 6.1, preparing your own program is a fairly easy six-step process.

Step 1. Prepare your own Weight-Control Program Work Sheet.
Step 2. Fill out your Weight-Control Program Contract.
Step 3. Get your contract approved.
Step 4. Implement the program and record your progress in the Weight-Control Program Progress Log in figure 6.2.
Step 5. Check your progress.
Step 6. Complete your contract.

To help you become familiar with these procedures, we will go through them step-by-step.

Weight-Control Program Contract

1. Name _____ Age _____ Sex _____

2. Present weight _____ Pounds to be lost _____ Target weight _____ Fitness category _____

3. Desired exercise(s) _____

4. Exercise heart rate training zone: _____ to _____

Week	Exercise	Duration	Weekly Exercise Periods	Weight to Be Lost (lbs.)	Desired Caloric Intake
1				2	
2				2	
3				2	
4				2	
5				2	
6				2	
7				2	
8				2	
9				2	

Signature: _____

Contract approval date: _____ Approved by: _____

Reassessment date: _____ Approved by: _____

Contract completion date: _____ Approved by: _____

Figure 6.1.

Weight-Control Program Progress Log

Name _____ Age _____ Sex _____

Current weight _____ Pounds to be lost _____ Target weight _____ Fitness category _____

Exercise(s) _____ Exercise heart rate
training zone: _____ to _____

Week	Day and Date	Exercise	Duration		Caloric Intake	Weight
			Time	Distance		

Figure 6.2.

Step 1: Preparing your own Weight-Control Program Work Sheet

You should have learned how to complete a personal Weight-Control Work Sheet while you were studying chapter 5. If you have not written a work sheet for yourself, write one now before going on with this unit.

Step 2: Filling out your Weight-Control Program Contract

The work copy of the Weight-Control Program Contract in figure 6.1 will help you implement your weight program. This contract is quite easy to fill out from your Weight-Control Work Sheet. With your work sheet in front of you, fill out your contract as follows:

Item 1. Write your name, age, and sex.

Item 2. Write your present weight and target weight. Take this information from item 2 of your Weight-Control Work Sheet. Record the number of pounds to lose by subtracting the target weight from your present weight. Also record your fitness category from item 4 of this work sheet.

Item 3. Write in your desired exercise. In the *Week* column are listed the numbers 1 through 9, representing nine weeks of a weight-control program. In the *Exercise* column, write the exercise you prefer. In the *Duration* column, write the number of minutes you plan to exercise during each exercise period. Take this information from item 8 of your Weight-Control Work Sheet. In the *Weekly Exercise Periods* column, write in the number of exercise periods you will engage in weekly. Take this information from item 9 of your Weight-Control Work Sheet. In the *Weight to Be Lost* column, you will notice that the number of pounds you will lose during each week has already been filled in. In the *Desired Caloric Intake* column, write the caloric intake you need to lose the specified weight and still sustain you in your exercise program. This information can be found from item 15 of your Weight-Control Work Sheet.

Item 4. Write in your exercise heart rate training zone. Take this information from item 2 of your Weight-Control Work Sheet.

Step 3: Getting your contract approved

When you have filled in every week of your program, you need to have it approved. If you are a student in a physical education class, it can be signed by your instructor. If you are not enrolled in some organized class, have it signed by a friend.

The reason for having your contract approved is to solidify your commitment to a life-style that will improve your personal fitness. It has been found that people are more likely to fulfill personal decisions if they involve another person.

Step 4: Implementing your program and recording your progress in the Weight-Control Program Progress Log

Begin your activity as soon as your contract has been approved. After each exercise period you should fill in your Weight-Control Program Progress Log. This log is found in figure 6.2. After every exercise period, write in the log the number of the week of your program (1–9), the day of the week and the date, the exercise you engaged in, and the duration of the exercise. In addition, you must record at the end of each day the number of calories you have consumed and your weight.

Your diet-exercise program requires you to select proper amounts of the foods listed in the food-selection guide in chapter 5. You do not need to count calories if you eat the specified amounts.

An easy way to keep track of the foods you eat on your food plan every day is to carry a card that states your desired daily caloric food plan for that day and spaces to check off each food when you eat it. Food-plan cards are illustrated in figure 6.3 for each daily caloric level from 1,200 to 2,500 calories. Simply get plain three-by-five-inch cards and make a set for your own daily caloric level (such as 1,200 calories or 1,500 calories, etc.). Carry a card in your pocket, purse, or other convenient place so that you can refer to it and check off the foods you eat daily. If at the end of the day you have eaten only those foods stipulated on your card, record the number of calories appearing at the top of your card under the appropriate date on your Weight-Control Program Progress Log. If you have eaten more or less than your daily food plan recommendation, determine how many additional or fewer calories you have eaten. Add or subtract this amount from the desired number of calories on your daily food plan, and record this on your Weight-Control Program Progress Log. You can figure the extra calories by checking the calorie count on the appropriate food exchange lists on the food-selection guide in chapter 5.

Daily Caloric Food Plan Guides

Daily Food Plan			1,200 Calories
Vegs.	(2)	1 2	
Breads	(5)	1 2 3 4 5	
Meats	(4)	1 2 3 4	
Milk	(2)	1 2	
Fruits	(4)	1 2 3 4	
Fats	(2)	1 2	

As you use each food exchange, cross off a number to remind yourself not to overeat.

Daily Food Plan			1,300 Calories
Vegs.	(2)	1 2	
Breads	(5)	1 2 3 4 5	
Meats	(5)	1 2 3 4 5	
Milk	(2)	1 2	
Fruits	(5)	1 2 3 4 5	
Fats	(2)	1 2	

As you use each food exchange, cross off a number to remind yourself not to overeat.

Daily Food Plan			1,400 Calories
Vegs.	(3)	1 2 3	
Breads	(6)	1 2 3 4 5 6	
Meats	(3)	1 2 3	
Milk	(3)	1 2 3	
Fruits	(4)	1 2 3 4	
Fats	(2)	1 2	

As you use each food exchange, cross off a number to remind yourself not to overeat.

Daily Food Plan			1,500 Calories
Vegs.	(3)	1 2 3	
Breads	(6)	1 2 3 4 5 6	
Meats	(5)	1 2 3 4 5	
Milk	(3)	1 2 3	
Fruits	(4)	1 2 3 4	
Fats	(2)	1 2	

As you use each food exchange, cross off a number to remind yourself not to overeat.

Daily Food Plan			1,600 Calories
Vegs.	(5)	1 2 3 4 5	
Breads	(7)	1 2 3 4 5 6 7	
Meats	(4)	1 2 3 4	
Milk	(3)	1 2 3	
Fruits	(4)	1 2 3 4	
Fats	(2)	1 2	

As you use each food exchange, cross off a number to remind yourself not to overeat.

Daily Food Plan			1,700 Calories
Vegs.	(4)	1 2 3 4	
Breads	(8)	1 2 3 4 5 6 7 8	
Meats	(5)	1 2 3 4 5	
Milk	(3)	1 2 3	
Fruits	(4)	1 2 3 4	
Fats	(2)	1 2	

As you use each food exchange, cross off a number to remind yourself not to overeat.

Figure 6.3.

```
Daily Food Plan                1,800 Calories

Vegs.      (6)      1 2 3 4 5 6

Breads     (8)      1 2 3 4 5 6 7 8

Meats      (5)      1 2 3 4 5

Milk       (3)      1 2 3

Fruits     (4)      1 2 3 4

Fats       (3)      1 2 3

As you use each food exchange, cross off a
number to remind yourself not to overeat.
```

```
Daily Food Plan                1,900 Calories

Vegs.      (6)      1 2 3 4 5 6

Breads     (8)      1 2 3 4 5 6 7 8

Meats      (4)      1 2 3 4

Milk       (4)      1 2 3 4

Fruits     (5)      1 2 3 4 5

Fats       (2)      1 2

As you use each food exchange, cross off a
number to remind yourself not to overeat.
```

```
Daily Food Plan                2,000 Calories

Vegs.      (7)      1 2 3 4 5 6 7

Breads     (8)      1 2 3 4 5 6 7 8

Meats      (6)      1 2 3 4 5 6

Milk       (3½)    1 2 3½

Fruits     (6)      1 2 3 4 5 6

Fats       (2)      1 2

As you use each food exchange, cross off a
number to remind yourself not to overeat.
```

```
Daily Food Plan                2,100 Calories

Vegs.      (8)      1 2 3 4 5 6 7 8

Breads     (8)      1 2 3 4 5 6 7 8

Meats      (6)      1 2 3 4 5 6

Milk       (4)      1 2 3 4

Fruits     (6)      1 2 3 4 5 6

Fats       (2)      1 2

As you use each food exchange, cross off a
number to remind yourself not to overeat.
```

```
Daily Food Plan                2,200 Calories

Vegs.      (8)      1 2 3 4 5 6 7 8

Breads     (8)      1 2 3 4 5 6 7 8

Meats      (6)      1 2 3 4 5 6

Milk       (4)      1 2 3 4

Fruits     (7)      1 2 3 4 5 6 7

Fats       (3)      1 2 3

As you use each food exchange, cross off a
number to remind yourself not to overeat.
```

```
Daily Food Plan                2,300 Calories

Vegs.      (9)      1 2 3 4 5 6 7 8 9

Breads     (9)      1 2 3 4 5 6 7 8 9

Meats      (6)      1 2 3 4 5 6

Milk       (4)      1 2 3 4

Fruits     (7)      1 2 3 4 5 6 7

Fats       (3)      1 2 3

As you use each food exchange, cross off a
number to remind yourself not to overeat.
```

Figure 6.3—*Continued.*

```
Daily Food Plan              2,400 Calories

Vegs.      (9)    1 2 3 4 5 6 7 8 9

Breads    (10)    1 2 3 4 5 6 7 8 9 10

Meats     (6)     1 2 3 4 5 6

Milk      (4)     1 2 3 4

Fruits    (8)     1 2 3 4 5 6 7 8

Fats      (3)     1 2 3

As you use each food exchange, cross off a
number to remind yourself not to overeat.
```

```
Daily Food Plan              2,500 Calories

Vegs.      (9)    1 2 3 4 5 6 7 8 9

Breads    (10)    1 2 3 4 5 6 7 8 9 10

Meats     (6)     1 2 3 4 5 6

Milk      (4½)   1 2 3 4½

Fruits    (8)     1 2 3 4 5 6 7 8

Fats      (3)     1 2 3

As you use each food exchange, cross off a
number to remind yourself not to overeat.
```

Figure 6.3—*Continued.*

Before moving on to the next week of your program, be sure you have (a) fulfilled the specified calorie-intake diet for seven consecutive days; (b) completed your weekly schedule of exercises; and (c) recorded your diet-exercise activities on the Weight-Control Program Progress Log. Maintain daily records in order to keep on your program.

To check your progress, weigh yourself daily on the same scales at about the same time of day and wear no clothing. The reducing diet is calculated to cause a weight reduction of 2 pounds per week, but this should be considered an average over one or two months' time. Individual metabolism and activity can cause the rate of weight loss to vary widely from one person to another. Often a rapid weight loss will occur in the first week, followed by from one to three weeks of no weight change at all. The body may temporarily retain water even though it is losing fatty tissue. Do not be too discouraged when you experience these "plateau" periods—weight loss will resume and you should be able to lose an overall average of 2 pounds per week.

GUIDELINES FOR FOLLOWING A DIET

Here are some guidelines to help you stay on your diet.

1. Beware of accepting invitations to dinner at which you might be tempted to go off your diet or to snack. It will take time to adjust to your new eating patterns. When you learn the basic food plan for your diet, you can accept invitations with the understanding that you might not be able to eat everything served.
2. Avoid boring or fatiguing situations that cause you to think of food or to nibble between meals.
3. Learn what tempts you to snack, and avoid the temptation.
4. Eat only the foods listed on your daily food plan.
5. Don't read or watch TV while eating. This leads to thoughtless overeating.
6. When shopping, be sure to (a) use a list; (b) shop only for what is on the list; (c) take only enough money for what is on the list; (d) avoid putting high-calorie foods on the list; and (e) never shop when you are hungry!
7. When eating, try the following: (a) chew the food in your mouth and swallow it before you take the next bite; (b) learn to savor the food you eat; and (c) measure your servings with measuring cups, spoons, and a small food scale. The eye is not a very good judge of serving size.
8. Cook vegetables in as little water as possible for as short a time as possible. They will look better, taste better, and be more nutritious.
9. Always eat three regular meals a day. If you try to cram all your daily calories into one or two meals, your body will not be able to handle all the nutrients at once and some calories will be stored as fat. In addition, waiting too long between meals affects blood-sugar level and causes undue fatigue and irritability. Be good to yourself. Eat good meals and acceptable snacks in between meals.
10. Never eat less than 1,200 calories a day if you are a woman and 1,500 calories if you are a man, unless you are under the care of a medical doctor. Even if your weight-control program calls for less, consume

1,200 or 1,500 calories a day until you have lost the desired amount of weight.

11. Plot your progress as you lose weight.

Step 5: Progress check

After a few weeks, make an appointment with the person who approved your contract. This progress check will help to reaffirm your decision to improve your body weight.

Step 6: Measuring percent body fat

When you reach your target weight, it is possible to make a final check to determine what percentage of your body is fat. The measurement procedures are explained in chapter 2. By using this information you will be able to obtain a good indication of what your body weight should be.

Step 7: Contract completion

When you reach your desired weight, have your contract approved by the person who originally signed it. Now you may increase your caloric intake. This can be accomplished by multiplying your target weight times 15 calories. Remember, however, that this may have to be adjusted to individual energy needs and expenditure. Keep weighing yourself at least once a week to make sure you are maintaining your desired weight. Exercise will help keep extra weight and body fat from creeping up on you. Daily exercise should be a part of your life-style!

SUGGESTIONS FOR FURTHER READING

1. Bjorntory, P., K. de Jounge, M. Krotkiewski, L. Sullivan, L. Sjostrom, and J. Stenberg. "Physical Training in Human Obesity: Effects of Long-Term Physical Training on Body Composition" *Metabolism* 22 (1973):1467.
2. Burton, Benjamin. "Food Facts and Fallacies: Nutritional Misinformation." *Health* 21 (1976):20.
3. DeLacerda, Fred. "The Pre-Game Meal." *The Athletic Journal* 56 (1976):66.
4. DeMoss, V. "Struggle Against Starvation." *Runner's World* 16 September (1981):no. 9, p. 60.
5. Galton, L. "The Truth about High-Fiber Diets." *Runner's World* 17 June (1982):no. 6, p. 31.
6. Girandola, Robert N. "Body Composition Changes in Women: Effects of High and Low Exercise Intensity." *Archives of Physical Medicine and Rehabilitation* 57 (1976):297.
7. Grollman, Arthur. "How Drugs Work: Vitamins." *Consultant,* March 1975.
8. Kendrick, M. M., M. F. Ball, and J. J. Canary. "Exercise and Weight Reduction and Obesity." *Archives of Physical Medicine and Rehabilitation* 53 (1972):323.
9. Kesselman, Judi. "Obesity: A Family Disease." *Weight Watchers,* May 1975.
10. Larson, R., and C. Johnson. "Anorexia Nervosa in the Context of Daily Experience." *Journal of Youth and Adolescence* 10 December (1981):455.
11. Lohmann, J. "Fight Against Fat." *School and Community* 67 May (1981):30.
12. Londeree, Ben. "Pre-Event Diet Routine." *Runner's World* 9 (1974):26.
13. McCunney, R. J. "Fitness, Heart Disease, and High-Density Lipoproteins." *The Physician and Sports Medicine* 15 February (1987):67.
14. Miller, A. J. "Sensible Snacking: A Guide to a Healthful Daily Eating Plan." *Forecast Home Economics* 26 May–June (1981):58.
15. Nelson, R. A. "Nutrition and Physical Performance: A Review." *The Physician and Sports Medicine* 10 April (1982):no. 4, p. 54.
16. Nelson, R. A. "What Should Athletes Eat? Unmixing Folly and Facts." *The Physician and Sports Medicine* 3 (1975):67.
17. Ryan, Allan J. "Charting the Factors of Fatness." *The Physician and Sports Medicine* 3 (1975):57.
18. Sherman, W. M. "Carbohydrate, Muscle Glycogen, and Improved Performance." *The Physician and Sports Medicine* 15 February (1987):157.
19. Smith, E. L. "Exercise for Prevention of Osteoporosis." *The Physician and Sports Medicine* 10 March (1982): no. 3, p. 72.
20. Smith, T. K. "Nutrition, Energy, and the Athlete." *Athletic Journal* 63 October (1982):38.
21. Stephan, Jerry. "Questions and Answers About Weight Control in Wrestling." *Scholastic Coach* 46 (1976):78; 46 (1976):38.
22. Thompson, J. K., and P. Blanton. "Energy Conservation and Exercise Dependence: A Sympathetic Arousal Hypothesis." *Medicine and Science in Sports and Exercise* 19 April (1987):p. 91.
23. Wallace, Janet P. "Responses of the Composition of Body Fat to Cardiovascular Training in College Women." *The Research Quarterly* 46 (1975):317.
24. Wesley, M. M., and S. G. Ruddy. "Fad Diets: Facts vs. Fallacies." *Forecast Home Economics* 27 November (1981):33.
25. Whigham, M. "Diet Pill Phenomenon." *Forecast Home Economics* 27 November (1981):46.
26. Williams, Melvin H. *Nutrition for Fitness and Sport.* Dubuque, Iowa: Wm. C. Brown Company Publishers, 1983.
27. Williams, P. T., R. D. Wood, and W. L. Haskell. "The Effects of Running Mileage and Duration on Plasma Lipoprotein Levels." *Journal of American Medical Association* 247 May (1982):2674.
28. Winick, Myron. "Childhood Obesity." *Nutrition Today* 9 (1974):6.

7

WRITING A STRENGTH PROGRAM

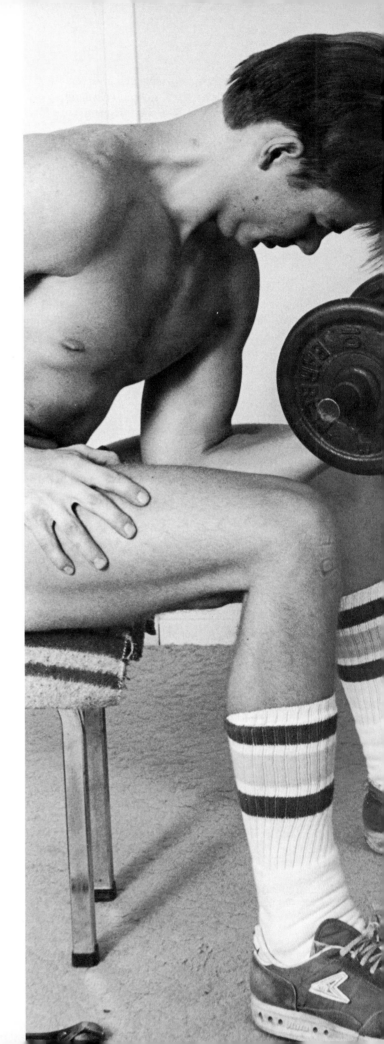

Objectives

After study of this chapter you should be able to

1. write a strength program, tailor-made to your choice of exercises;
2. pass a multiple-choice mastery self-check involving the selection of appropriate strength programs for persons desiring various choices of exercises.

Strength is defined as the ability to exert force against resistance. Strength is important in overall body performance, not only for athletes, but also for people engaging in ordinary daily activities like walking, lifting, sitting, and running. It is an important factor in child-bearing, doing housework, and engaging in recreational activities. The overall efficiency of the body depends upon the condition of the large muscles of your legs, arms, and trunk, especially abdominal and back muscles. In fact, if you wish to pursue the "good life," adequate strength levels are imperative. If all else remains equal, an increase in strength will contribute to an improvement in the performance of the human body.

Following a program of progressive resistance is the most effective method for achieving strength gains. Hit-and-miss programs are doomed to failure. Although it may take several weeks before observable changes in strength and general appearance are apparent in some people, those individuals who are muscularly weak may show dramatic strength gains in a short period of time.

Sometimes when strength programs are discussed, women express concern that strength exercises will make them less feminine. Some young girls are afraid that training will produce unsightly bulging muscles.

Research indicates that this is false. Inherent endocrinological factors, such as the secretion of the hormones testosterone and estrogen, and morphological characteristics, not physical activity, determine femininity and masculinity.

Before puberty, there is little difference between the muscular size and strength of boys and girls. With the onset of puberty, however, testosterone from the boys' testes and estrogen from the girls' ovaries enter the bloodstream and trigger the development of the appropriate secondary sexual characteristics.

The majority of women could not develop large muscles under any circumstances; however, strength training will develop and bring about sufficient changes in a woman's muscles so that she is better prepared to perform her daily activities. The end result will be better muscle tone, a replacement of fatty tissue with firm muscles, and improved fitness.

Another misconception concerning strength training is that it will make you inflexible or **"muscle-bound."** There is no evidence that participating in strength training reduces range of movement or agility, or that it causes loss of coordination or timing. In fact, proper strength programs may contribute to these components of fitness.

MUSCLE MASS AND BODY FAT

The relation between the amount of **muscle mass** in the body and body fat is often overlooked. The amount and size of muscle tissue decreases in many older persons because of the lack of proper exercise, sometimes called the rocking-chair syndrome. As the muscle mass decreases, a person uses less energy and a larger percentage of the body weight becomes fat. Fat tissue does not burn nearly as many calories as muscle tissue does when the body is at rest, and many people become too fat. In other words, many people become fat because they are using fewer calories as a result of the loss of muscle mass caused by a lack of activity. Since people spend more time sitting than they do in activity (the average American spends more than four hours a day watching television), this is obviously an important factor in weight control.

Ancel Keys, a researcher in weight control, showed that the decrease in calories in different age groups at rest was related to the change in muscle mass rather than to age. For example, at age sixty a person will use approximately 15 calories less per hour than a person who is twenty-six years of age; over a twenty-four-hour period this would be a total of 360 unused calories per day. The sixty-year-old individual, therefore, must increase activity, decrease caloric intake, or put on more fat.

If that person desires to continue to have the same eating habits but not put on fat, it will be necessary to walk approximately 6 miles each day to expend the 360 calories, since the energy used in walking one mile is about 60 calories.

You can help eliminate the problem of overfatness by using a strength development program to maintain your muscle mass so that you won't have to increase your exercise so extensively to combat fat. Your body will continue to use more calories if you maintain your muscle mass.

COMMON TERMS FOR STRENGTH PROGRAMS

In order to write a strength program, there are some terms that you must become familiar with.

barbell A six-foot-long iron bar with iron plates attached.

dumbbell A hand weight.

guestimate A guess at the resistance to be used in a strength exercise.

isokinetic resistance An attempt to produce a maximal resistance to all joint angles through a full range of motion. Requires a special machine to provide the resistance and control the speed of movement.

isometric contraction A muscle contraction with little or no movement.

isotonic contraction A muscle contraction with movement.

maximum resistance Maximum weight lifted in one repetition of the exercise.

minimum resistance to gain strength Approximately 60 percent of the maximum resistance that a muscle group can exert.

muscular endurance The ability to perform repeated muscle movements for a given period of time.

muscular strength The ability to exert force against resistance.

progressive resistance Increasing the number of repetitions in timed calisthenics; the resistance in weight training.

range of motion The distance through which a limb can travel at a given joint.

recovery period The rest interval time between sets.

repetitions In timed calisthenics, the number of times each exercise is repeated; in weight training, the number of complete muscle contractions.

resistance In timed calisthenics, the weight of the body; in weight training, the weight moved by a muscle contraction.

set A given number of repetitions.

time The length of the period within which repetitions can be done; equivalent to one set.

variable resistance An attempt to produce a maximal resistance to all joint angles through a full range of motion. Speed of movement is not controlled but a special machine is required to provide the resistance.

OVERLOAD PRINCIPLE

In any physical fitness program, the **overload principle** is the basic concept that is necessary to improve the condition of the body. All that it entails is subjecting the selected systems of the body to loads greater than those to which they are accustomed; this overload causes the body to adjust and increase its capacity to perform physical work.

It should be emphasized that specific body systems require **specific overloads,** and thus an overload for the cardiovascular system is different from that necessary to bring about strength gains. We controlled the overload for cardiovascular endurance by using the variables of duration, intensity, and frequency, and monitoring heart rate and caloric expenditure for various activities. We will use duration, intensity, and frequency for a strength program also, but they will be different types from those used in an endurance program.

The enlargement of a muscle in training is the result of an increase in the cross-sectional area of the individual muscle cells rather than an increase in the number of muscle cells. In an untrained muscle, the individual diameters of the cells vary considerably. The objective of strength development is to bring the smaller muscle cells up to the size of the larger ones. The increase in muscle cell size is termed **hypertrophy;** a decrease is referred to as **atrophy.**

A systematic overloading of a muscle increases the strength of the muscle. In most cases the degree of improvement in strength is related to the amount of overload. Once a muscle has adapted to the higher resistance, an additional increase in resistance is necessary to produce further gains. This is why strength programs are sometimes referred to as *progressive resistance programs.*

There are four possible methods that you can use to increase the difficulty of a strength workout.

1. Increase the resistance.
2. Increase the repetitions.
3. Increase the number of sets.
4. Decrease the recovery period or rest intervals between sets.

The greatest strength gains seem to be obtained when the resistance is increased and the other variables are held constant.

STRENGTH PROGRAMS

The physiological causes of increased strength are not presently known. Increased strength may be a combination of changes in the muscular, skeletal, and nervous systems.

There are many types of training programs that can be utilized to develop strength. Isotonic training is the most common type used to increase strength. Some advantages of this program are that it allows you to develop strength through a full range of motion, and it may also have a training effect on the nervous system.

Because isotonic training allows you to observe the gains made in strength and muscle development, it can be very satisfying psychologically. This type of program causes a greater muscle hypertrophy in males and a firming and toning effect in females. This is a very significant plus, because the cosmetic effects of a strength program are quite important to many people.

Some advantages ascribed to an isometric training program are that it requires less equipment and usually causes little muscle soreness. Two major disadvantages are that strength is not developed throughout the full range of motion of the muscle lever system. In addition, isometric contractions produce high systolic and diastolic blood pressures that might be dangerous to the heart and circulatory system.

SYSTEMS OF TRAINING

Set System

The set system is the most popular type of training to develop strength. In this system, the person does an exercise for a given number of repetitions (a set), then rests, and then performs another set. A variation of this system is referred to as **supersets,** in which an exercise set for a particular muscle group is followed immediately by an exercise set for the antagonist muscle. An example of this training system would be to do a set of arm curls for the biceps and then do a set of triceps extensions for the triceps. This combination would be one superset.

Another variation of this type of training is known as the **super multiple set system.** In this training system, the lifter completes all of the sets for a given muscle group and then follows this exercise with the same number of sets for the opposite muscle group.

Split Routine

The **split routine** method exercises every major muscle group in the body and requires a great amount of time and work. To obtain the maximum development, the major body parts are split into groups, and the lifter works out six days a week but exercises the selected body parts on alternate days. For example, the arms, legs, and midsection might be exercised on Monday, Wednesday, and Friday, and the chest, shoulders, and back would be exercised on Tuesday, Thursday, and Saturday. This system is one of the most popular types of training used by bodybuilders.

A variation of the split routine system is known as the **blitz method.** This is often utilized when the bodybuilder is preparing for a contest and wishes to obtain the maximum size and muscle definition so important in competition. In this system, a person would perform all the arm exercises one day, the next day engage in just chest exercises, the legs on the next day, and follow each day with another body part. This is a very strenuous and tiring method of training and is usually recommended only for a few weeks at a time.

Burns

Some individuals include sets of rapid half contractions, or **burns,** in their workout. The reason is to produce a burning sensation in the muscle, which is thought to be due to the forcing of blood into the muscle area to produce the so-called **muscle pump.** The lifter is trying to achieve a greater increase in the size of the musculature.

Forced Reps

The **forced-reps** method of training requires the use of a partner who assists the lifter so that more repetitions with greater resistance can be accomplished. The partner can push the individual far beyond the normal point of fatigue, the result being more strength and muscle-building stimulation. For example, an individual might do ten repetitions on the lat pulldown without assistance. When the person reaches the normal point of fatigue on the tenth repetition, the partner would assist the lifter through the sticking point for three to five more forced reps.

Preexhaustion

Most exercises in strength training are accomplished by a large muscle group working in conjunction with a smaller muscle group. For example, the back muscles work with the biceps of the arms in pull-ups. The small muscle may fatigue before the large muscle group, and as a result, the large muscle group does not receive the optimum resistance to bring about physiological changes, such as an increase in size.

The **preexhaustion** system is based on the idea of doing a preliminary isolation exercise to overload the large muscle group before doing the exercise that uses both the large and small muscle groups together. This technique theoretically fatigues the larger group to make it weaker than the smaller muscle group and, thus, the lifter can push the basic combination exercise to a point where both muscle groups develop.

Pyramid System

The pyramid system consists of adding weight until the lifter can only complete one repetition. For example, a person may start doing the bench press with a set of ten maximum repetitions, then add enough weight to do nine maximum repetitions, then eight maximum repetitions, and so on until the final set would consist of one maximum repetition.

In the first type of pyramid, the lifter went from light to heavy resistance. There is another pyramid system where one goes from heavy to light resistance. After a warm-up set, the lifter does a set of one to two maximum repetitions, removes (for example) five pounds, then does the maximum number of repetitions, and continues to do this until only the weight of the bar or a small resistance remains.

MACHINES VERSUS FREE WEIGHTS

In the past few years, as interest in the development of strength has increased, there has appeared on the market a dazzling array of exercise machines. Each advertisement, in very convincing language, explains why this specific machine is best and why all other machines and training methods will soon be obsolete. Many times the advertisement contains testimonies from prominent athletes or coaches.

With the development of these machines have come two new terms in strength training, isokinetic and variable resistance. They are based on the fact that as a muscle goes through a range of motion, the ability of the lever system to exert force changes at different angles. Thus, the amount of weight that can be lifted is limited by the weakest point in the range of motion. Therefore, many manufacturers of equipment have developed machines that theoretically have the ability to adjust the resistance of the machine to the muscle's ability to exert force. The claim is that these machines will bring about a faster and greater increase of strength through the full range of motion.

The other type of training devices is sometimes referred to as **free weights.** Free weights include barbells, dumbbells, and other related equipment. In the early 1900s Alan Calvert developed adjustable barbells with weighted plates that could be added or removed to change the resistance. In over eighty years, there have been few changes to alter his basic design.

There have been many discussions regarding the merits of the "machines versus free weights" question, and in the judgment of some observers, it may never be answered.

The authors take the stand that it is not an "either or" problem. Any method of training has some advantages and some disadvantages. As long as the basic principles regarding strength development are observed, it is possible to make strength gains and body changes with either machines or free weights. Being consistent in your training in the program you choose is probably more important than the type of equipment you select. It is recommended that each person should experiment with different exercises and various types of training equipment and use them to develop a program that is tailored to his or her needs.

Regardless of the training method, the overload principle must be utilized to obtain strength gains.

When selecting a strength program, there are three basic questions that you should ask.

Mode: What type of equipment and exercises should be used?

Quantity: How much training will be required to produce the desired results?

Quality: How should the intensity of the training be established?

The two strength programs selected for *Fitness for Life* are weight training and timed calisthenics. Weight training uses equipment that increases the resistance progressively and thus develops strength.

Many people are in locations where weight-training facilities are not available, so a second program, called **timed calisthenics,** has been developed for *Fitness for Life.* As previously indicated, it is possible to increase the difficulty of an exercise bout by increasing the number of repetitions and the number of sets comprising the exercise.

Timed calisthenics utilize the weight of the body as resistance, and the intensity can be controlled by how fast you do the repetitions in each set of an exercise. This program consists of eight exercises that stimulate all of the major muscle groups of the body. Each set of an exercise is followed by a ten-second rest period, and after each exercise you walk for two minutes before beginning the next exercise. As your fitness improves, you are able to increase the number of repetitions in each set, thus you continue to overload your body and bring about improvement.

One of the advantages of timed calisthenics is that the program not only improves strength but also improves cardiovascular endurance. If a person's time to exercise is limited, this type of training will accomplish the two objectives at the same time. Timed calisthenics strength programs have the following advantages:

1. A minimum of inexpensive equipment is needed.
2. Only simple, easy-to-learn skills are involved.
3. A large variety of strength exercises allows you to change your program from time to time.
4. Specific muscle groups of the body can be developed.
5. Engaging in a strength-training program can be very satisfying because you can easily observe the gains made in strength and muscular development.

In this unit you will learn how to write a strength program.

All the exercises used in the strength program are described and illustrated in the sections Weight-Training Exercises, and Timed Calisthenics Exercises, located at the end of this chapter. Each description gives an explanation of the body areas and muscles affected by the exercise; the starting position; the action to be used in performing the exercise; any precautions that you need to be aware of while performing the exercise; and the number of sets and repetitions to be used.

By using the Strength Program Work Sheet located in Appendix C, writing a strength program is a simple two-step process.

Step 1. Fill in the general information on the work sheet.
Step 2. Write a weight-training program or a timed calisthenics program.

To help you become familiar with these steps, we will write a strength program for a sample case.

CASE
Dan Barton

Dan is interested in pursuing a program to help him gain strength and improve his muscle tone. He prefers weight training to doing timed calisthenics, and he has time to weight train on Mondays, Wednesdays, and Fridays. Using the Strength Program Work Sheet and the step-by-step instructions that follow, write his program. He is in *Strength Fitness Category IV*.

Step 1: Filling in the general information on the work sheet

Item 1. Fill in Dan's full name and the date.

Item 2. Since Dan prefers weight training to doing timed calisthenics, check *Weight Training* to the right of item 2 on the work sheet.

Item 3. A weight-training program is most effective if it requires exercise every other day, three days a week. Since Dan has time to exercise on Mondays, Wednesdays, and Fridays, circle *M W F* to the right of item 3 on the work sheet. In order to obtain the desired training effects from timed calisthenics, it is necessary to work out five days a week. If a person selects this program, he or she should circle five days per week next to timed calisthenics.

Item 4. Check the *Strength Fitness Category* that Dan is in *(IV—Good)*. This information can be obtained by taking the strength appraisal in

chapter 2. If you do not know the fitness category of your subject, then you would check *0—Beginner*.

Item 5. If Dan had chosen a timed calisthenics program, he would be required to rest for ten seconds between the sets of an exercise and for two minutes between each exercise. The weight-training program Dan has chosen, however, requires only that he rest ninety seconds between the sets of an exercise. Another method is alternating the selected exercises rather than taking a rest period. For example, Dan could do one set of exercise 1 and a set of exercise 10, and then repeat this process until the required number of sets are completed. So, check *90 Seconds* or *Alternating Exercises* to the right of item 5 on the work sheet.

Step 2: Writing a weight-training or a timed calisthenics program

To write Dan's strength program, we will use chart I on the work sheet labeled Weight Training.

The first column on the chart is labeled *Body Parts*. Listed under this heading are the various muscle group areas that Dan must exercise in order to develop strength and muscle tone.

The second column on the chart is labeled *Exercise*. Listed under this heading are numerals. These refer to exercises of the selected training programs.

The Arabic numerals refer to the weight-training exercises. The Roman numerals refer to the timed calisthenic exercises.

Look at the first line of the *Body Parts* column. It is labeled *Shoulders*. To the right, in the *Exercise* column, you will find the numbers 1, 2, 3. These numbers refer to weight-training exercises for developing strength in the shoulder muscles. By turning to the weight-training exercises, you will find that exercises 1, 2, and 3 refer to (1) the seated overhead press, (2) upright rowing, and (3) dips on the parallel bars. Dan chooses one of these three for his shoulder exercise. He decides on exercise 1. Circle 1 on the chart and in the *Exercise Preference* column write the name of the specific exercise Dan has selected (the seated overhead press). If a person wishes, he or she may increase the number of exercises chosen for any body part. One exercise is the minimum program only.

By following this same procedure, Dan should select one exercise for each muscle-group area listed in the *Body Parts* column. Dan decides that he will select weight-training exercises 1, 10, 7, 11, 13, 14, 5, 4, and 6 for his program. Locate Dan's other exercise choices in the charts and record the names of these exercises in the *Exercise Preference* column.

Be sure that Dan, in making his selection, has not chosen the same exercise twice. Exercise 1 is good for developing shoulder muscles as well as back muscles. If Dan has chosen exercise 1 for his shoulders, however, he must choose another exercise (5 or 8) for his back. He should not use the same exercise to develop two different muscle-group areas.

To fill in the *Sets and Repetitions* columns, refer again to Dan's preferred exercises in the description of the strength exercises. There you will find the proper number of sets and repetitions to do. In order to develop muscle strength, muscle endurance, and muscle hypertrophy, three sets of ten repetitions bring about good results in a weight-training program. With the exception of curl-ups, all of the weight-training exercises follow this recommendation for sets and repetitions. Since Dan is seeking to develop both strength and muscle endurance, he chooses to do three sets of ten repetitions. For weight training, this information is already written in the *Sets and Repetitions* columns on the work sheet.

Filling in the *Resistance* column is difficult because there are no set rules to guide you. Resistance refers to the weight to be lifted in the exercise. There is no way to determine exactly how much weight a person should be lifting during his exercises before starting a program. It is basically a process of trial and error.

1. Guess how many pounds you can lift.

2. Try this weight for the given number of repetitions for one set.

3. If the exercise seems too easy and you can do more than the recommended number of repetitions, increase the resistance for the next set. Note that most weights come in 5-pound increments.

4. If the exercise is too hard and you cannot do the recommended number of repetitions, decrease the resistance for the next set.

5. Remember to increase the weight whenever you can do more than the recommended number of repetitions on the last set.

By using this method you do not have to measure your maximum repetition for any given exercise. Doing a one-repetition maximum can be time consuming and also dangerous for beginners.

By trial and error, Dan has determined the proper amount of resistance for each of his exercises. He finds that he will use the following resistance:

Exercise	Resistance
1	60 lbs.
10	body weight
7	120 lbs.
11	20 lbs.
13	30 lbs.
14	100 lbs.
5	body weight
4	70 lbs.
6	150 lbs.

(Note: Usually the weight given in the *Resistance* column of the work sheet is written in pounds. Sometimes an exercise will require no weight or will use the body's weight as in timed calisthenics and the chin-up and curl-up.)

When you have completed the work sheet, compare your copy with the one in figure 7.1.

Instructions: Following are cases of two individuals requesting strength programs. Read each one carefully and answer the multiple-choice items related to the case by circling the letter of the best answer. You may use the exercise charts and your Strength Program Work Sheet to help you find the correct answers.

A. Ron is a thirty-two-year-old food inspector who wants to add weight training to his fitness program. He prefers *not* to use strength exercises 4, 6, 8, 9, and 12.

1. For exercise 5, Ron will do
   a. 4 sets of 6 repetitions.
   b. 3 sets of 10 repetitions.
   c. 2 sets of 20 repetitions.
   d. 3 sets of 30 repetitions.

Strength Program Work Sheet

1. Name: __Dan Barton__   Date: _____

2. Program Preference: Weight Training __X__   Timed Calisthenics _____

3. Exercise Days for Weight Training: (M)   T   (W)   Th   (F)   S

   Exercise Days for Timed Calisthenics: 5 days per week

4. Strength Fitness Category: __ 0. Beginner   __ II. Poor   **X** IV. Good   __ VI. Excellent
                             __ I. Very Poor   __ III. Fair   __ V. Very Good   __ VII. Superior

5. Rest Periods:

   Weight Training: 90 seconds or alternating exercise __X__

   Timed Calisthenics: 10 seconds and 2 minutes _____

I. WEIGHT TRAINING*

Body Parts	Exercise	Exercise Preference	Sets	Repetitions	Resistance
Shoulders	① 2, 3	seated overhead press	3	10	60 lbs
Abdomen	⑩	curl-up	3	30	body weight
Chest	6 ⑦ 9	incline bench press	3	10	120 lbs
Hamstrings	⑪	leg curl	3	10	20 lbs
Quadriceps	12, ⑬	quad lift	3	10	30 lbs
Legs (calves)	⑭	heel raise	3	10	100 lbs
Back	⑤ 1, 8	chin-up	3	10	body weight
Biceps	④ 2, 5	arm curl	3	10	70 lbs
Triceps	7, 1, 3 ⑥	bench press	3	10	150 lbs

*Arabic numerals refer to charts in the weight-training program.

II. TIMED CALISTHENICS†

Shoulders	IV	four-count burpee			
Abdomen	VI	curl-up			
Chest	VII	push-up			
Hamstrings	II	treadmill			
Quadriceps	I, V	run in place/shuffle			
Legs (calves)	III	high jumper			
Back	VIII	chin-up			
Biceps	VIII	chin-up			
Triceps	VII	push-up			

†Roman numerals refer to charts in the timed calisthenics program.

Figure 7.1.

2. Ron will need to do his weight-training exercises
   a. Mon., Wed., Fri.
   b. Tues., Thurs., Fri., Sat.
   c. daily.
   d. Mon., Tues., Wed., Thurs.
3. Ron's rest periods for weight training will be
   a. 10 seconds and 2 minutes.
   b. 90 seconds.
   c. 2 minutes.
   d. 10 minutes.
4. Ron's exercises could include
   a. 1, 10, 6, 11, 13, 14, 5, 4, 3.
   b. 3, 10, 7, 11, 13, 14, 1, 5, 1.
   c. 1, 10, 7, 11, 13, 14, 5, 2, 3.
   d. 3, 10, 7, 11, 13, 14, 1, 4, 3.

B. Carol is a twenty-six-year-old dress designer. She has requested help in organizing a strength program. She has selected timed calisthenics. She is in *Fitness Category III.*
   1. For exercise VI, Carol will do
      a. 4 sets of 10 seconds.
      b. 7 sets of 10 seconds.
      c. 10 sets of 10 seconds.
      d. any of these.
   2. Carol will do her timed calisthenics
      a. Mon., Wed., Fri.
      b. Tues., Thurs., Sat.
      c. Mon., Tues., Wed., Thurs., Fri.
      d. daily.
   3. The resistance for Carol's timed calisthenics will be
      a. barbells.
      b. dumbbells.
      c. her own body.
      d. the number of exercises done in 10 seconds.
   4. Carol's rest periods for timed calisthenics will be
      a. 10 seconds and 2 minutes.
      b. 90 seconds.
      c. alternating exercises.
      d. 2 minutes.

C. Brittany chooses to do 3 sets of 10 bench presses in her weight-training program. She tries a 40-pound weight and discovers that it is too heavy. A 20-pound weight proves to be too light.
   1. Brittany's original "guestimate" was
      a. 10 pounds.
      b. 20 pounds.
      c. 30 pounds.
      d. 40 pounds.
   2. She tried her first guestimate for
      a. 1 repetition.
      b. 1 set of 10 repetitions.
      c. 3 sets of 6 repetitions.
      d. 3 sets of 10 repetitions.
   3. What solution would you give Brittany at this time (after using the 20-pound weight)?
      a. Use a ten-pound weight.
      b. Use a twenty-pound weight.
      c. Use a thirty-pound weight.
      d. Use a forty-pound weight.
   4. When should Brittany increase her resistance?
      a. every Tuesday, Thursday and Saturday
      b. every Tuesday
      c. when she exceeds the number of repetitions listed on the exercise chart

D. 1. Exercise 4 strengthens which of the following muscles?
      a. abdominals
      b. biceps
      c. latissimus dorsi
      d. trapezius

Answers:

A. 1. b   B. 1. b   C. 1. d   D. 1. b
   2. a   2. c   2. b
   3. b   3. c   3. c
   4. c   4. a   4. c

If you responded correctly to each item, you are ready to proceed with the next unit.

WEIGHT-TRAINING EXERCISES

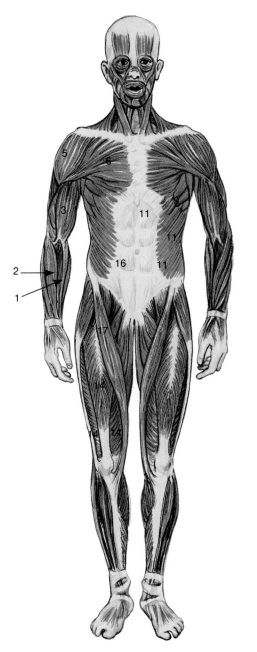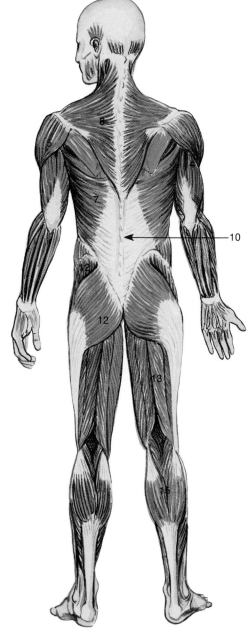

1. Forearm flexors
2. Brachioradialis
3. Biceps
4. Triceps
5. Deltoid
6. Pectoral muscles
7. Latissimus dorsi
8. Trapezius
9. Serratus anterior
10. Erector spinae
    (spinal extensors)
11. Abdominal muscles
12. Gluteal muscles
13. Hamstrings
14. Quadriceps muscles
15. Gastrocnemius, soleus
    muscles
16. Psoas major (under
    abdominal muscles)
17. Sartorius

Figure 7.2. Major muscle groups of the body. *(From John W. Hole, Jr., Human Anatomy and Physiology, 4th ed. © 1987 Wm. C. Brown Publishers, Dubuque, Iowa. All Rights Reserved. Reprinted by permission.)*

STRENGTH—WEIGHT TRAINING
Seated Overhead Press

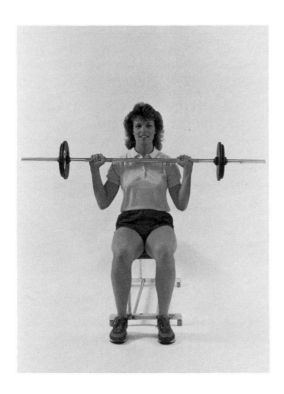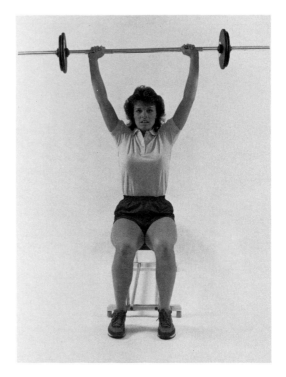

Body areas strengthened: Shoulders, back, upper chest, back of upper arms.

Muscles strengthened: Triceps, deltoids, pectoral muscles, trapezius, serratus anterior.

Starting position: Seated on bench with eyes facing straight ahead. Bar will be at midline of chest.

Action: Push the bar overhead until arms are extended. Lower bar to chest position to complete the repetition.

Precautions: Keep head up and back straight.

Sets and repetitions: 3 sets–10 repetitions.

STRENGTH—WEIGHT TRAINING
Upright Rowing

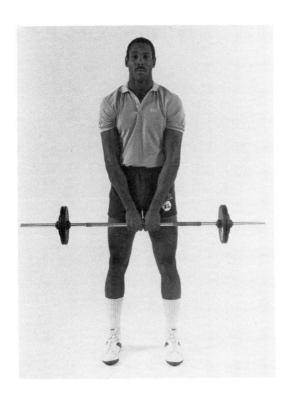 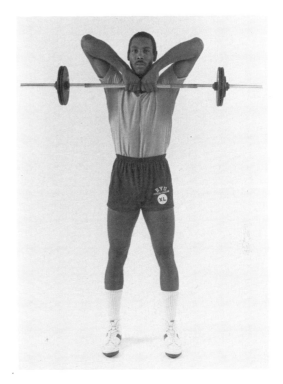

Body areas strengthened: Shoulders, back, front of upper arms.

Muscles strengthened: Brachioradialis, biceps, deltoids, trapezius.

Starting position: In a standing position, grasp the bar with hands approximately four inches apart. Use a palms-down grip and allow the bar to touch thighs.

Action: Keep eyes straight ahead and chest high. Raise the bar until it touches chin. Lower the bar to starting position to complete the repetition.

Precautions: Keep body in an erect position throughout movement. Keep the bar close to body with elbows higher than hands, and don't jerk to start exercise.

Sets and repetitions: 3 sets–10 repetitions.

STRENGTH—WEIGHT TRAINING
Dip

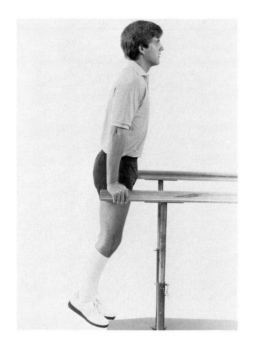

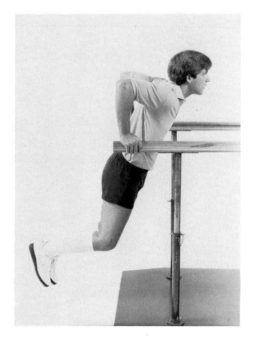

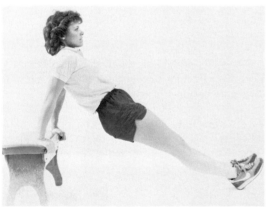

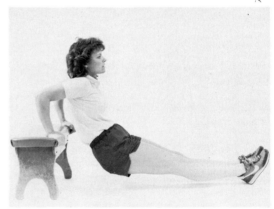

Body areas strengthened: Shoulders, forearms, back of upper arms.

Muscles strengthened: Triceps, deltoids, pectoral muscles, forearm flexors.

Starting position: Body is supported in a suspended position between the parallel bars.

Action: Dip downward as far as possible and return to the starting position to complete the repetition.

Precautions: Avoid unnecessary body swing.

Sets and repetitions: 3 sets–10 repetitions. In order to add resistance, weights placed on a rope and hooked to a belt can be used.

NOTE: If you cannot do the dip as described, it is possible to decrease the resistance. Check the picture description for this alternative dip.

STRENGTH—WEIGHT TRAINING
Arm Curl

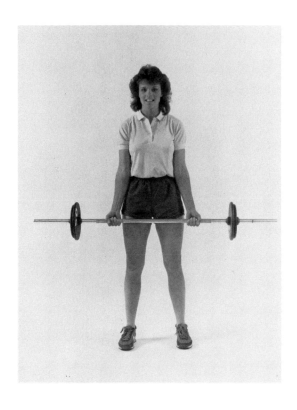 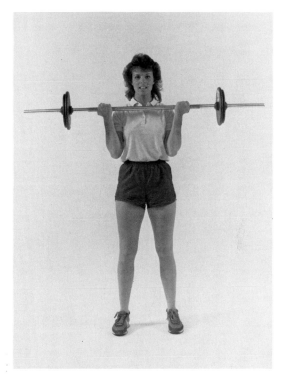

Body areas strengthened: Front of upper arms and front of forearms.

Muscles strengthened: Forearm flexors, brachioradialis, biceps.

Starting Position: Use a palms-up grip, approximately the width of shoulders, with arms extended. The bar rests against thighs.

Action: Curl the bar up to shoulder-neck area, touch, and then return to the starting position to complete the repetition.

Precautions: Elbows should be kept close to the sides of body. Keep body erect, eyes forward. Avoid unnecessary body movement.

Sets and repetitions: 3 sets–10 repetitions.

STRENGTH—WEIGHT TRAINING
Chin-Up

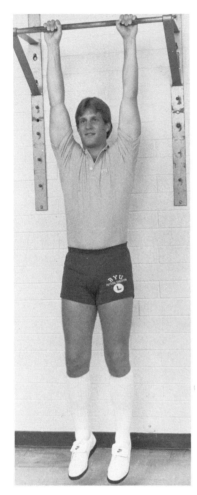
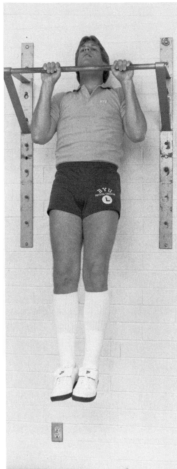
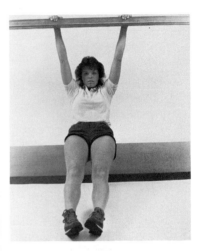
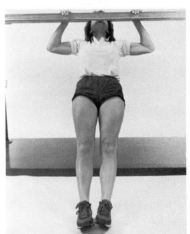

Body areas strengthened: Forearms, front of upper arms, back.

Muscles strengthened: Forearm flexors, brachio-radialis, biceps, latissimus dorsi, trapezius.

Starting position: Use a palms-down grip, approximately the width of shoulders, with arms extended to support body suspended from the chinning bar.

Action: Pull body upward toward the bar until chin is above the bar; then return to the starting position to complete the repetition.

Precautions: Straighten out arms on each repetition. Avoid unnecessary body swing and movement.

Sets and repetitions: 3 sets–10 repetitions. In order to add resistance, weights placed on a rope and hooked to a belt can be used.

NOTE: If you cannot do the chin-up as described, it is possible to decrease the resistance. Check the picture description for this alternative chin-up.

STRENGTH—WEIGHT TRAINING
Bench Press

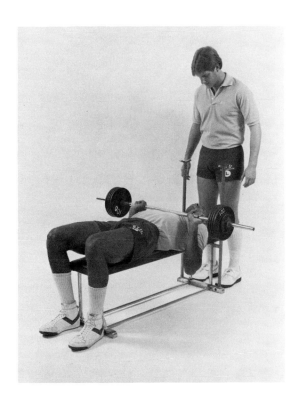 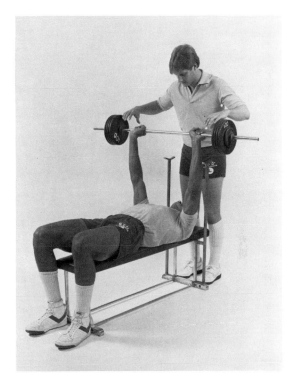

Body areas strengthened: Chest, shoulders, back of upper arms.

Muscles strengthened: Triceps, deltoids, pectoral muscles.

Starting position: Lie flat on bench with knees bent and feet flat on the floor. Use a palms-down grip, approximately the width of shoulders. Hold the bar in a chest-rest position.

Action: Press the bar directly upward until arms are extended and then return to the starting position to complete the repetition.

Precautions: Have partner assist as spotter during exercise. Do not arch back or raise buttocks during movement. Do not bounce weight off chest. Avoid pushing with feet to lift weight.

Sets and repetitions: 3 sets–10 repetitions.

STRENGTH—WEIGHT TRAINING
Inclined Bench Press

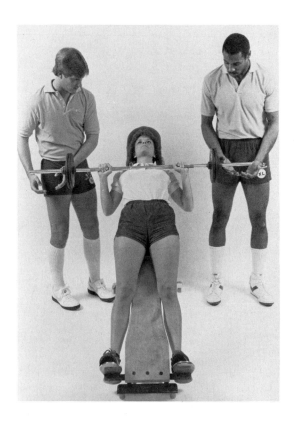 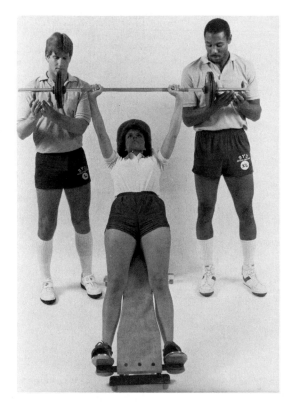

Body areas strengthened: Chest, shoulders, backs of upper arms.

Muscles strengthened: Triceps, deltoids, pectoral muscles.

Starting position: Lie flat on inclined bench, with legs straight and feet flat against supports. Use a palms-down grip, approximately the width of shoulders. Hold the bar in a chest-rest position.

Action: Press the bar upward until arms are extended and then return to the starting position to complete the repetition.

Precautions: Have partners assist as spotters during exercise. Do not arch back or raise buttocks during movement. Do not bounce weight off chest.

Sets and repetitions: 3 sets—10 repetitions.

STRENGTH—WEIGHT TRAINING
Lat Machine Pulldown

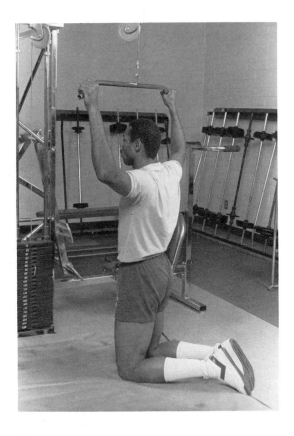 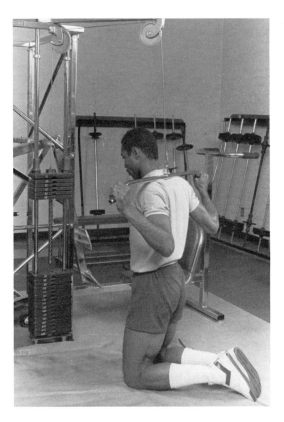

Body areas strengthened: Forearms, back, upper chest.

Muscles strengthened: Latissimus dorsi, trapezius, brachioradialis, pectoral muscles.

Starting position: Start in a kneeling or seated position. Grasp the bar in a wide palms-down grip with arms fully extended.

Action: Pull the bar down until it touches the base of neck and then return to the starting position to complete the repetition.

Precautions: Keep upper body straight. Do not jerk or raise body to assist in the movement.

Sets and repetitions: 3 sets–10 repetitions.

STRENGTH—WEIGHT TRAINING
Bent-Arm Pullover

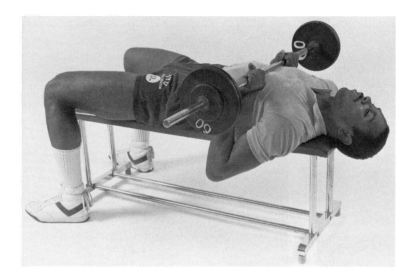

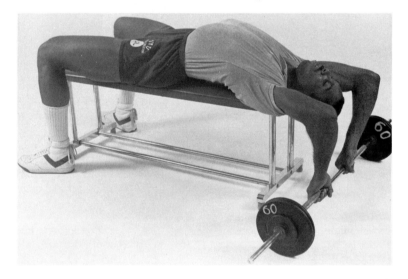

Body areas strengthened: Chest, back of upper arms.

Muscles strengthened: Deltoids, pectoral muscles, serratus anterior, latissimus dorsi.

Starting position: Lie flat on bench with knees bent and feet flat on the floor. Allow head to hang over the end of the bench. Use palms-down grip, with hands approximately 12 inches apart. Hold the bar in a chest-rest position.

Action: Lower the bar back over head, with elbows bent, as far as possible. Pull the weight back to the starting position to complete the repetition.

Precautions: Keep elbows close to head and pointing toward the ceiling during the exercise. Avoid unnecessary arching of back. Do not jerk or make unnecessary body movements. Keep the bar close to face during the exercise movement.

Sets and repetitions: 3 sets–10 repetitions.

STRENGTH—WEIGHT TRAINING
Curl-Up

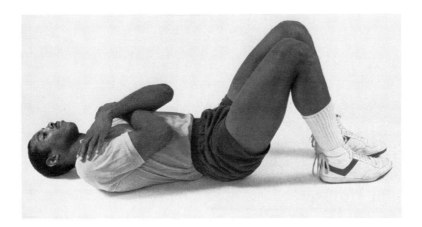

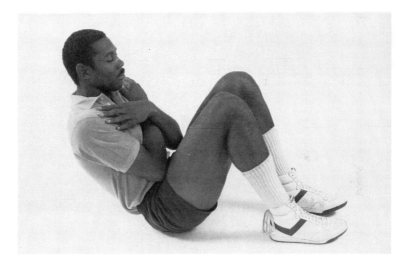

Body areas strengthened: Abdomen.

Muscles strengthened: Abdominal muscles.

Starting position: Lie flat on floor, with legs bent at knees, feet flat on the floor. Hands are folded over chest.

Action: Curl up to approximately a 30° angle and then return to the starting position to complete the repetition.

Precautions: Do not stabilize feet unless absolutely necessary. Do not arch back during the exercise. Keep arms flat against chest. Avoid any jerking or unnecessary body movement. Be sure to start by bending head forward and then progressing down the back until you curl up to approximately a 30° angle. Curl back to starting position by touching lower back, then upper back, and finally head. A good check is to have someone place his or her hand under lower back. You should press down on the hand until lower back is curled forward.

Sets and repetitions: 3 sets–30 repetitions.

NOTE: If you cannot do the curl-up as described, it is possible to decrease the resistance by placing hands alongside hips. Follow the same procedure as described above.

STRENGTH—WEIGHT TRAINING
Leg Curl

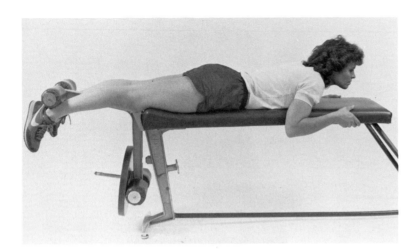

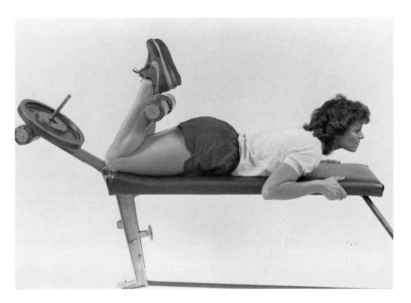

Body areas strengthened: Back of upper legs.

Muscles strengthened: Gluteal muscles, hamstrings.

Starting position: Lie face downward, with legs extended and backs of heels against the bar.

Action: Lift feet upward until they are over or touching buttocks and then return to the starting position to complete the repetition.

Precautions: Movement should be entirely in knee joint. Avoid unnecessary jerking or body movement.

Sets and repetitions: 3 sets—10 repetitions.

STRENGTH—WEIGHT TRAINING
Squat

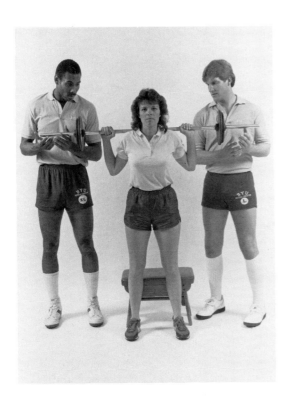 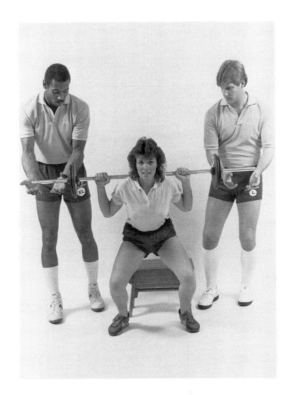

Body areas strengthened: Legs, lower and upper back.

Muscles strengthened: Quadriceps, erector spinae, gluteal muscles, hamstrings, gastrocnemius, soleus, trapezius.

Starting position: Place bar across shoulders, with body in an erect position. Keep head up and back flat. Feet are placed in a parallel position approximately 14 inches apart.

Action: Lower body until thighs are parallel with the floor. Rise to the starting position by extending knees and hips to complete the repetition.

Precautions: Have partners assist as spotters during exercise. Keep back straight and chest high throughout the movement. Rounding the back can place stress on spine and cause injury. Do not bounce at bottom of exercise. As a safety device, place a bench behind you that will allow you to sit down if you lose your balance.

Sets and repetitions: 3 sets–10 repetitions.

STRENGTH—WEIGHT TRAINING
Quad Lift

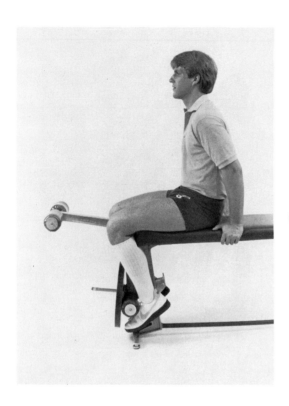 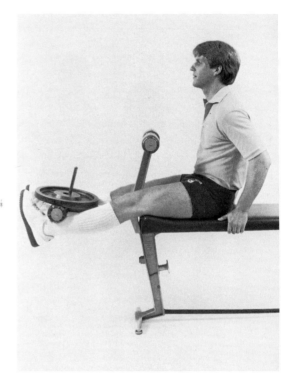

Body areas strengthened: Front of thigh and knee joint.

Muscles strengthened: Quadriceps.

Starting position: Sitting position with lower legs at right angles to thighs and fronts of ankles against the bar. Elevate thighs, if necessary, so they are parallel to the floor.

Action: Extend knee until lower leg is parallel to the floor. Return to starting position to complete the repetition.

Precautions: Keep trunk straight at all times. Do not jerk or bounce weight at bottom of the exercise. Make sure leg is extended at top of the exercise, but do not lock the knee joint as this increases stress to the joint.

Sets and repetitions: 3 sets–10 repetitions.

STRENGTH—WEIGHT TRAINING
Heel Raise

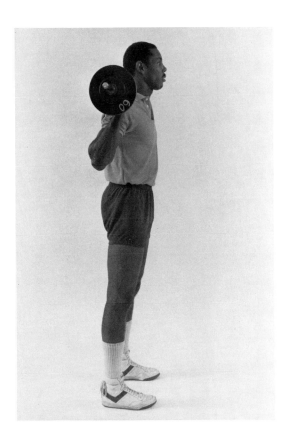 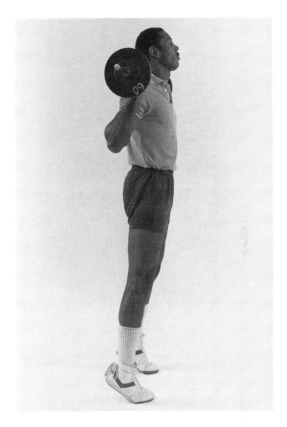

Body areas strengthened: Lower legs, ankles, feet.

Muscles strengthened: Gastrocnemius, soleus.

Starting position: Place bar across shoulders with body in an erect position. Feet should be pointed straight ahead and approximately 8 inches apart.

Action: Rise up on toes as far as possible and then return to starting position to complete the repetition.

Precautions: Keep body in a straight line and do not bend knees during the exercise. Avoid any jerky or unnecessary movements.

Sets and repetitions: 3 sets–10 repetitions.

TIMED CALISTHENICS EXERCISES

Exercise Chart I

STRENGTH—TIMED CALISTHENICS
Running in Place

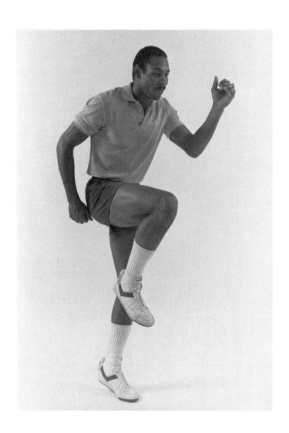 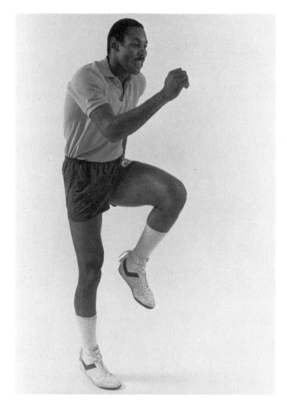

Body areas strengthened: Legs, hips, buttocks.

Muscles strengthened: Gluteal muscles, hamstrings, quadriceps, gastrocnemius, soleus.

Starting position: Standing in an erect position.

Action: Run in place as rapidly as possible.

Precautions: Avoid running on hard surfaces that might bruise feet.

Sets and repetitions for selected strength fitness categories:

0, I	4 sets–10 seconds in each set. Do as many repetitions as possible in each set.
II, III	7 sets–10 seconds in each set. Do as many repetitions as possible in each set.
IV, V, VI	10 sets–10 seconds in each set. Do as many repetitions as possible in each set.

STRENGTH—TIMED CALISTHENICS
Treadmill

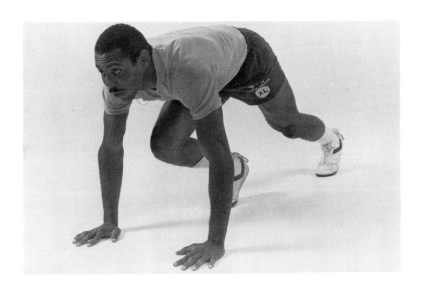

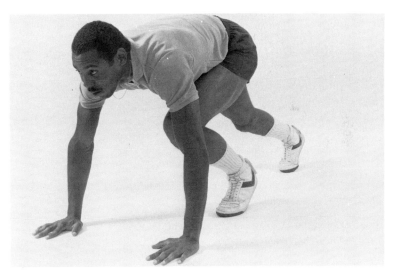

Body areas strengthened: Back of upper arms, shoulders, chest, buttocks, legs.

Muscles strengthened: Triceps, deltoids, pectoral and gluteal muscles, hamstrings, gastrocnemius, soleus.

Starting position: In a front-leaning position with arms extended, one leg extended, and one leg drawn up under chest.

Action: Alternate the position of legs as rapidly as possible.

Precautions: Keep arms straight during exercise and move legs through a full range of motion.

Sets and repetitions for selected strength fitness categories:

0, I	4 sets–10 seconds in each set. Do as many repetitions as possible in each set.
II, III	7 sets–10 seconds in each set. Do as many repetitions as possible in each set.
IV, V, VI	10 sets–10 seconds in each set. Do as many repetitions as possible in each set.

STRENGTH—TIMED CALISTHENICS
High Jumper

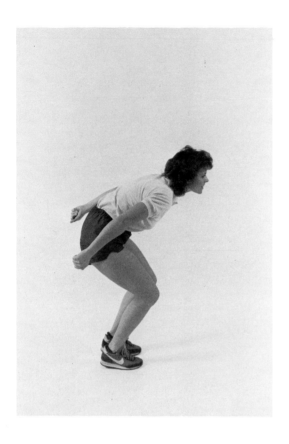
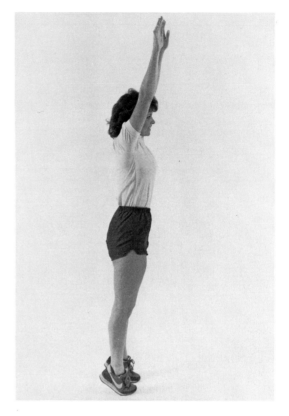

Body areas strengthened: Legs, buttocks.

Muscles strengthened: Gluteal muscles, hamstrings, quadriceps, gastrocnemius, soleus.

Starting position: A crouched position, with knees bent and arms extended backward.

Action: Jump as high as possible into the air and extend arms upward over head.

Precautions: Avoid hitting the ceiling.

Sets and repetitions for selected strength fitness categories:

0, I	4 sets–10 seconds in each set. Do as many repetitions as possible in each set.
II, III	7 sets–10 seconds in each set. Do as many repetitions as possible in each set.
IV, V, VI	10 sets–10 seconds in each set. Do as many repetitions as possible in each set.

STRENGTH—TIMED CALISTHENICS
Four-Count Burpee

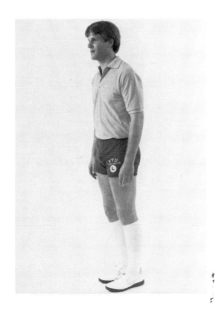
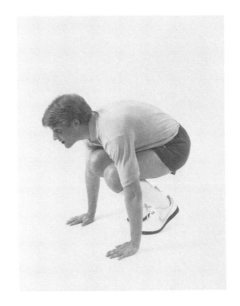
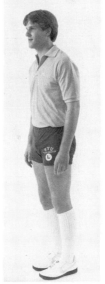
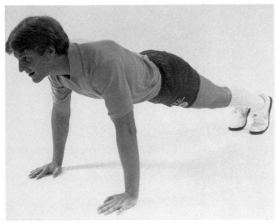
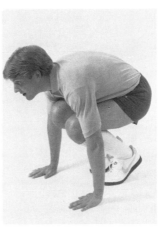

Body areas strengthened: Forearms, back of upper arms, shoulders, chest, stomach.

Muscles strengthened: Forearm flexors, triceps, deltoids, pectoral and abdominal muscles.

Starting position: Standing in an erect position with arms at sides.

Action: (1) Drop down to a squat position with hands flat on the floor, about shoulder-width apart. (2) Throw back legs, keeping them together, to a fully extended position. Support your weight on extended arms and toes. (3) Pull up legs to the squat position. (4) Return to starting position and repeat.

Precautions: None.

Sets and repetitions for selected strength fitness categories:

0, I	4 sets–10 seconds in each set. Do as many repetitions as possible in each set.
II, III	7 sets–10 seconds in each set. Do as many repetitions as possible in each set.
IV, V, VI	10 sets–10 seconds in each set. Do as many repetitions as possible in each set.

STRENGTH—TIMED CALISTHENICS
Shuffle Step

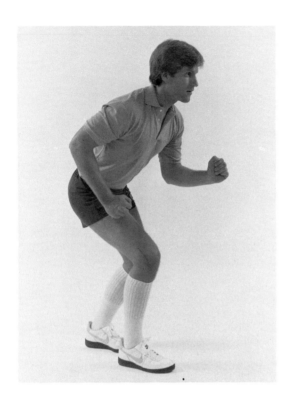 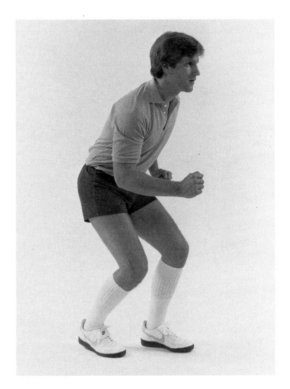

Body areas strengthened: Buttocks, legs.

Muscles strengthened: Gluteal muscles, quadriceps, gastrocnemius, soleus.

Starting position: In an erect position with knees slightly bent. Toe of left foot should be near heel of right foot.

Action: Shuffle feet back and forth as rapidly as possible.

Precautions: Keep knees bent and feet flat on the floor. You should feel the resistance in upper thigh.

Sets and repetitions for selected strength fitness categories:

0, I	4 sets–10 seconds in each set. Do as many repetitions as possible in each set.
II, III	7 sets–10 seconds in each set. Do as many repetitions as possible in each set.
IV, V, VI	10 sets–10 seconds in each set. Do as many repetitions as possible in each set.

STRENGTH—TIMED CALISTHENICS
Curl-Up

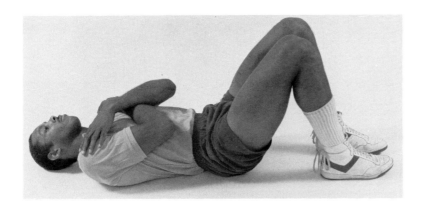

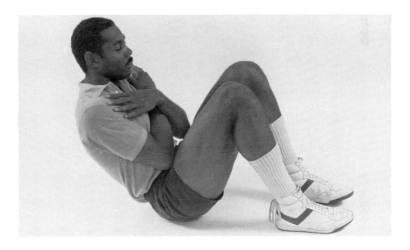

Body areas strengthened: Abdomen.

Muscles strengthened: Abdominal muscles.

Starting position: Lie flat on floor, with legs bent at knees and feet flat on the floor. Hands are folded over chest.

Action: Curl up to an angle of 30° and then return to starting position.

Precautions: Do not arch back during exercise. Keep arms flat against chest. Start by bending head forward and then progressing down the back as you curl up to approximately a 30° angle. Curl back to starting position by touching lower back, then upper back, and finally head. A good check is to have someone place his or her hand under lower back. You should press down on the hand until lower back is curled forward.

It is important to do this exercise properly. Good form is more important than the number performed in each set.

Sets and repetitions for selected strength fitness categories:

0, I	4 sets–10 seconds in each set. Do as many repetitions as possible in each set.
II, III	7 sets–10 seconds in each set. Do as many repetitions as possible in each set.
IV, V, VI	10 sets–10 seconds in each set. Do as many repetitions as possible in each set.

NOTE: If you cannot do the curl-up as described, it is possible to decrease the resistance by placing hands alongside hips. Follow the same procedures as described above.

STRENGTH—TIMED CALISTHENICS
Push-Up

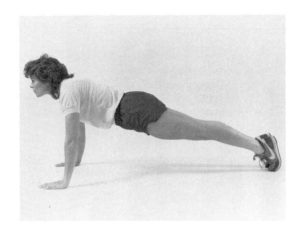
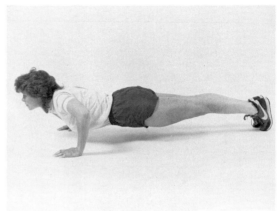
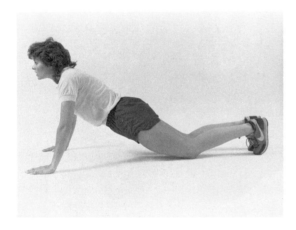
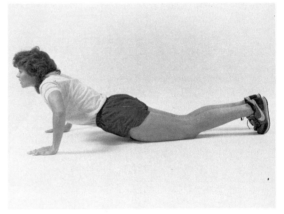

Body areas strengthened: Forearms, back of upper arms, chest, stomach.

Muscles strengthened: Forearm flexors, triceps, pectoral and abdominal muscles.

Starting position: In a front-leaning position with both legs extended. Hands are approximately shoulder-width apart. Weight will be supported on hands and toes.

Action: Lower body by bending arms until chest is within an inch of the floor and then return to starting position.

Precautions: Keep body line straight during the movement. Do not touch the floor with chest.

Sets and repetitions for selected strength fitness categories:

0, I	4 sets–10 seconds in each set. Do as many repetitions as possible in each set.
II, III	7 sets–10 seconds in each set. Do as many repetitions as possible in each set.
IV, V, VI	10 sets–10 seconds in each set. Do as many repetitions as possible in each set.

NOTE: If you cannot do the push-up as described, it is possible to decrease the resistance. Check the picture description for this alternative push-up.

STRENGTH—TIMED CALISTHENICS
Chin-Up

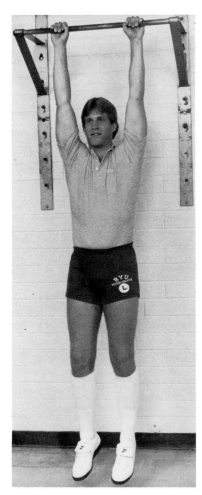
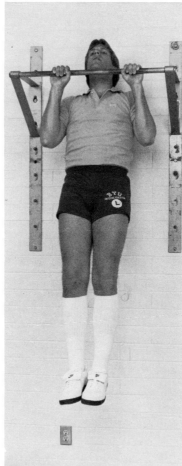
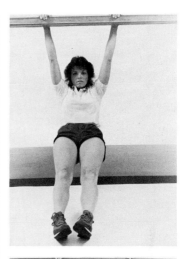
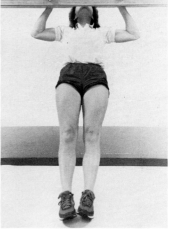

Body areas strengthened: Forearms, front of upper arms, back.

Muscles strengthened: Forearm flexors, brachioradialis, biceps, latissimus dorsi, trapezius.

Starting position: Use a palms-down grip, approximately the width of shoulders, with arms extended to support body suspended from the bar.

Action: Pull body upward toward the bar until chin is above the bar and then return to the starting position.

Precautions: Straighten out arms on each repetition. Avoid unnecessary body swing and movement.

Sets and repetitions for selected strength fitness categories:

0, I	4 sets–10 seconds in each set. Do as many repetitions as possible in each set.
II, III	7 sets–10 seconds in each set. Do as many repetitions as possible in each set.
IV, V, VI	10 sets–10 seconds in each set. Do as many repetitions as possible in each set.

NOTE: If you cannot do the chin-up as described, it is possible to decrease the resistance. Check the picture description for this alternative chin-up.

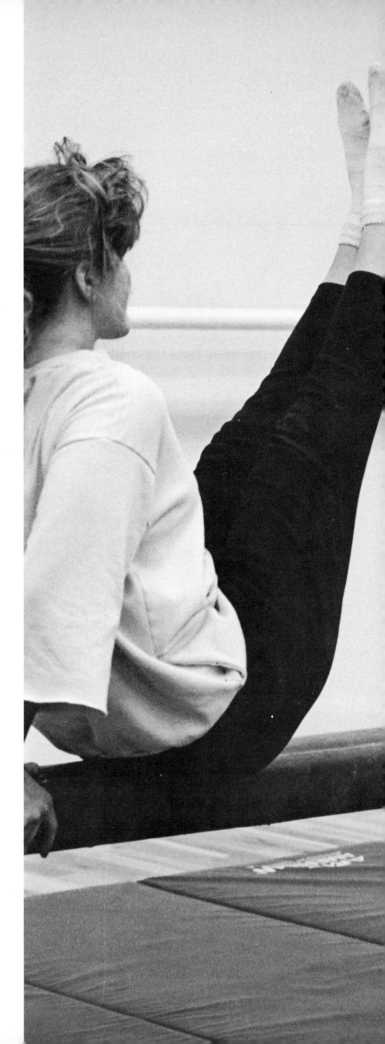

8

APPLYING A STRENGTH PROGRAM

Objective

After study of this chapter you should be able to

• use your own written strength program and contract to engage in an appropriate strength program.

Now that you have completed the chapter "Writing a Strength Program," you are ready to start your own individualized program. Before you begin your program you should read the following suggestions.

SAFETY TIPS

Warm-up

All exercise programs should either be preceded by a warm-up period or have warm-up exercises as a part of the program. This will reduce the chance of muscle and joint injury. Warm-up also prepares the systems of the body for more demanding exercise. A good warm-up for your strength program is to engage in the flexibility exercises you have chosen and to run in place for two to three minutes. The best indicator that you are warmed up is the onset of sweating.

Spotting

Spotting is the term given to the use of a partner or partners to assist in the exercise program. This is especially important in certain weight-training programs in which dropping a weight on the body might cause an injury.

Correct Body Position

All of the suggested exercises in this text stress the correct body position and proper movement. By placing the body in awkward and unnatural positions, you increase the chances of injury. When lifting a weight, the movements are relatively slow with the weight under control.

Breathing

For most individuals, proper breathing during strength development programs is not a problem. If you find you are having problems, inhale as the weight is lowered and exhale as the weight is lifted. The important thing is not to hold the breath during the complete exercise, as this causes increased pressure that might result in dizziness or light-headedness.

Dangerous Exercises

Almost any exercise can be potentially dangerous if done incorrectly. Following is a list of specific exercises that might cause problems in an exercise program.

1. Toe-touching, done with the knees in a locked position and with a rapid, bouncing action, which causes tremendous pressure to be applied to the lumbar vertebrae (lower back). This could be a factor in causing low-back pain.
2. Leg lifts, performed while lying on the back and raising both legs at the same time. This exercise can cause the pelvis to rotate and can increase the problem of low-back lordosis (swayback).
3. Deep knee bends, performed so that the buttocks touch the heels, causing a stretching of the ligaments of the knee. In some cases, the cartilage of the knee can be injured by deep squatting. Bending the knees so that the thighs are parallel to the floor is acceptable and will not cause injury to the knees.
4. Body arch, performed by attempting to arch the head and feet as high off the floor as possible. This can contribute to or aggravate the problem of lordosis (swayback).
5. Sit-ups performed improperly can contribute to an increased curvature of the lower back. This results in part from the improper utilization of the iliopsoas muscle. When doing the sit-up, it is recommended that the knees be bent and the arms folded over the chest to prevent giving a forward swing with the arms. Then curl up to only a thirty-degree angle. In this way the abdominal muscles will do a major share of the work.

The important point to remember is that any repeated movement in an unnatural position can create problems. Two key areas of the body to be concerned with are the lower back and the knees.

COMMONLY ASKED QUESTIONS

Why do I exercise only three or four times a week instead of every day to get strength gains? There is very little difference in strength gains resulting from a weight-training program requiring daily exercise and one requiring exercise three times per week. This is not necessarily true in timed calisthenics programs because the resistance is less. For this reason we recommend five exercise sessions per week when utilizing timed calisthenics.

What happens if I lift weights every day? There will not be any injury to the body tissues, but little additional gain will result from the extra time spent in weight training. A three-times-per-week schedule, with a day of rest between each workout, provides an opportunity for the body to recuperate and the muscle tissue to develop.

How can I tell if I am progressing? The best indicator of progress will be the amount of weight you can lift in your selected exercises or the increased number of sets and repetitions you can perform in the timed calisthenics program. In addition, your body composition will probably change, with a decrease in body fat and an increase in muscle tissue or lean body tissue.

How much strength do I need? This question cannot be answered specifically, because all individuals are different. Strength is very important in sports skills and daily activity; by increasing our strength, we become much more efficient in both skills and daily activity.

How can I maintain strength once I have it? Strength can be maintained by having a strength workout only once a week. Each body part must be exercised, using a close-to-maximum repetition. A workout schedule of this type, however, might contribute to muscle soreness.

Are there other exercises for problem areas? If so, where can I find out about them? Yes. Additional information can be obtained by consulting a reputable physical educator, or you can get books on weight training and/or flexibility at the library. The books will contain many additional exercises; be careful to select only those recommended by a knowledgeable person. Check on the authors to determine their expertise in the field.

*What is **circuit training**?* Basically, it is an organized course of exercises at a series of exercise stations placed around a room or gymnasium. You do a certain number of repetitions of each exercise at each station, in a prescribed amount of time. The intensity of the exercise can be increased by decreasing the amount of time allotted to complete the repetitions.

What are anabolic steroids? Certain synthetic derivatives of the male hormone testosterone, the ingestion of which it is hoped will stimulate increased growth of muscle and increased strength gains, are known as *anabolic steroids*. The American College of Sports Medicine has issued a position statement against the use of these drugs, as there is no conclusive scientific evidence that they either aid or hinder performance. There are potential dangers in taking certain forms of these substances, especially in large doses, for prolonged periods of time. The complete statement, with the supporting research review, can be obtained from the American College of Sports Medicine, 401 West Michigan Street, Indianapolis, Indiana, 46202.

If I increase my muscle mass, will it turn to fat when I stop exercising? Muscle tissue and fat tissue are entirely different from one another, and it is not possible to change a muscle cell to a fat cell or vice versa. It is the amount of calories that you take in that determines fat increases. If a person stops exercising and eats more calories than are expended, the fat content will increase in the fat cells.

When I start a strength program, should I increase my intake of protein in order to get stronger? There is no scientific evidence that supports the belief that people engaging in strength programs require increased amounts of protein. The National Research Council recommends that both men and women consume one gram of protein per kilogram (2.2 lbs.) of body weight. Excess protein will probably be passed as a waste product or changed to fat, in order to be stored by the body.

What are isometrics? Are they worthwhile in developing strength? Isometric contractions are muscle contractions with little or no movement. They can contribute to strength development. In isometrics, however, only that specific angle at which the muscle contraction takes place is usually strengthened; the rest of the range of motion will not be greatly affected.

Will weight training reduce flexibility and make me muscle-bound? No. Being muscle-bound means the inability to take a muscle through its normal range of motion. In a fitness program, we emphasize going through a full range of motion. This will increase flexibility and reduce the tendency to be muscle-bound.

What causes sore muscles? What can I do to relieve them? Sore muscles may be caused when waste products, given off during chemical reactions in the body, begin to collect in the muscle tissues and circulatory system. These waste products stimulate the pain receptors. The best way to relieve the soreness is to do slow, rhythmic stretching exercises to stimulate the blood flow through the sore areas. In most exercise programs this soreness will disappear after the first few workouts. Much muscle soreness can be prevented by avoiding quick, jerky, bouncing movements during exercise.

What will happen to my strength if I stop exercising? Since the effects of all exercise are temporary, your level of strength will drop if you stop exercising regularly.

What is the difference between muscular strength and muscular endurance? In the strict sense of the definition, muscular strength is the ability to exert maximal force for one contraction; muscular endurance is the ability to exert a force for a series of repeated contractions. The question becomes whether you need separate programs to develop each factor. Research reported by Clarke and Stull[1, 2] leads to speculation that the main result of both muscle strength and muscle endurance training is an increase in strength.

1. David H. Clarke and C. Alan Stull, "Endurance Training as a Determinant of Strength and Fatigability," *Research Quarterly* 41 (1970):19.
2. C. Alan Stull and David H. Clarke, "High Resistance, Low Repetition Training as a Determiner of Strength and Fatigability." *Research Quarterly* 41 (1970):189.

Endurance changes may be a secondary outgrowth. A simple rule that works well in planning a program is as follows:

1. If you want to emphasize strength, then increase the resistance and decrease the number of repetitions.
2. If you want to emphasize muscular endurance, then decrease the resistance and increase the number of repetitions.

The *Fitness for Life* program is devised to obtain both muscular strength and muscular endurance.

Is the muscle in women different from the muscle in men? When the quality of muscle in men and women is measured, the ability to exert force is almost identical. The reason that men usually have greater total body strength is that they are larger and have a greater quantity of muscle tissue.

APPLYING A STRENGTH PROGRAM

By using the Strength Program Contract in figure 8.1, preparing your own fitness program is a fairly easy six-step process.

Step 1. Prepare your own Strength Program Work Sheet.
Step 2. Fill out your Strength Program Contract.
Step 3. Get your contract approved.

Step 4. Implement the program and record your progress on the Strength Program Progress Log in figure 8.2.
Step 5. Check your progress.
Step 6. Complete your contract.

To help you become familiar with these procedures, we will go through them step-by-step.

Step 1: Preparing your own Strength Program Work Sheet

You should have learned how to complete a personal Strength Program Work Sheet as you studied chapter 7. If you have not already written a work sheet for yourself, do it now before going on with this unit.

Step 2: Filling out your Strength Program Contract

The Strength Program Contract in figure 8.1 will help you implement your fitness program. This contract is quite easy to fill out if you have completed a Strength Program Work Sheet, as explained in chapter 7. With your work sheet in front of you, fill out your contract as follows:

Item 1. Fill in your full name, age, and sex.

Item 2. Check your *Strength Fitness Category.* This information can be found in item 4 of your Strength Program Work Sheet.

Item 3. Write your body measurements in the blanks. This information will be important to use as a comparison in determining what happens to your body as a result of your program.

Item 4. Place a check in the blank beside your desired program. If you have selected *Weight Training,* list the days you will exercise each week (i.e., Monday, Wednesday, Friday). A program utilizing *Timed Calisthenics* requires that you work out five days each week.

Item 5. Fill in the number of weeks you will engage in your *Strength* program.

Step 3: Getting your contract approved

When you have filled in your program, you should have it approved. If you are a student in a physical education class, the contract can be signed by your instructor. If you are not in some organized class, then have it signed by a friend.

Step 4: Implementing your program and recording your progress on the Strength Program Progress Log

Begin your activity as soon as your contract has been approved. After each exercise period fill in your Strength Program Progress Log in figure 8.2. It will help you keep an accurate account of your work in the program. During each exercise session, write the date and day of your workouts in the log. Check the exercises you engaged in and note the resistance and/or repetitions. This will help you to observe the gains that come with a strength program.

Strength Program Contract

1. Name _____ Age _____ Sex _____

2. Strength Fitness Category: ___ 0. Beginner   ___ II. Poor   ___ V. Very Good
                                   ___ I. Very Poor   ___ III. Fair   ___ VI. Excellent
                                                     ___ IV. Good   ___ VII. Superior

3. Body Measurements: Weight _____ Waist _____ Chest _____

           Hips _____ Biceps: Right _____ Left _____

           Calf: Right _____ Left _____

4. Selected Program: Weight Training _____ Days _____

                       Timed Calisthenics _____

5. Number of Weeks for Program _____

Signature: _____

Contract approval date: _____ Approved by: _____

Reassessment check date: _____ Approved by: _____

Contract completion date: _____ Approved by: _____

Figure 8.1.

Strength Program Progress Log

Name _____   Beginning Strength Category _____

Date	Day	Exercise	TIMED CALISTHENICS								WEIGHT TRAINING													
			I	II	III	IV	V	VI	VII	VIII	1	2	3	4	5	6	7	8	9	10	11	12	13	14
		Reps																						
		Resistance																						
		Reps																						
		Resistance																						
		Reps																						
		Resistance																						
		Reps																						
		Resistance																						
		Reps																						
		Resistance																						
		Reps																						
		Resistance																						
		Reps																						
		Resistance																						
		Reps																						
		Resistance																						
		Reps																						
		Resistance																						
		Reps																						
		Resistance																						
		Reps																						
		Resistance																						
		Reps																						
		Resistance																						
		Reps																						
		Resistance																						

Figure 8.2.

Step 5: Checking your progress

At the completion of five weeks of your program, it is recommended that you take a progress check by retaking the Strength Test, as explained in the unit on Measuring Strength in chapter 2. The check will give you some idea of how you are progressing in your fitness program. If you wish to make changes in your fitness program after your progress check, you may do so. Make sure you have the progress check approved in order to reaffirm your decision to improve your strength.

Step 6: Completing your contract

When you have completed your strength program for the selected number of weeks, have your contract approved by the person who originally signed it.

This does not mean that you will stop engaging in a strength program; it only indicates that you have started a new life-style. You must continue to exercise for the rest of your life either to improve or to maintain your strength. Strength is reversible and will decline if you do not continue to work out.

SUGGESTIONS FOR FURTHER READING

1. Allsen, P. *Strength Training: Beginners, Bodybuilders, and Athletes.* Glenview, Illinois: Scott, Foresman and Company, 1987.
2. American Academy of Pediatrics. "Weight Training and Weight Lifting: Information for the Pediatrician." *The Physician and Sports Medicine* 11 March (1983):157.
3. American College of Sports Medicine. "Position Stand on the Use of Anabolic-Androgenic Steroids in Sports." Indianapolis, Indiana: American College of Sports Medicine, 1984.
4. Baechle, Thomas R. "Resistance Training for Women." *Journal of Health, Physical Education and Recreation* 45 (1974):28.
5. Berger, Richard A. "Development of Speed, Coordination, and Accuracy Through Strength Training." *The Athletic Journal* 53 (1972):21.
6. "Determining Factors of Strength—Parts I and II." *National Strength and Conditioning Association Journal* 7 February–March and April–May (1985).
7. Fardy, P. S. "Isometric Exercise and the Cardiovascular System." *The Physician and Sports Medicine* 9 September (1981):no. 9, p. 42.
8. Foran, B. "Advantages and Disadvantages of Isokinetics, Variable Resistance and Free Weights." *National Strength and Conditioning Association Journal* 7 February–March (1985):24.
9. Gambetta, V. "How Much Strength is Enough?" *National Strength and Conditioning Association Journal* 9 June–July (1987):51.
10. Gettman, L. "Circuit Weight Training: A Critical Review of its Physiological Benefits." *The Physician and Sports Medicine* 9 January (1981): no. 1, p. 44.
11. Hakkinen, K. "Factors Influencing Trainability of Muscular Strength During Short Term and Prolonged Training." *National Strength and Conditioning Association Journal* 7 April–May (1985):32.
12. Herling, J. "It's Time to Add Strength Training to Our Fitness Programs." *Journal of Physical Education and Programs* 79 Spring (1981):17.
13. Humphrey, L. D. "Flexibility." *Journal of Physical Education, Recreation, and Dance* 52 September (1981):41.
14. Lamb, David R. "Androgens and Exercise." *Medicine and Science in Sports* 7 (1975):1.
15. National Strength and Conditioning Association. "Position Paper on Prepubescent Strength Training." *National Strength and Conditioning Association Journal* 7 August–September (1985):27.
16. O'Shea, J. P. "Interval Weight Training—A Scientific Approach to Cross-Training for Athletic Strength Fitness." *National Strength and Conditioning Association Journal* 9 April–May (1987):53.
17. O'Shea, J. P. "Power Weight Training and the Female Athlete." *The Physician and Sports Medicine* 9 June (1981): no. 6, p. 109.
18. Pauletto, B. "Strength Training for the Multi-Sport Athlete." *National Strength and Conditioning Association Journal* 9 June–July (1987):70.
19. Prokop, D. "Relieving Pain with Weights." *Runner's World* 17 April (1982): no.4, p. 16.
20. Rasch, Philip J. "The Present Status of Negative (Eccentric) Exercise: A Review." *American Corrective Therapy Journal* 28 (1974):77.
21. Redding, Norman. "Weight Training: Are Low Reps With Heavy Weights Best for Strength Increment?" *Journal of Physical Education* 70 (1973):148.
22. "Relative Strength in Males and Females." *Athletic Training* 10 (1975):189.
23. Research Consortium—AAHPERD. "The Value of Strength Training for Athletic Success." Reston, Virginia: American Alliance for Health, Physical Education, Recreation, and Dance, 1987.
24. Sobey, E. "Aerobic Weight Training." *Runner's World* 16 August (1981):no.8, p. 43.
25. Stanford, B. "The Difference Between Strength and Power." *The Physician and Sports Medicine* 13 July (1985):155.
26. Stern, William H. "Weight Training for Children." *The Athletic Journal* 55 (1974):80.
27. Wilmore, Jack H. "Body Composition and Strength Development." *Journal of Physical Education and Recreation* 46 (1976):38.
28. Wilmore, J. H., R. B. Parr, T. J. Pipes, P. A. Vodak, P. Ward, and P. Leslie. "Circuit Weight Training." *Scholastic Coach* 46 (1976):7.

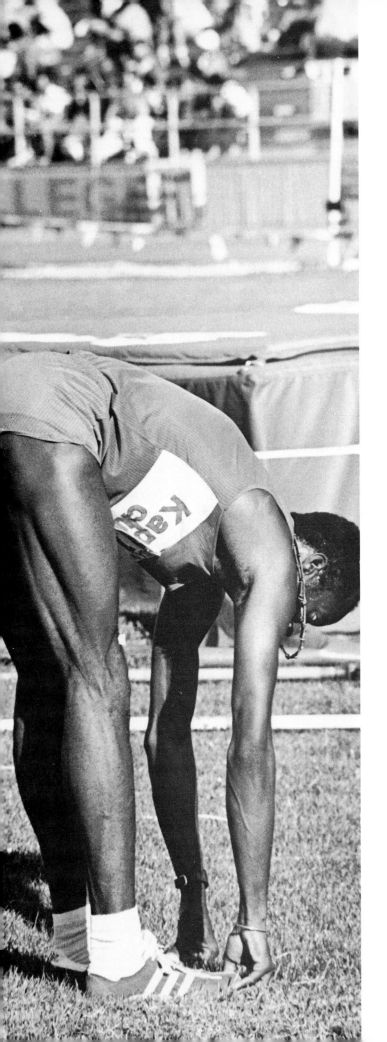

9

WRITING A FLEXIBILITY PROGRAM

Objectives

After study of this chapter you should be able to

1. write a flexibility program, tailor-made to your choice of exercises;
2. pass a multiple-choice mastery self-check involving the selection of appropriate flexibility programs for persons desiring various choices of exercises.

Flexibility refers to the range of motion possible at a joint or a series of joints. A certain amount of flexibility is necessary for body movement. Muscles move the body levers by shortening and lengthening muscle tissue and the resistance caused by a lack of flexibility during movement has an effect on body performance.

FACTORS AFFECTING FLEXIBILITY

Flexibility is influenced by three major factors: (1) the bone structure of the joint; (2) the amount of tissue surrounding the joint; and (3) the extensibility of ligaments, tendons, and muscle tissue that cross over the joint. Of these factors, the third component is the one that can be most affected by a proper flexibility program.

Sedentary living habits and increased inactivity are the major contributors to a loss of flexibility. Inactivity causes muscles and connective tissue to lose extensibility. An increase in body fat often accompanies inactivity and contributes to decreased flexibility.

Physical therapists tell us that insufficient flexibility is frequently the cause of improper body movement. Thus, insufficient flexibility can contribute to improper sitting, walking, running, and other body movements.

Flexibility tends to be specific to particular movements and to particular joints of the body. This means that a person might be flexible in the shoulder girdle but inflexible in the lower limbs. Most people tend to lack flexibility in the posterior thigh, anterior hip, lower back, neck, and shoulders. In order to increase overall body flexibility, it is necessary to engage in basic flexibilty exercises that will affect the large muscle groups of these areas. These exercises should be performed on a daily basis to ensure that increases in flexibility will not be lost again because of inactivity. The nice thing about a flexibility program is that once a good degree of flexibility is obtained, it only takes a few minutes each day to maintain it.

TYPES OF STRETCHING

Increased flexibility of the body can be achieved through the proper use of stretching exercises. Muscular tissue, ligaments, tendons, and other tissues that limit joint movement can be affected by properly stretching them. Most stretching techniques are either of a ballistic nature (a fast, jerky, bobbing movement) or a static stretch (a slow, sustained movement).

In order to determine which type of stretching procedure is best, you must understand that certain sensory receptors located in the muscles and joints are stimulated by specific kinds of stretching movements. When a muscle is stretched suddenly, sensory receptors within that muscle are stimulated and the muscle shortens. This, of course, is counterproductive since the muscle you are attempting to lengthen is now shorter.

If the muscle is stretched slowly, other sensory receptors are activated that override the initial stretch response and inhibit muscle contraction. Thus, the muscle will relax and you can lengthen the muscle without stress of movement. The more relaxed a muscle is, the less chance there will be of an injury during the stretching movement.

Ballistic stretching causes the muscle you are attempting to stretch to contract at the same time. This reduces the effectiveness of your stretching and often causes muscle soreness. The slow, sustained movements of **static stretching** help cause the muscle to relax and lengthen and, thus, increase flexibility. Much muscle soreness is prevented or alleviated by using static stretching. When performing the recommended flexibility exercises in your flexibility program use a slow, sustained stretch.

An important element of any flexibility program is the proper use of stretching exercises and warm-up. Flexibility exercises should not be done at the beginning of the warm-up period. The temperatures in the muscles, ligaments, tendons, and other tissues are relatively low at this time and it appears that the tissues are less flexible and more vulnerable to injury through overstretching, especially if stretching is of a ballistic nature. Spend some time doing light exercise such as brisk walking, slow jogging, or cycling to increase the tissue temperature. A good rule is to warm up until you begin to perspire. This increase in body temperature will ensure that the stretching is safer and much more productive in obtaining increased flexibility.

The question sometimes arises as to how long a person should hold the various stretches when engaging in a flexibility program. There is no research data that indicates an optimal time to hold a specific stretch. It takes at least six seconds of slow, sustained static stretching to stimulate the sensory receptors that bring about muscle relaxation. In the *Fitness for Life* program we suggest that you hold the stretch position for ten or more seconds. As you progress with your flexibility program, it will become easier to hold the stretch position for a longer period of time. The specific recommended procedure to obtain the stretch position is to go through the movement slowly until the muscles and connective tissue stretch far enough to experience the so-called **stretch stress**. This is a feeling of stress, but with no undue pain. Hold this position for ten or more seconds while consciously relaxing the muscles of the body. Then release the body slowly and return to the starting position. Repeat this procedure for the given number of repetitions as called for in the selected flexibility exercise.

GUIDELINES FOR STRETCHING

The following are some guidelines to use in your flexibility program.

1. You must have a daily stretching program because it takes time to make progress in flexibility.

2. Select simple exercises to begin stretching a muscle group.

3. Be sure to warm up the muscles gradually before doing any stretching exercises.

4. Move into the stretching position slowly and continue until stretch on the muscle is felt. Remember that excessive pain is not part of a good stretching program.

5. After reaching a good stretch position, hold that position for ten or more seconds.

6. As the muscles are being stretched, always try to relax the muscle that is being placed in a stretched position.

7. When the stretching exercise is complete, release the body slowly from the exercise position.

8. It is important to remember that stretching exercises are not meant to be competitive. Trying too hard can lead to injury and a loss of flexibility.

Developing a safe and effective flexibility program requires careful planning. Proper use of flexibility in the conditioning program is important in the development of total fitness.

WRITING A FLEXIBILITY PROGRAM

In this unit you will learn how to write a flexibility program. All the exercises used in the flexibility program are described and illustrated in the Flexibility Exercises section located at the end of this chapter. Each description gives an explanation of the muscles stretched by the exercise; the starting position; the action to be used in performing the exercise; any precautions that you need to be aware of while performing the exercise; and the number of sets and repetitions to be used.

By using the Flexibility Program Work Sheet located in Appendix C, writing a flexibility program is a simple two-step process.

Step 1. Fill in the general information on the work sheet.
Step 2. Write a flexibility program.

To help you become familiar with these steps, we will write a flexibility program for a sample case.

CASE
Sally Norton

Sally is interested in developing a program to help her increase her flexibility. Using the Flexbility Program Work Sheet and the step-by-step instructions that follow, write her program. Her *Flexibility Fitness Category* is *Good* for the Sit-and-Reach and *Very Good* for the Shoulder Lift.

Step 1: Filling in the general information on the work sheet

Item 1. Fill in Sally's full name and date.

Item 2. Check the *Flexibility Fitness Category* that Sally is in for the flexibility tests. This information can be obtained by taking the flexibility appraisal in chapter 2. Sally has the following flexibility test scores: *Good* for the Sit-and-Reach and *Very Good* for the Shoulder Lift. Write this information next to the blanks in item 2.

Item 3. For Sally's flexibility program circle *daily,* which indicates that she must engage in her flexibility exercises every day of the week.

Step 2: Writing a flexibility program

Now that you have filled out the flexibility information, you can write a flexibility program for Sally. To do this, use the flexibility chart at the bottom of the work sheet.

The first column on this chart is labeled *Body Parts.* Listed under this heading are the various muscle-group areas Sally should stretch in order to develop flexibility.

The second column on the chart is labeled *Exercise.* Under this heading are a series of letters corresponding to the flexibility exercises. For each body part there is an exercise or a selection of exercises. A description of each exercise is explained in the Flexibility Exercises section at the end of the chapter. Sally selects exercises D, A, G, I, K, M, and J to increase her flexibility. Look up the specific exercises and write their names in the *Exercise Preference* column. The number of sets and repetitions are already given. Remember to do slow, sustained stretching in order to prevent sore muscles.

When you have completed the work sheet, compare your copy with the one in figure 9.1.

Flexibility Program Work Sheet

1. Name _____ *Sally Norton* _____ Date _____

2. Flexibility Fitness Category
   A. Sit-and-Reach _____ *Good* _____
   B. Shoulder Lift _____ *Very Good* _____

3. Exercise Days for Flexibility: (Daily)

FLEXIBILITY

Body Parts	Exercise	Exercise Preference	Sets	Repetitions
Low back muscles	C Ⓓ E	Sitting curl	1	10
Hamstrings	Ⓐ B	Sitting toe touch	1	10
Trunk rotators	F Ⓖ	Leg-over	1	10
Hip flexors	H Ⓘ	Table-lying knee-pull	1	10
Pectoral muscles	Ⓚ L	Door frame stretch	1	10
Heel cords	Ⓜ N	Heel cord stretch	1	10
Pelvic muscles	Ⓙ	Billig stretch	1	10

*Letters refer to charts in the flexibility program.

Figure 9.1.

Instructions: Following are cases of two individuals requesting flexibility programs. Read each one carefully and answer the multiple-choice items related to the case by circling the letter of the best answer. You may use the flexibility exercise charts and your Flexibility Program Work Sheet to help you find the correct answers.

A. Peter is a twenty-nine-year-old accountant who wants to include flexibility exercises in his fitness program. He would like to use exercises D, B, F, I, J, K, and M.
   1. Peter will need to do his flexibility exercises
     a. Mon., Wed., Fri.
     b. Tues., Thurs., Sat.
     c. daily.
     d. Mon., Tues., Wed., Thurs.
   2. Exercise M will stretch
     a. pectoral muscles.
     b. heel cords.
     c. pelvic girdle.
     d. hip flexors.
   3. Exercise F is called
     a. cross-legged curl.
     b. sitting twist.
     c. leg-over.
     d. lying knee-pull.

B. Norma is an eighteen-year-old college student. She has requested help in organizing a flexibility program. She has selected flexibility exercises D, B, F, H, L, M, and J.
   1. Exercise B will stretch
     a. hamstrings.
     b. back extensors.
     c. trunk rotators.
     d. hip flexors.
   2. Norma will perform how many repetitions of exercise H?
     a. 6 to each side
     b. 8 to each side
     c. 10 to each side
     d. 12 to each side
   3. While doing exercise L, she will hold the stretch position for
     a. 2+ seconds.
     b. 3+ seconds.
     c. 4+ seconds.
     d. 10+ seconds.

Answers:

A. 1. c   B. 1. a
   2. b   2. c
   3. b   3. d

If you responded correctly to each item, you are ready to proceed with the next unit.

FLEXIBILITY EXERCISES

FLEXIBILITY
Sitting Toe-Touch

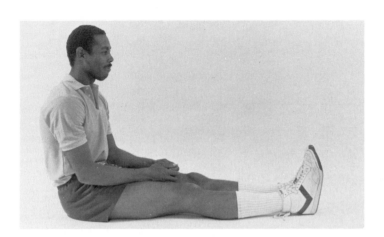

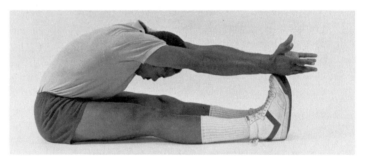

Muscles stretched: Hamstrings.

Starting position: Sit on the floor with legs straight and together.

Action: Extend arms forward toward toes, palms up. Stretch to or beyond toes until stretch pain is felt. Hold 10+ seconds. Return to starting position.

Precautions: Do not bob. Keep legs straight.

Repetitions: 10.

FLEXIBILITY
Hamstring Stretch

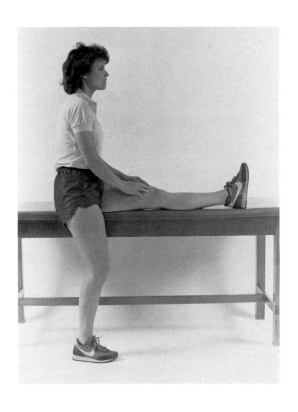 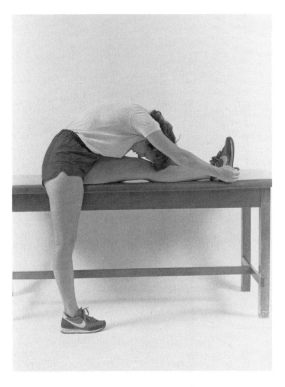

Muscles stretched: Hamstrings.

Starting position: Sit with one leg extended on table, opposite leg hanging.

Action: Bend forward at waist and attempt to touch toes or beyond. Hold 10+ seconds. Return to starting position.

Precaution: Do not bob. Keep extended leg straight.

Repetitions: 10 times each side.

FLEXIBILITY
Cross-Legged Curl

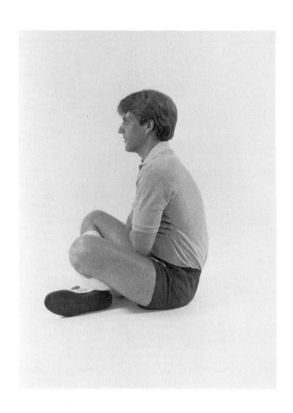 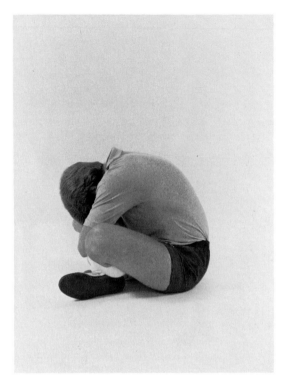

Muscles stretched: Back extensors.

Starting Position: Sit with legs crossed and arms folded or relaxed.

Action: Tuck in chin and curl forward attempting to touch forehead to knees. Hold 10+ seconds. Return to starting position.

Precautions: Do not bob. Keep buttocks on the mat.

Repetitions: 10.

FLEXIBILITY
Sitting Curl

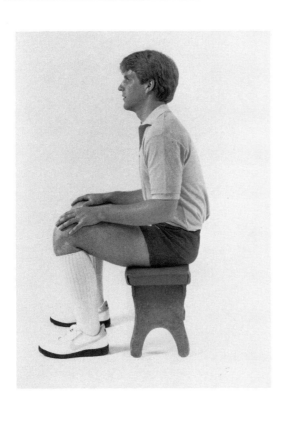 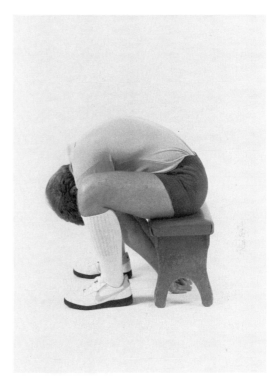

Muscles stretched: Low back extensors.

Starting position: Sit on chair with hips back, feet flat on floor and spread slightly apart.

Action: Tuck in chin and curl forward between knees with arms hanging toward the floor. Continue until a stretch pain is felt in lower back. Hold 10+ seconds. Return to starting position.

Precautions: Keep hips well back in the chair. Keep feet flat.

Repetitions: 10.

FLEXIBILITY
Knee-Chest Curl

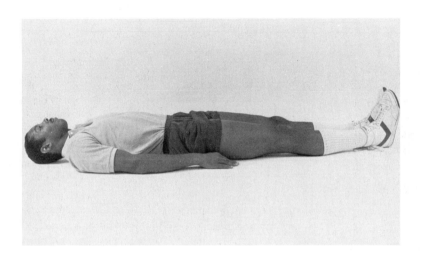

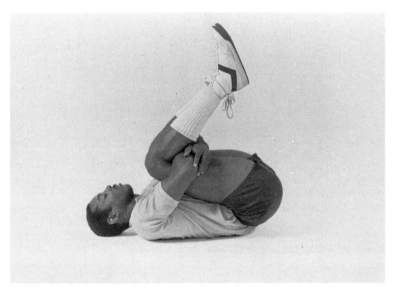

Muscles stretched: Low back extensors.

Starting position: Lie on back.

Action: Bring both knees to chest, grabbing just under knees and pulling knees toward armpits. Hold 10+ seconds. Return to starting position.

Precautions: Avoid placing excess weight on back of the neck.

Repetitions: 10.

FLEXIBILITY
Sitting Twist (on floor)

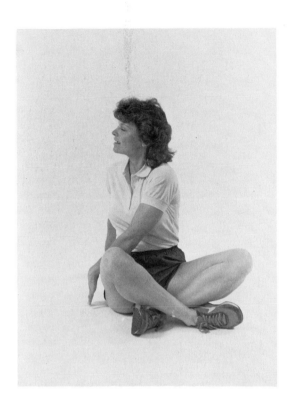
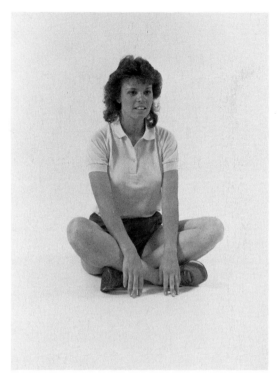

Muscles stretched: Trunk rotators.

Starting position: Sit with legs crossed.

Action: Twist body to right. Place hands on right side of thigh and pull. Hold 10+ seconds. Return to starting position. Repeat to opposite side.

Precautions: Keep trunk straight and sit tall.

Repetitions: 10 to each side.

FLEXIBILITY
Leg-Over

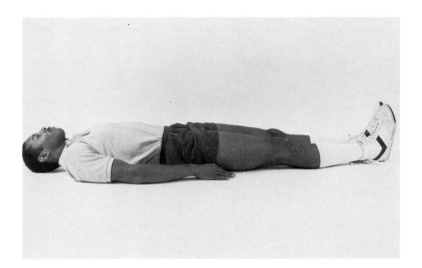

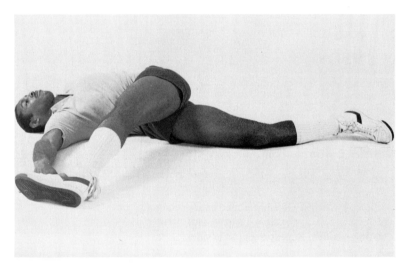

Muscles stretched: Trunk rotators and gluteal muscles.

Starting position: Lie on back with arms extended to the sides at shoulder level.

Action: Raise left leg to a vertical position, keeping leg straight. Twist body to touch left leg to right hand. Hold 10+ seconds. Return to starting position. Repeat to opposite side.

Precautions: Keep knees straight. Keep arms and trunk on the mat.

Repetitions: 10 to each side.

FLEXIBILITY
Lying Knee-Pull

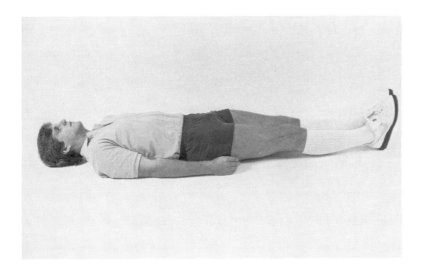

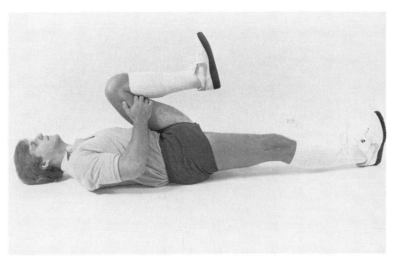

Muscles stretched: Hip flexors, hamstrings, and lower-back muscles.

Starting position: Lie on back with legs extended.

Action: Bring left knee to chest, grabbing just under knee with both hands. Pull until a stretch pain is felt. Hold 10+ seconds. Return to starting position. Repeat to opposite side.

Precaution: Keep extended leg straight and on the floor. Stretch slowly.

Repetitions: 10 to each side.

FLEXIBILITY
Table-Lying Knee-Pull

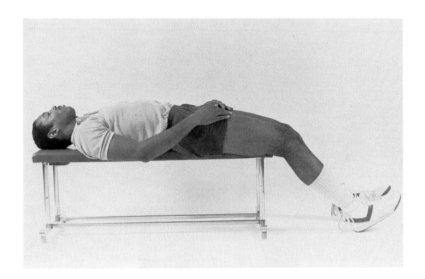

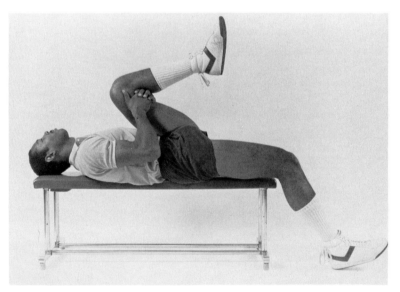

Muscles stretched: Hip flexors, hamstrings, and lower-back muscles.

Starting position: Lie on back on a table with legs over the edge.

Action: Bring left knee to chest, grabbing just below knee with both hands. Let left leg hang freely over the table edge. Hold 10+ seconds. Return to starting position. Repeat to opposite side.

Precautions: Make sure free leg hangs relaxed over the table edge. Stretch only one leg at a time. Bring knee toward armpit rather than chest.

Repetitions: 10 to each side.

FLEXIBILITY
Billig Stretch

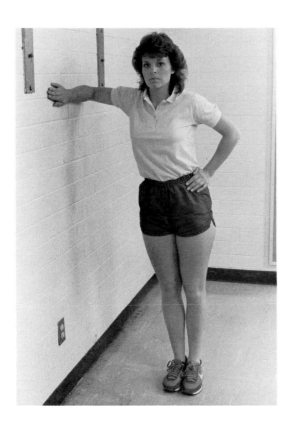 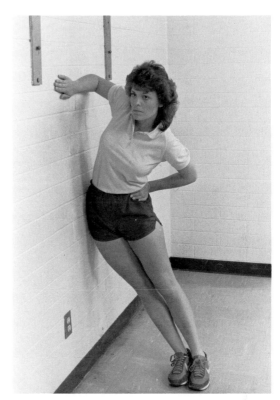

Muscles stretched: Muscles of pelvic girdle.

Starting position: Stand with feet together and right side to wall, about 18 inches from the wall. Place right hand and forearm against the wall at shoulder level. Place heel of left hand on buttocks.

Action: Keeping body straight and facing forward, move hips forward and inward to the wall below hand by contracting abdominal and gluteal (buttock)

muscles and pushing with left hand. Hold for 10+ seconds. Return to starting position. Repeat to opposite side.

Precautions: Keep knees straight. Keep hips and shoulders facing forward.

Repetitions: 10 to each side. 3 times daily to avoid menstrual cramps.

FLEXIBILITY
Doorframe Stretch

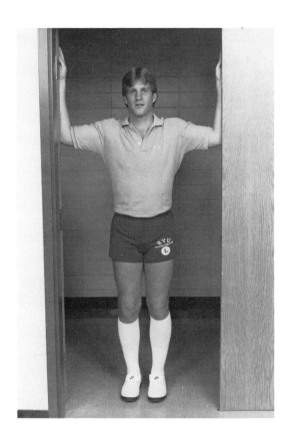 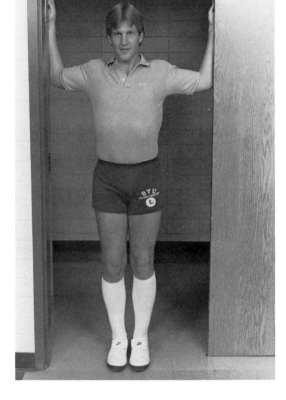

Muscles stretched: Pectoral muscles.

Starting position: Stand facing doorway, hands on wall on either side with upper arms straight out and elbows bent.

Action: Walk through doorway until stretch pain is felt. Hold 10+ seconds. Repeat with arms at 45° angle upward.

Precautions: Maintain good standing posture.

Repetitions: 10.

FLEXIBILITY
Chair Stretch

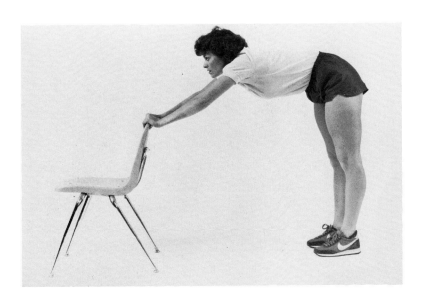

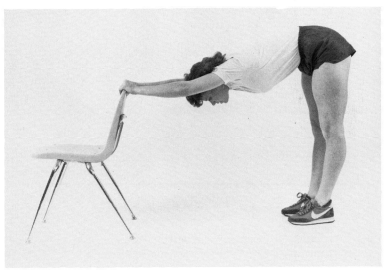

Muscles stretched: Pectoral muscles.

Starting position: Stand with feet apart (sideways) facing the back of the chair. Reach forward and place both hands on the chair back.

Action: Draw head and chest downward by contracting abdominal muscles. Hold 10+ seconds. Return to starting position.

Precautions: Keep feet spread and well back from the chair. Keep lower back flat with no arch.

Repetitions: 10.

FLEXIBILITY
Heel-Cord Stretch

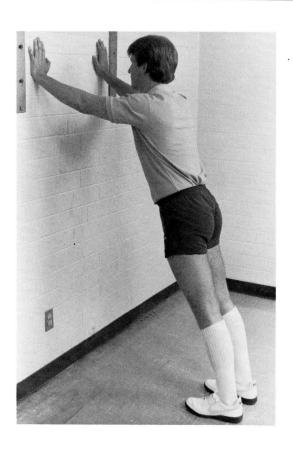 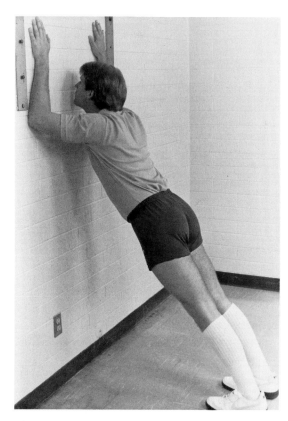

Muscles stretched: Heel cord, gastrocnemius, soleus.

Starting position: Stand facing the wall with palms against the wall and body at arm's length. Spread feet apart slightly.

Action: Keeping feet flat and body in a straight line, lean forward allowing elbows to bend slightly until a stretch pain is felt in calf muscles. Hold 10+ seconds. Return to starting position.

Precautions: Keep knees and body straight and feet flat. For more stretch, put a book under balls of feet.

Repetitions: 10.

FLEXIBILITY
Sitting Heel-Cord Stretch

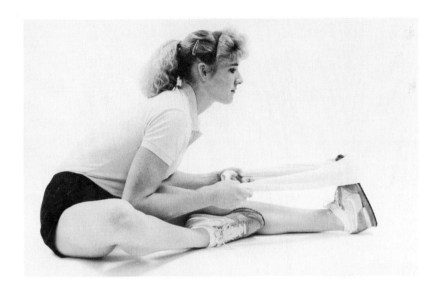

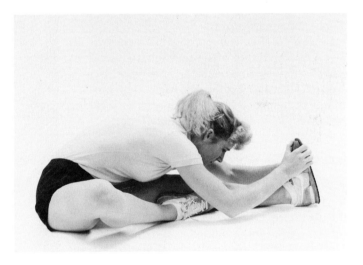

Muscles stretched: Heel cord, gastrocnemius, soleus.

Starting position: Sit on the floor with one leg extended and the opposite leg bent with the foot against the inside of the thigh.

Action: Hook a towel around the ball of the foot and pull the toes toward the knee. If flexible enough, the hand can be used to pull the toes toward the knee. Hold for 10+ seconds and return to the starting position.

Precautions: Keep knee straight. If necessary, lean forward at the waist and hips to increase the stretch.

Repetitions: 10 times each leg.

10

APPLYING A FLEXIBILITY PROGRAM

Objective

After study of this chapter you should be able to

- use your own written flexibility program and contract to engage in an appropriate flexibility program.

A person can maintain good joint mobility, decrease the chance of injury, enhance body posture, and improve the development of motor skills by engaging in a regular flexibility program.

Although it takes time to improve or maintain flexibility, this is time well spent. Now that you have completed chapter 9, you are ready to start your own individualized program. Before you begin your program, it will be helpful to read the answers to some commonly asked questions about flexibility.

COMMONLY ASKED QUESTIONS

Will strength-training exercises that employ a full range of motion of a joint be as effective as regular flexibility exercises in increasing flexibility? As long as a full range of motion is used, proper strength-training techniques will promote and help maintain a functional range of motion. Strength exercises are usually performed not more than three days per week and flexibility exercises are recommended on a daily basis; therefore, you would want to supplement your strength program with specific flexibility exercises.

What are the uses of flexibility exercises in an athletic training program? Flexibility exercises allow the athlete to improve the range of joint motion and, thus, contribute to athletic skill. Increased flexibility may also reduce muscle soreness and the chance of injury.

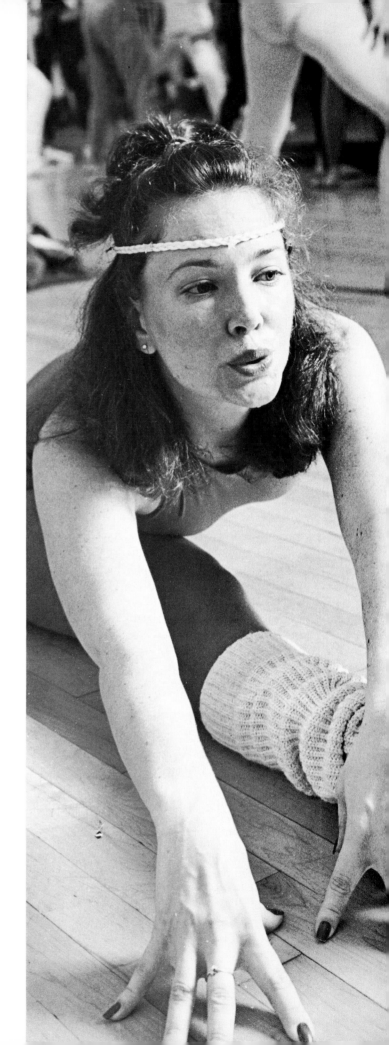

Should I stretch before or after an activity? It is suggested that you stretch before an activity, but remember to warm up before starting your stretching routine. Postactivity stretching is a good way to offset muscle tightness and reduce the soreness that might follow a workout. Flexibility can be increased with a proper stretching program regardless of the time of day.

How can I avoid having lower-back pain? Most of the people in the United States will suffer from lower-back pain sometime in their life. It is estimated that over 75 million Americans suffer from chronic lower-back pain each year. This problem costs employers millions of dollars in lost income and production due to sick leave from work and medical expenses. Unfortunately, in many cases, this problem could have been prevented. Lower-back pain is caused by physical inactivity, poor posture and body mechanics, and excessive body fat, all of which contribute to increased stress on the body parts.

Weak abdominal muscles, combined with tight lower-back muscles, cause an unnatural forward tilt of the pelvis. This imbalance can place undue pressure on the lower back and cause pain. Excessive fat around the midsection of the body can also contribute to the forward tilt of the pelvis and, thus, cause lower-back pain.

Figure 10.1 contains some excellent information on your back and how to care for it. By following these suggestions you can reduce the chance of lower-back pain. The incidence of lower-back pain can also be reduced by including flexibility and strength exercises in your fitness program. Specific exercises can be found in the units on strength and flexibility.

Why do you suggest that I stretch every day? Since the purpose of a flexibility program is to relieve muscle tension and tightness, a daily stretching helps not only to relax muscles used in activity, but also to relax muscles that tighten due to the stresses of daily life. The few minutes spent each day in stretching can be a tremendous aid in stress management.

If my legs are flexible, why can't I assume the rest of my body is flexible? Research results have established that flexibility tends to be highly specific to a particular movement or body part. A person might have excellent range of motion in some areas and below normal range in other movements. This indicates that in order to obtain extensibility of the muscles and connective tissue surrounding each of the joints, you must engage in a total body flexibility program.

Why can't I just use my stretching exercises as the only means of warm-up? The components that make up muscle and connective tissue are less stretchable and more vulnerable to injury if they are not warmed up previous to activity. Since stretching exercises usually elongate the tissue to a greater extent than normal, a warm-up before doing stretching exercises is beneficial.

What is PNF? **PNF** stands for **proprioceptive-neuromuscular-facilitation** and is a stretching procedure that utilizes a partner to assist in the flexibility routine. It involves the contraction and relaxation of both the muscle being stretched and the opposing muscles. If both people have been trained in PNF techniques, it can be a very effective means of increasing flexibility, but if the partner is overzealous and doesn't know proper procedures, there is some danger of injury to the joint and muscles.

How can I tell if I am overstretching? To ensure safe stretching, pay attention to the feeling in the body part or parts being stretched. Do not stretch the tissues to the point where you feel pain. Remember, a flexibility program is not meant to be competitive or to cause injury or pain.

Since I am a runner, should I just stretch the backs of my legs? A flexibility program should be designed to stretch the entire body. In body movement you operate as a linked system with the various segments functioning together; thus, a comprehensive flexibility program is essential. Flexibility is specific to a joint and so you must use specific exercises for the various parts of the body.

Can I use external heat to increase the temperature and thus aid my stretching program? External heat applied to the body might increase circulation to an area and thus increase the elasticity of the tissues. If a person has an injury and is using flexibility exercises in the rehabilitation program, the application of external heat would prove beneficial.

I get abdominal pains during my period. Is there a specific flexibility exercise you might suggest? The use of the Billig stretch demonstrated in the section on flexibility exercises has proven to be an excellent exercise to aid in this problem.

Do people lose flexibility as they get older? Research indicates that there is a steady decrease in flexibility from childhood through old age. The connective tissue especially seems to be affected

Your Back and How to Care For It

HOW TO STAY ON YOUR FEET WITHOUT TIRING YOUR BACK

To prevent strain and pain in everyday activities, it is restful to change from one task to another before fatigue sets in. Housewives can lie down between chores, others should check body position frequently, drawing in the abdomen, flattening the back, bending the knees slightly.

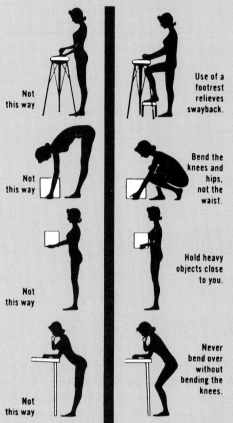

Not this way

Use of a footrest relieves swayback.

Not this way

Bend the knees and hips, not the waist.

Hold heavy objects close to you.

Not this way

Not this way

Never bend over without bending the knees.

HOW TO PUT YOUR BACK TO BED

For proper bed posture, a firm mattress is essential. Bedboards, sold commercially, or devised at home, may be used with soft mattresses. Bedboards, preferably, should be made of ¾ inch plywood. Faulty sleeping positions intensify swayback and result not only in backache but in numbness, tingling, and pain in arms and legs.

Incorrect:
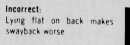
Lying flat on back makes swayback worse

Correct:
Lying on side with knees bent effectively flattens the back. Flat pillow may be used to support neck, especially when shoulders are broad

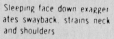
Use of high pillow strains neck, arms, shoulders

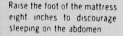
Sleeping on back is restful and correct when knees are properly supported

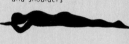

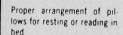

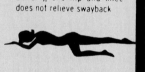
Sleeping face down exaggerates swayback, strains neck and shoulders

Raise the foot of the mattress eight inches to discourage sleeping on the abdomen

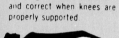
Bending one hip and knee does not relieve swayback

Proper arrangement of pillows for resting or reading in bed.

HOW TO SIT CORRECTLY

A back's best friend is a straight, hard chair. If you can't get the chair you prefer, learn to sit properly on whatever chair you get. To correct sitting position from forward slump: Throw head well back, then bend it forward to pull in the chin. This will straighten the back. Now tighten abdominal muscles to raise the chest. Check position frequently.

Relieve strain by sitting well forward, flatten back by tightening abdominal muscles, and cross knees.

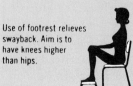

Use of footrest relieves swayback. Aim is to have knees higher than hips.

Correct way to sit while driving, close to pedals. Use seat belt or hard backrest, available commercially.

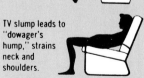

TV slump leads to "dowager's hump," strains neck and shoulders.

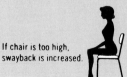

If chair is too high, swayback is increased.

Keep neck and back in as straight a line as possible with the spine. Bend forward from hips.

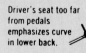

Driver's seat too far from pedals emphasizes curve in lower back.

Strained reading position. Forward thrusting strains muscles of neck and head.

Figure 10.1.

by the aging process and, thus, loses flexibility. It should be emphasized that a major factor that decreases flexibility is inactivity. Exercise programs have been found to be effective in the improvement of flexibility in elderly subjects.

Are females normally more flexible than males? Some studies have found that elementary school girls are more flexible than boys and this difference appears to exist throughout life. Even though there may be a difference, both sexes can still benefit from a proper flexibility program.

Is it possible to be too flexible? Some data indicates that muscles and joints that are too loose or too flexible may be more susceptible to injury than muscles with an average range of motion, especially if a person is engaging in a contact sport such as football. This can be offset by combining a strength program with the flexibility program and thus decreasing the chance of injury. A person should adjust the conditioning program to obtain flexibility but not so much as to place the muscles and joints in a vulnerable position.

APPLYING A FLEXIBILITY PROGRAM

By using the Flexibility Program Contract in figure 10.2, preparing your own flexibility fitness program is a fairly easy six-step process.

Step 1. Prepare your own Flexibility Program Work Sheet.

Step 2. Fill out your Flexibility Program Contract.

Step 3. Get your contract approved.

Step 4. Implement the program and record your progress on the Flexibility Program Progress Log in figure 10.3.

Step 5. Check your progress.

Step 6. Complete your contract.

To help you become familiar with these procedures, we will go through them step-by-step.

Step 1: Preparing your own Flexibility Program Work Sheet

You should have learned how to complete a personal Flexibility Program Work Sheet in chapter 9. If you have not already written a work sheet for yourself, do it now before going on with this unit.

Step 2: Filling out your Flexibility Program Contract

The Flexibility Program Contract in figure 10.2 will help you implement your flexibility program. This contract is quite easy to fill out if you have completed a Flexibility Program Work Sheet as explained in chapter 9. With your work sheet in front of you, fill out the contract as follows:

Item 1. Fill in your full name, age, and sex.

Item 2. Record your *Flexibility Fitness Category* for each of the flexibility tests. This information can be found in item 2 of your Flexibility Program Work Sheet.

Item 3. Fill in the number of weeks you will engage in your flexibility program.

Step 3: Getting your contract approved

When you have filled in your program, you should have it approved. If you are a student in a physical education class, the contract can be signed by your instructor. If you are not in some organized class, then have it signed by a friend.

Step 4: Implementing your program and recording your progress on the Flexibility Program Progress Log

Begin your flexibility program as soon as your contract has been approved. After each exercise period, fill in your Flexibility Program Progress Log in figure 10.3. It will help you keep an accurate account of your work in the program. During each exercise session, write the date and day of your workouts in the log. Check the exercises you engaged in.

Step 5: Checking your progress

After completing five weeks of your program, is is recommended that you take a progress check by retaking the flexibility tests explained in chapter 2. The check will give you some idea of how you are progressing in your flexibility program. If you wish to

Flexibility Program Contract

1. Name _____ Age _____ Sex _____

2. Flexibility Fitness Category

    A. Sit-and-Reach _____

    B. Shoulder Lift _____

3. Number of Weeks for Program _____

Signature _____

Contract approval date _____ Approved by _____

Reassessment check date _____ Approved by _____

Contract completion date _____ Approved by _____

Figure 10.2.

Flexibility Program Progress Log

Name _____

Beginning Flexibility Category

    A. Sit-and-Reach _____

    B. Shoulder Lift _____

Flexibility Exercises

Date	Day	A	B	C	D	E	F	G	H	I	J	K	L	M

Figure 10.3.

make changes in your program after your progress check, you may do so. Make sure you have the progress check approved in order to reaffirm your decision to improve your flexibility.

Step 6: Completing your contract

When you have completed your flexibility program for the selected number of weeks, have your contract approved by the person who originally signed it. You may want to retake the flexibility tests in chapter 2 to determine your improvement.

This does not mean that you will stop engaging in a flexibility program. If you do not make stretching a part of your fitness program, the gains in flexibility will be lost.

SUGGESTIONS FOR FURTHER READING

1. Allers, Vern. "Flexibility Stretching." *The Athletic Journal* 56 (1975):34.
2. Anderson, B. *Stretching.* Bolinas, California: Shelter Publications, 1980.
3. Beaulieu, J. E. "Developing a Stretching Program." *The Physician and Sports Medicine* 9 November (1981):59.
4. Beaulieu, J. E. *Stretching For All Sports.* Pasadena, California: The Athletic Press, 1980.
5. Cooper, D. H., and J. Fair. "Developing and Testing Flexibility." *The Physician and Sports Medicine* 10 Oct (1978):137.
6. Corbin, C. B., and L. Noble. "Flexibility: A Major Component of Physical Fitness." *Journal of Physical Education and Recreation* 6 (1980):23.
7. DeVries, H. A. "Evaluation of Static Stretching Procedures for Improvement of Flexibility." *Research Quarterly* 33 (1962):222.
8. Etnyre, B. R., and L. D. Abraham. "Changes in Range of Ankle Dorsiflexion Using Three Popular Stretching Techniques." *American Journal of Physical Medicine* 65 (1986):189.
9. "Flexibility—Round Table" *National Strength and Conditioning Association Journal* 6 August–September (1984):10.
10. Hardy, L. "Improving Active Range of Hip Flexion." *Research Quarterly for Exercise and Sport* 56 (1985):111.
11. Hardy, L., and D. Jones. "Dynamic Flexibility and Proprioceptive Neuromuscular Facilitation." *Research Quarterly for Exercise and Sport* 57 (1986):150.
12. Holt, L. E., and R. Smith. "The Effect of Selected Stretching Programs on Active and Passive Flexibility." Del Mar, California: Research Center for Sport, 1983.
13. Holt, L. E., T. M. Travis, and T. Okita. "Comparative Study of Three Stretching Techniques." *Perceptual and Motor Skills* 31 (1970):611.
14. Hutinger, Paul. "How Flexible Are You?" *Aquatic World Magazine,* January, 1974.
15. Ishii, D. K. "Flexibility Strexercises for Co-ed Groups." *Scholastic Coach* 45 (1976):31.
16. Johns, R. J., and V. Wright. "Relative Importance of Various Tissues in Joint Stiffness." *Journal of Applied Physiology* 17 (1962):824.
17. Knortz, K. "Flexibility Techniques." *National Strength and Conditioning Coaches Association Journal* 7 April–May (1985):50.
18. Kottke, F. J., D. L. Pauley, and K. A. Ptak. "The Rationale for Prolonged Stretching for Correction of Shortening of Connective Tissue." *Archives of Physical Medicine Rehabilitation* 47 (1966):345.
19. Lucas, R. C., and R. Koslow. "Comparative Study of Static, Dynamic, and Proprioceptive Neuromuscular Facilitation Stretching Techniques on Flexibility." *Perceptual and Motor Skills* 58 (1984):615.
20. McKenzie, R. *Treat Your Own Back.* Lower Hutt, New Zealand: Spinal Publications, 1980.
21. Moore, M. A., and R. S. Hutton. "Electromyographic Investigation of Muscle Stretching Techniques." *Medicine and Science in Sports and Exercise* 12 (1980):322.
22. Sapega, A. A., T. C. Quedenfeld, R. A. Moyer, and R. A. Butler. "Biophysical Factors in Range of Motion Exercise." *The Physician and Sports Medicine* 12 December (1981):57.
23. Shellock, F. "Physiological, Psychological and Injury Prevention Aspects of Warm-up." *National Strength and Conditioning Association Journal* 8 October–November (1986):24.
24. Weaver, N. "Ten Easy Exercises to Prevent Injuries." *Runner's World* 17 November (1982):no. 11, p. 40.
25. Wilkerson, G. B. "Buddy Up and Stretch." *Scholastic Coach* 52 September (1982):62.
26. Wishchina, B. "First Hand Facts on the Benefits of Massage." *Runner's World* 16 September (1981):no. 9.
27. Wright, V., and R. J. Johns. "Physical Factors Concerned With the Stiffness of Normal and Diseased Joints." *Johns Hopkins Medical Journal* 106 (1960):215.

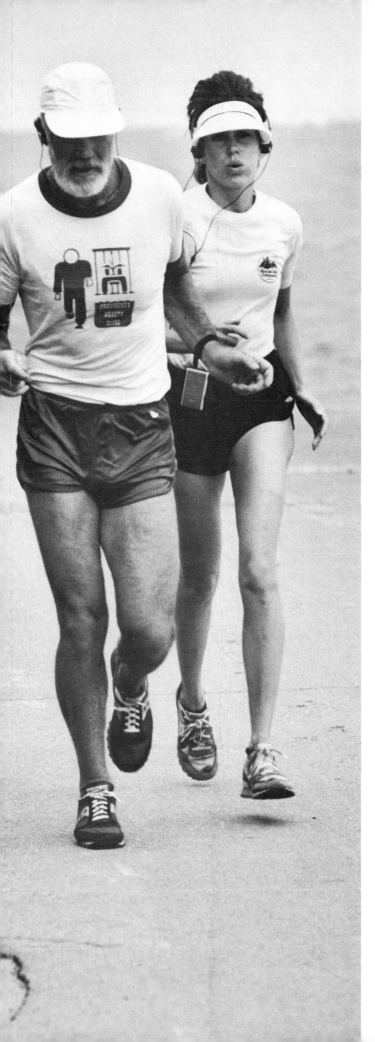

11

WRITING AND APPLYING A RELAXATION PROGRAM

Objective

After study of this chapter you should be able to

- write and engage in a personalized relaxation program to combat stress and tension.

There is one thing that is certain in our society: we face a great deal of stress and tension during the course of each day. With the large amount of political and economic uncertainty that exists in the world today, it is not surprising that we are sometimes referred to as the "uptight generation." A great amount of time is devoted to the conservation of our natural resources; in the long run, however, it might be the preservation of human resources that will be of most benefit in bringing about significant changes in the world.

The word **stress** is used continually in our society, but it is not an easy concept to define. The late Dr. Hans Selye, who was associated with Montreal's Institute of Experimental Medicine and Surgery and considered one of the world's greatest authorities on stress, defined it as the nonspecific response of the human organism to any demand that is placed upon it. In simple terms, he explained stress as the rate of wear and tear on the body. It is impossible to escape from the stresses of life, but by learning to cope with and adapt to stress, people can begin to control stress rather than have stress control them.

Today, we face an extremely complex environment. The invention of machines and their use in all aspects of our lives require many types of adjustment that were not needed in more primitive times. We also must adjust to the activities of a great number of social institutions. Emotional tension, accidents, fire hazards, crime, juvenile delinquency, unemployment, retirement from work, old age, security, illness, dying, and the high cost of living are but a few of our worries.

According to Dr. Selye, it is the continual adaptation of the body to various stresses that ultimately exhausts its ability to adapt, wears out vital organs, and leads to a variety of illnesses.

The symptoms of stress include headaches; feelings of tenseness, restlessness, fatigue; lack of concentration; difficulty in relaxing and falling asleep at night; lack of appetite; and unreasonable irritability.

In the previous chapters, it has been possible to quantify the amount of activity needed to affect the selected physical fitness variables such as cardiovascular endurance, body composition, strength, and flexibility. It is not that simple to write an individualized program for stress management. We are all unique individuals and what one person might perceive as a negative stressor could easily be a positive form of stress for another person.

It is known that physical activity can be used to control and reduce the effects of stress in daily life. Data from various studies indicate that exercise does produce relaxation and elevation in mood states. The physiological cause of these changes is not known, but the results are observable. Dr. Herbert DeVries reviewed the research and concluded that, "A close examination of the available data suggests substantial agreement among researchers that there is a tranquilizer effect from exercise. Although more corroborative evidence is needed, we should draw a cautious conclusion that appropriate types, intensities, and duration of exercise can bring about a significant tranquilizer effect." It may be that physical activity reduces muscle tension and helps eliminate some of the chemicals produced by a reaction to stress.

Another way exercise may help reduce stress is by diverting the stress from one body system to another. Selye explains that when a specific task becomes difficult, a change of activity might be better than even rest. For example, if you are having difficulty in studying for a final exam, it might be advantageous to jog, swim, or play racquetball for fifteen or more minutes than to just sit and become more frustrated and increase the stress on certain systems of the body. By engaging in physical activity, you might divert the mental stress to the circulatory and muscular systems; thus, you would reduce negative stress and obtain beneficial results from a cardiovascular endurance stimulus.

You might wish to consider one of the various physical fitness programs explained in this book as a form of stress management.

In the *Fitness for Life* program, the emphasis so far has been on the contracting of muscle and the vigorous movement of the body. There is also a need, however, to learn how to relax muscle tissue. Relaxation is a neuromuscular accomplishment that results in a reduction of tension in the skeletal musculature.

As the human body reacts to stress, adrenalin is released from the adrenal glands, and it brings about different responses in the various body systems. One of the responses is the tightening and contraction of muscle tissue. When the large muscle groups, located in the stomach, neck, chest, upper and lower back, and the extremities, contract for extended periods of time, pain is the result. The way to get rid of this pain is to learn to relax these muscle groups.

Many years ago the outstanding psychiatrist, William James, recognized the importance of muscle tension and its effect on the human body when he stated, "If muscular contraction is removed from emotion, then no emotion is left." This concept is the basis of any muscle-relaxing program that attempts to relieve tension by reducing muscular activity.

You are told to relax, but it is not as easy as it sounds to bring the human body into a state of relaxation. Even at rest there is always some tension in the muscles of your body. This occurs because gravity acts on the body and causes a reflex mechanism within the muscles whenever they are stretched.

Dr. Edmund Jacobsen used relaxation in the practice of psychiatry for years. He has shown that people can be taught to relax away the residual tensions, regularly present in the normal, quiet resting stage, to the point where muscle tonus virtually disappears. One study indicated that the muscle tension in people could be reduced as much as 30 percent following the use of relaxation techniques. Some of the other results of a relaxation program are:

1. a reduction of previously elevated blood pressure;
2. reduction of insomnia;
3. relief from nervous headaches;
4. lowered sensitivity to loud noises and pain-causing stimuli, including menstrual distress;
5. relief from some forms of stomach distress;
6. ability to rest the mind for a few minutes in the course of a busy day, and to return to difficult tasks with renewed energy and a clearer mind.

It should be emphasized that relaxation is not a panacea for all of the ills that beset people, but it can be used to help us increase our ability to cope with the stresses of day-to-day living.

RELAXATION TECHNIQUES

The following techniques, developed by Dr. Jacobsen, have been used by many people in organizing relaxation programs. To start, make certain that you are warm and the room is well ventilated. A warm bath is sometimes helpful as a beginning activity for your relaxation routine. The object of the program is to concentrate on the "feeling" of muscle tenseness as it appears when a muscle contracts, and how tenseness disappears when you allow a muscle to relax.

The starting position for the relaxation exercises is on the back with the legs straight, arms at the sides, and eyes closed. Begin by slowly and deeply inhaling and exhaling four to five times. Try to put your mind at rest by repeating to yourself: "Breathe and let go, breathe and let go." Attempt to make your mind as blank as possible and then let yourself go limp.

Relaxation of Arms (Time: 4–5 min.)

First

Settle back as comfortably as you can. Let yourself relax to the best of your ability. Now clench your right fist, tighter and tighter, and study the tension as you do so. Keep it clenched and feel the tension in your right fist, hand, and forearm. Relax. Let the fingers of your right hand become loose, and observe the contrast in your feelings. Let yourself become more relaxed all over.

Second

Clench your right fist very tightly. Hold it and notice the tension again. Now let go. Relax your fingers. Straighten them out and you will notice the difference once more.

Third

Repeat with your left fist. Clench your left fist while the rest of your body relaxes; clench that fist tighter and feel the tension. Now relax. Repeat that once more, enjoying the contrast. Clench the left fist; it is tight and tense. Now do the opposite: relax and feel the difference. Continue relaxing for a while.

Fourth

Clench both fists more and more tightly; both fists are tense; forearms are tense. Study the sensations. Relax. Straighten out your fingers and feel the relaxation. Continue relaxing your hands and forearms more and more.

Fifth

Bend your elbows and tense your biceps; tense them harder and study the tense feelings. Straighten your arms; let them relax and feel the difference. Let the relaxation develop. Tense your biceps again; hold the tension and observe it carefully. Straighten your arms and relax. **Pay close attention to your feelings each time you tense up and relax.**

Sixth

Straighten your arms until you feel tension in the triceps muscles along the backs of your arms. Stretch your arms and feel the tension; then relax. Get your arms back into a comfortable position. Let the relaxation proceed on its own. The arms should feel comfortably heavy as you allow them to relax. Straighten the arms once more so that you feel the tension. Relax.

Seventh

Concentrate on pure relaxation in the arms without any tension. Make your arms comfortable and let them relax more and more. Continue relaxing your arms further. Even when your arms seem fully relaxed, try to go that extra bit farther, and try to achieve deeper and deeper levels of relaxation.

Relaxation of Facial Area, Neck, Shoulders, and Upper Back (Time: 4–5 min.)

First

Let all your muscles go loose and heavy. Settle back quietly and comfortably. Wrinkle up your forehead; wrinkle it more tightly. Now stop wrinkling your forehead; relax and smooth it out. Picture the entire forehead and scalp becoming smoother as the relaxation increases.

Second

Frown and crease your brows and study the tension. Let go of the tension again. Smooth out the forehead once more. Close your eyes more and more tightly. Feel the tension. Relax your eyes. Keep your eyes closed, gently, comfortably, and notice the relaxation.

Third

Clench your jaws, bite your teeth together; study the tension throughout the jaws. Relax your jaws now. Let your lips part slightly. Appreciate the relaxation.

Fourth

Press your tongue hard against the roof of your mouth. Feel the tension. Let your tongue return to a comfortable and relaxed position.

Fifth

Now purse your lips; press your lips together more and more tightly. Relax the lips. Note the contrast between tension and relaxation. Feel the relaxation all over your face, forehead and scalp, eyes, jaws, lips, tongue, and throat. The relaxation progresses further and further.

Sixth

Now attend to your neck muscles. Press your head back as far as it can go and feel the tension in the neck; roll it to the right and feel the tension shift; now roll it to the left. Straighten your head and bring it forward; press your chin against your chest. Let your head return to a comfortable position, and study the relaxation. Let the relaxation develop.

Seventh

Shrug your shoulders, and hold the tension. Drop your shoulders and feel the relaxation. Relax your neck and shoulders. Shrug your shoulders again and move them around. Bring your shoulders up and forward and back. Feel the tension in your shoulders and in your upper back. Drop your shoulders once more and relax. Let the relaxation spread deeply into the shoulders, right into your back muscles; relax your neck and throat and your jaws and other facial areas as the pure relaxation takes over and grows deeper and deeper.

Relaxation of Chest, Stomach, and Lower Back (Time: 4–5 min.)

First

Relax your entire body to the best of your ability. Feel that comfortable heaviness that accompanies relaxation. Breathe easily and freely in and out. Notice how the relaxation increases as you exhale. As you breathe out, feel that relaxation.

Second

Breathe in and fill your lungs; inhale deeply and hold your breath. Study the tension. Now exhale; let the walls of your chest grow loose, and push the air out automatically. Continue relaxing and breathe freely and gently. Feel the relaxation and enjoy it.

Third

With the rest of your body as relaxed as possible, fill your lungs again. Breathe in deeply and hold it again. Breathe out and appreciate the relief. Just breathe normally. Continue relaxing your chest and let the relaxation spread to your back, shoulders, neck, and arms. Simply let go and enjoy the relaxation.

Fourth

Now pay attention to your abdominal muscles; make your stomach hard. Notice the contrast. Once more, press and tighten your stomach muscles. Hold the tension and study it. Relax. Notice the general well-being that comes with relaxing your stomach.

Fifth

Draw your stomach in; pull the muscles in and feel the tension. Now relax again. Let your stomach out. Continue breathing normally and easily, and feel the gentle massaging action all over your chest and stomach. Pull your stomach in again and hold the tension. Now push out and tense your muscles in that position; hold the tension. Pull in once more and feel the tension.

Sixth

Relax your stomach fully. Let the tension dissolve as the relaxation grows deeper. Each time you breathe out, notice the rhythmic relaxation in both your lungs and your stomach. Notice how your chest and stomach relax more and more. Try to let go of all contractions anywhere in your body.

Seventh

Now direct your attention to your lower back. Arch up your back, make your lower back quite hollow, and feel the tension along your spine. Settle down comfortably again, relaxing the lower back. Arch your back up and feel the tension as you do so. Try to keep the rest of your body as relaxed as possible. Try to localize the tension throughout your lower back area. Relax once more, relaxing further and further.

Eighth

Relax your lower back, relax your upper back, spread the relaxation to your stomach, chest, shoulders, arms, and facial area. Relax these parts further and further and even deeper.

Relaxation of Hips, Thighs, and Calves, Followed by Complete Body Relaxation

First

Let go of all tensions and relax. Now flex your buttocks and thighs. Flex your thighs by pressing down your heels as hard as you can. Relax and note the difference. Straighten your knees and flex your thigh muscles again. Hold the tension. Relax your hips and thighs. Allow the relaxation to proceed on its own.

Second

Press your feet and toes downward, away from your face, so that your calf muscles become tense. Study the tension. Relax your feet and calves.

Third

This time bend your feet toward your face so that you feel tension along your shins. Bring your toes right up. Relax again. Keep relaxing for a while. Now let yourself relax further all over. Relax your feet, ankles, calves, shins, knees, thighs, buttocks, and hips. Feel the heaviness of your body as you relax still further.

Fourth

Now spread the relaxation to your stomach, waist, lower back. Let go more and more. Feel that relaxation all over. Let it proceed to your upper back, chest, shoulders, and arms, and right to the tips of your fingers. Keep relaxing more and more deeply. Make sure that no tension has crept into your throat; relax your neck and your jaws and all your facial muscles. Keep relaxing your whole body for a while.

Fifth

Now you can become twice as relaxed as you are by taking a deep breath and slowly exhaling. With your eyes closed so that you become less aware of objects and movements around you and thus prevent any surface tensions from developing, breathe in deeply and feel yourself becoming heavier. Take in a long, deep breath and let it out very slowly. Feel how heavy and relaxed you have become.

Sixth

In a state of perfect relaxation you should feel unwilling to move a single muscle in your body. Think about the effort that would be required to raise your right arm. As you *think* about raising your right arm, see if you can notice any tensions that might have crept into your shoulder and arm. Now you decide not to lift the arm but to continue relaxing. Observe the relief and the disappearance of tension.

Seventh

Continue to relax. When you want to get up, count backward from four to one. You should then feel fine and refreshed, wide awake and calm.

After learning the relaxation techniques, you must practice them. Set aside a regular period of time once a day for positive relaxation. By being aware of the signs of muscle tenseness that may develop during the day, you can learn to apply relaxation techniques and thus prevent tension before it creates a problem.

MEDITATION

In the past few years the art of **meditation** has received a lot of publicity, especially with the introduction of transcendental meditation (T.M.). The basic principle behind all forms of meditation is the attempt to "clear" the mind, and thus remove the stimuli that might be causing stress and tension within the body.

This form of relaxation is one that can be learned quite easily and then utilized during the course of the day to obtain a quick release from increased muscular tension.

The steps to utilize to achieve relaxation through meditation follow.

1. Choose a place that is comfortable and free from noise. You will need at least ten minutes of uninterrupted time.
2. Sit quietly in a chair in an upright position with your hands resting on the thighs. Close your eyes or turn out the lights to reduce the visual stimulation. Reduce or eliminate as much of the outside stimulation as possible.
3. Starting at the feet and progressing to the head, relax all of the body parts.
4. Now pay attention to your breathing.
5. Count ten breaths and then as you breathe out, silently say the word *two*. Attending to your breathing and the word *two* helps keep other disturbing thoughts from entering into your mind.
6. Continue to breathe easily and slowly for ten minutes.

As you learn to relax and enjoy the act of meditation, you will be able to block out the external environment and thus obtain a relaxed calm attitude any time or any place you might have the need to relax. This can prove to be time well spent; it will provide you with the stimulus for a longer, happier, and healthier life.

SUGGESTIONS FOR FURTHER READING

1. Bartlett, J. C. "Emotional Mood and Memory in Young Children." *Journal of Experimental Child Psychology* 34 August (1982):59.
2. Bartley, D. A. R., and F. Z. Belgrave. "Physical Fitness and Psychological Well-being in College Students." *Health Education* June–July (1987):57.
3. Blumenthal, J., R. S. Williams, R. B. Williams, and A. Wallace. "Effects of Exercise on the Type A Behavior Pattern." *Psychosomatic Medicine* 42(1980):289.
4. Boland, J. M. "Relaxation Exercises." *School and Community* 68 October (1981):34.
5. Bortz, W., P. Angwin, I. Mefford, M. Boarder, N. Neyce, and J. Barchas. "Catecholamines, Dopamine, and Endorphin Levels During Extreme Exercises." *New England Journal of Medicine* 305(1981):466.
6. "Coping with Stress." *NASSP Bulletin* 65 December (1981):1.
7. Daniels, R. L. "Life Change Unit Rating Scale for College Students." *Health Educator* 13 July/August (1982):29.
8. Danish, S., and B. Hale. "Toward an Understanding of Sport Psychology." *Journal of Sport Psychology* 3(1981):90.
9. Deffenbacher, J. L. "Anxiety Management Training and Self Control Desensitization 15 Months Later." *Journal of Counseling Psychology* 28 September (1981):459.
10. DeVries, H. "Tranquilizer Effects of Exercise: A Critical Review." *The Physician and Sports Medicine* 9 November (1981):53.
11. DeVries, H. A., R. Wirswell, R. Bubulian, and R. Moritani. "Tranquilizer Effects of Exercise." *American Journal of Physical Medicine* 60(1981):57.
12. Folkins, C., B. Lynch, and M. Gardener. "Psychological Fitness As A Function of Physical Fitness." *Archives of Physical Medicine and Rehabilitation* 53(1982):503.
13. Garner, R. "When Breaking Point Comes to a Head." *Times Education Supplement* 3412 November 20 (1981):7.
14. Greenberg, J. S. "Study of Stressors in the College Student Population." *Health Educator* 12 July/August (1982):8.
15. Griffiths, T. J., D. J. Steele, P. Vaccaro, and M. B. Karpman. "The Effects of Relaxation Techniques on Anxiety and Underwater Performance." *International Journal of Sport Psychology* 12(1981):176.
16. Hinskelwood, M. "Burnout—Fact, Fad, or Fiction?" *Momentum* 12 October (1981):16.
17. "How to Fight Stress on the Job." *Mademoiselle* 88 August (1982):98.
18. "How Well Are You Handling Stress in Your Life?" *Health* 14 August (1982):52.
19. Jacobson, E. *Progressive Relaxation.* Chicago, Illinois: University of Chicago Press, 1938.
20. Jobin, J. "Nine Minutes of Exercise: Better than a Nap." *Redbook* 158 January (1982):84.
21. McGeer, P. H., and E. G. McGeer. "Chemistry of Mood and Emotion." *Annual Review of Psychology* 31(1980):273.
22. "Meditation—Medicine?" *Health* 14 July (1982):16.
23. Morgan, W. P. "Psychological Benefits of Physical Activity." In F. J. Nagle and H. J. Montoye (Eds.), *Exercise in Health and Disease.* Springfield, Illinois: Charles C. Thomas Publisher, 1981.
24. Neal, N. D. "Mental Imagery and Relaxation in Skill Rehearsal." *Scholastic Coach* 51 December (1981):48.
25. Pauly, J., J. Palmer, C. Wright, and G. Pfeiffer. The Effect of a 14-Week Employee Fitness Program on Selected Physiological and Psychological Parameters." *Journal of Occupational Medicine* 249(1982):457.
26. Ross, M., and L. Pyott. "Stress Management: A Workshop for College Students." *Journal of National Association of Women's Deans, Administrators, and Counselors* (1981).
27. Selye, H. *Stress Without Distress.* New York: Signet, 1974.
28. Selye, H. *The Stress of Life.* New York: McGraw-Hill Book Company, 1978.
29. Sime, W. E. "A Comparison of Exercise and Meditation in Reducing Physiological Response to Stress." *Medicine and Science in Sports* 9(1977):55.
30. Wheeler, E. "Body Alive! Flexibility: Why You Need It, How to Get It." *Essence* 12 January (1982):96.
31. "Youngsters Under Stress—What Parents Can Do." *U.S. News & World Report* 93 August 9 (1982):58.

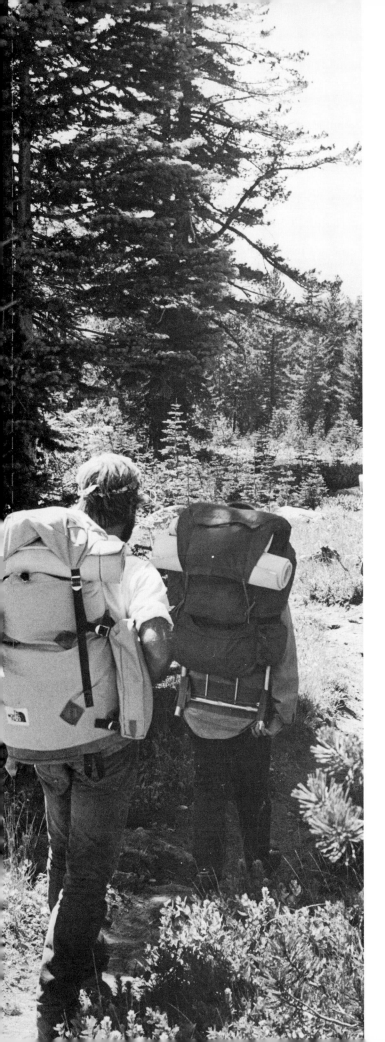

12

WHERE DO WE GO FROM HERE?

Objective

After study of this chapter you should

- reaffirm your decision to make physical fitness an important part of your life-style.

To look good and feel good are the end results of a planned exercise program. Your body was built to work, and it can be kept in good working order by making exercise a part of your way of life.

A planned program of physical exercise can bring about the following benefits:

1. increase your endurance for specific tasks;
2. increase the capacity and health of your circulatory and respiratory systems;
3. increase the strength and flexibility of your muscle-joint systems;
4. decrease the chance of lower-back disorders;
5. increase the strength of the skeletal system;
6. provide a means to control body weight and a method of decreasing body fat;
7. increase your ability to cope with physical emergencies that are dependent on strength and endurance;
8. have a positive effect upon the internal organs of your body;
9. possibly help delay the physiological aging process;
10. provide you with a foundation upon which to build physical skills and thus improve your physical performance;
11. decrease the onset of fatigue by decreasing the energy expenditure for specific tasks;
12. provide a means to relieve stress and tension;
13. probably help in the stimulation of increased mental activity.

When we started the *Fitness for Life* program, the goal was to convince people to adopt a style of fitness that they would follow for the rest of their life. But fitness can also be a means of saving a person's life. The following letter (written by Dr. Barbara Vance, one of the authors) dramatically explains how personal fitness can literally be a means of saving a life.

Dear Phil,

I'm not sure how you came up with the title for our book, *Fitness for Life*. In my case, the title is literally true.

Now begins the story. I went to Israel on leave during winter semester as a visiting scholar at the University of Haifa. During semester break in Israel in early February I took a bus to Jerusalem to visit with some of the leaders at our Jerusalem campus. While boarding a bus to return to Haifa on February 10, I had a massive brain hemorrhage. I didn't know it was a hemorrhage at the time. I just thought I had pulled a muscle in my neck when I lifted my overnight bag onto the seat beside me. This was 11:00 A.M. Monday morning. I remember feeling very fatigued at the time of the "pulled muscle," but I slumped down in my seat to relax on the two-and-one-half-hour journey back to Haifa.

When I got off the bus in the central bus terminal in Haifa, I still had another bus trip and a walk ahead of me before I arrived at the apartment where I was living with an Israeli family. I had such a headache I seriously thought of taking a cab to the apartment. However, I lugged my overnight bag and a loaded bookpack up a couple of flights of stairs to the city bus stop outside the terminal. My bus was waiting for me there, so I climbed on instead of taking a taxi. I carried my heavy overnight bag and bookpack to the back of the bus, still feeling headachy and terribly fatigued.

I had trouble getting my bags off the bus when we arrived at Mt. Carmel. My halting Hebrew wasn't enough to get the attention of the bus driver, so I went a stop beyond my normal stop before I was able to get off the bus. At that point I tied my bags to my luggage carrier (which I had carried with me to Jerusalem) and hauled them behind me about a half mile before I collapsed. Fortunately, I was still conscious when a women who could speak flawless English came up to me and asked me how she could help me. I gave her my name and address and a telephone number to call at the apartment. Lunch is the main meal of the day in Israel and I hoped that family members would still be home when the woman called for help. Within five minutes my Israeli friends were on the scene and they rushed me to Carmel Hospital only a mile away.

I don't know how much you know about brain hemorrhages, but they usually kill (by asphyxiation) their victims within a few seconds after they occur. It was at least three and one-half hours after my hemorrhage before I arrived at Carmel Hospital. I remember arriving at the hospital emergency room and then I lost consciousness.

Apparently, medical personnel at Carmel could tell immediately that I had had a brain hemorrhage. They called Rambam Hospital, just twenty minutes by ambulance away from Carmel, on the shore of the Mediterranean Sea in Haifa, where the only neurosurgery unit in Israel is located. Fortunately, the chief of neurosourgery and his entire surgical team (each man with an international reputation) were at the hospital when the call about my condition was put through from Carmel Hospital. I was transferred by ambulance to Rambam, but I was clinically dead (i.e., no vital signs) when I arrived there at the emergency room. Apparently, life-saving attempts in the ambulance were not successful. Dr. Feinsod, the chief neurosurgeon, directed Dr. Levy, another member of the surgical team, to relieve the pressure on my brain by drilling two small holes through the top of my skull and evacuating some of the hemorrhage. My vital signs started immediately after that brief surgery. I was wheeled in for a CAT scan X ray and the next morning I had an angiogram. My family was also notified.

Thirty hours after I arrived at Rambam I was wheeled into surgery, where surgeons repaired the aneurysm that caused the hemorrhage and resected most of the vascular system on the surface of my cerebellum, the most plastic part of the adult human brain, where the hemorrhage had first occurred. The cerebellum, as you know, is the master control panel for all body movement plus many other bodily functions.

My surgeons consider me their miracle patient because I survived a massive brain hemorrhage and ten hours of neurosurgery. The mortality rate for such hemorrhages is extremely high, not only in Israel, but in this country as well. I have a 10-inch incision down the back of my skull and neck as a memento of my surgery. Obviously, miracles cannot be explained; however, my surgeons later informed me that my body could not have survived such a lengthy trauma if I had not been in such excellent physical cardiovascular condition. Dr. Feinsod told me my heart pumped away during ten hours of surgery like that of a twenty-one-year-old athlete (I am in my early fifties). I haven't been able to jog since 1977 because of knee problems, but have always walked briskly at least an hour a day since then. While living in Israel, I went for long walks (about four miles each day) in the evenings. During that long bus ride from Jerusalem to Haifa, other parts of my vascular system took over that of the brain because they were in excellent condition.

I'm writing this so you can have another bit of evidence that physical fitness really pays off. I have continued to engage in cardiovascular fitness activities because I hate diets with a mad purple passion and would rather get the rewards of feeling good from good cardiovascular exercise. I got started on fitness activities in 1971 when I returned from a six-week trip to Europe, during which I gained 15 pounds. Ugh!! No diet for me. I peeled those extra pounds off by jogging them away. I have stayed with a CV program since then, even though I had to switch to walking, to stave off fat and a heart attack (heart problems run in our family) Little did I know that my many years of CV conditioning would literally save my life when I had a brain hemorrhage.

No one expects to have a brain hemorrhage, or a heart attack. I surely didn't. I didn't even know at the time that I had experienced a brain hemorrhage. College students think they are immortal. So did I. Boy, did I ever find out how really mortal I am!

When I returned to the states from Israel I had lost all my conditioning due to six long weeks of recovery, mostly lying in bed. My muscles had atrophied. Thanks to a very wise and experienced physical therapist who could see that it would be important to regain my physical fitness, I worked hard on regaining it during five weeks of HARD physical therapy at Utah Valley Regional Medical Center. It felt wonderful to feel energy and strength come back. I have learned to ignore signals from the brain that would pull me to the ground, and can pick up my canes now and walk for an hour a day again. I get tired easily. Walking an hour a day for me is like running a marathon daily! Imagine running a marathon every day of your life.

I'm sure my cardiovascular conditioning is the secret to my sense of well-being now. I have a few "inconveniences" because of the hemorrhage, but being physically fit has made all the difference in the world to my ability to cope with disability and live a quality life-style. I hope your students can catch the vision of the benefits of good cardiovascular conditioning.

Few of your students, most likely, must struggle as I do to maintain cardiovascular conditioning. However, I'll keep up the struggle because it makes the difference for me between being an invalid and simply being disabled. Besides, CV conditioning (fifteen years of it) and God saved my life.

Much love,
Barbara

Since the time this letter was written, Dr. Vance is now able to walk without a cane and carry on an active physical fitness program. Her doctors are amazed and consider her a medical marvel. She is certainly a living testimony of the benefits of a physical fitness program.

One of the most important aspects of a regular fitness program is that it should be fun. If somebody forces you to participate, you will take time to go through a boring, uninteresting, and unpleasant exercise program. In most cases, however, human nature is such that you won't devote any time to something that you don't want to do. Choose your lifetime activities to maintain cardiovascular endurance, proper weight, strength, flexibility, and relaxation, but also engage in physical activity for the enjoyment it provides. Exercise is not an end in itself. Companionship and enjoyment also are beneficial by-products of activity. Your goal should be to develop a life-style that will improve the quality of all of your everyday experiences because of your participation in physical activity.

"To feel better" is the response given by many people when asked why they participate in regular vigorous exercise. When people feel better, they behave in a more positive manner and thus receive more from living. This sense of accomplishment seems to fill people with a feeling of well-being and a new vigor and zest for life. It may be that those people who adopt the habit of regular activity will become new persons emotionally as well as physically.

Whenever you feel like quitting your physical fitness program, think of its positive aspects and concentrate on your success. You can keep track of your success by maintaining a progress chart. This type of chart enables you to compete with yourself rather than with someone else; it gives you the means to compare your current status with your standing in the past. It does not have to be a complicated, record-keeping device; rather, it can be a simple method of writing down such things as calories expended, minutes exercised, and how you felt. You may also want to record periodically some body measurements, percent body fat, and body weight so that you have a standard of comparison by which to determine how much you have achieved. This kind of record can become a matter of pride for you, and the result will be a lot fewer missed exercise sessions.

If you set building a more beautiful body as a goal, take photographs of yourself so that you can see the progress that you are making. It is difficult to remember how you looked a year or two years ago, but by taking photographs, you can see the transformation to a fine physique.

In this book, we have attempted to provide a road map to start you on the way to increased physical fitness. We have provided you with simple, easy-to-follow procedures for improving your level of fitness. Now that you are engaging in a personalized program of physical fitness, you are undoubtedly experiencing the benefits of such a program. You probably feel better, have a more positive self-image, and are more productive in your daily activities. Perhaps others around you have noticed the changes resulting from your exercise program.

Since you are now convinced of the value of physical fitness programs, you will most likely want to share your experiences with others. Why not challenge members of your family or your friends to join you in your fitness endeavors? It will be much more fun to exercise with others and you will be less inclined to procrastinate about your daily exercise session if you have others depending on you. Remember to have them begin with an appropriate medical examination and fitness appraisal. Perhaps you will want to work together for a Presidential Sports Award.

The President's Council on Physical Fitness and Sports has sponsored the Presidential Sports Award Program to motivate the average citizen to a life of activity. The award is offered for most popular sports, including a number that develop a high level of cardiovascular fitness, such as swimming, jogging, bicycling, wrestling, and handball.

The Presidential Sports Award Program is designed to encourage regular participation in activity. The basic qualification is a minimum of fifty hours of participation spread over at least fifty activity sessions within a four-month period of time. Some concessions are made in activities for which seasons are short or access to facilities is limited. The program is open to all men and women. You do not have to be highly skilled to qualify; participation is the important thing.

If you qualify for the Presidential Sports Award, you will receive a handsome enameled pin, a colorful embroidered emblem, and a certificate bearing the President's signature and seal. The President's Council on Physical Fitness and Sports has named the Amateur Athletic Union as the administrator of its nationwide award program. Information on the program, including qualifying standards, application forms, and personal log books, can be obtained free by writing to the Amateur Athletic Union address below.

Presidential Sports Award,
AAU House
P.O. Box 68207
Indianapolis, Indiana 46268

Another outstanding organization is the American Running and Fitness Association. This is a nonprofit organization that is dedicated to the promotion of fitness in the United States. They publish a monthly newsletter that contains up-to-date information concerning fitness, nutrition, and stress management. They also have a question and answer service that utilizes sports specialists to answer questions about diet, training, injuries, exercise programs, or any other topic of sports medicine. Information can be obtained from:

American Running and Fitness Association
2001 S. Street, N.W., Suite 540
Washington, D.C. 20009

The way to stay active is to be active. You should prepare yourself now for retirement with an investment in physical vitality, just as you plan for future financial security. With a well-planned road map for physical fitness, you can be off and running toward a happier, healthier, and more effective working mind and body, with *Fitness for Life.*

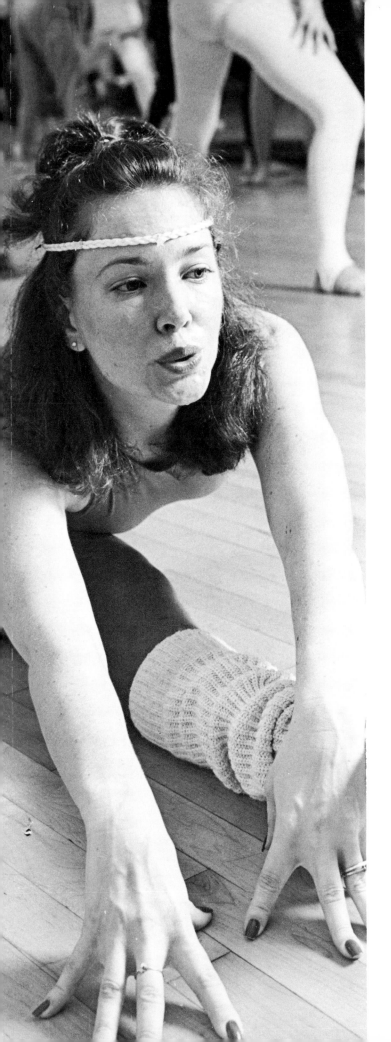

AMERICAN COLLEGE OF SPORTS MEDICINE POSITION STATEMENTS

1. The Recommended Quantity and Quality of Exercise for Developing and Maintaining Fitness in Healthy Adults

2. Proper and Improper Weight Loss Programs

The Recommended Quantity and Quality of Exercise for Developing and Maintaining Fitness in Healthy Adults

Increasing numbers of persons are becoming involved in endurance training activities and thus, the need for guidelines for exercise prescription is apparent.

Based on the existing evidence concerning exercise prescription for healthy adults and the need for guidelines, the American College of Sports Medicine makes the following recommendations for the quantity and quality of training for developing and maintaining cardiorespiratory fitness and body composition in the healthy adult:

1. Frequency of training: 3 to 5 days per week.

2. Intensity of training: 60% to 90% of maximum heart rate reserve or 50% to 85% of maximum oxygen uptake (Vo_2 max).

3. Duration of training: 15 to 60 minutes of continuous aerobic activity. Duration is dependent on the intensity of the activity, thus lower intensity activity should be conducted over a longer period of time. Because of the importance of the "total fitness" effect and the fact that it is more readily attained in

longer duration programs, and because of the potential hazards and compliance problems associated with high intensity activity, lower to moderate intensity activity of longer duration is recommended for the non-athletic adult.

4. Mode of activity: Any activity that uses large muscle groups, that can be maintained continuously, and is rhythmical and aerobic in nature, e.g. running-jogging, walking-hiking, swimming, skating, bicycling, rowing, cross-country skiing, rope skipping, and various endurance game activities.

Rationale and Research Background

The questions, How much exercise is enough? and What type of exercise is best for developing and maintaining fitness? are frequently asked. It is recognized that the term "physical fitness" is composed of a wide variety of variables included in the broad categories of cardiovascular-respiratory fitness, physique and structure, motor function, and many histochemical and biochemical factors. It is also recognized that the adaptive response to training is complex and includes peripheral, central, structural, and functional factors. Although many such variables and their adaptive response to training have been documented, the lack of sufficient in-depth and comparative data relative to frequency, intensity, and duration of training make them inadequate to use as comparative models. Thus, in respect to the above questions, fitness will be limited to changes in Vo_2 max, total body mass, fat weight (FW), and lean body weight (LBW) factors.

Exercise prescription is based upon the frequency, intensity, and duration of training, the mode of activity (aerobic in nature, e.g. listed under No. 4 above), and the initial level of fitness. In evaluating these factors, the following observations have been derived from studies conducted with endurance training programs.

1. Improvement in Vo_2 max is directly related to frequency (2,23,32,58,59,65,77,79), intensity (2,10,13,26,33,37,42,56,77), and duration (3,14,29,49,56,77,86) of training. Depending upon the quantity and quality of training, improvement in Vo_2 max ranges from 5% to 25% (4,13,27,31,35,36,43,45,52,53,62,71,77, 78,82,86). Although changes in Vo_2 max greater than 25% have been shown, they are usually associated with large total body mass and FW loss, or a low initial level of fitness. Also, as a result of leg fatigue or a lack of

motivation, persons with low initial fitness may have spuriously low initial Vo_2 max values.

2. The amount of improvement in Vo_2 max tends to plateau when frequency of training is increased above 3 days per week (23,62,65). For the non-athlete, there is not enough information available at this time to speculate on the value of added improvement found in programs that are conducted more than 5 days per week. Participation of less than two days per week does not show an adequate change in Vo_2 max (24,56,62).

3. Total body mass and FW are generally reduced with endurance training programs (67), while LBW remains constant (62,67,87) or increases slightly (54). Programs that are conducted at least 3 days per week (58,59,61,62,87), of at least 20 minutes duration (48,62,87) and of sufficient intensity and duration to expend approximately 300 kilocalories (Kcal) per exercise session are suggested as a threshold level for total body mass and FW loss (12,29,62,67). An expenditure of 200 Kcal per session has also been shown to be useful in weight reduction if the exercise frequency is at least 4 days per week (80). Programs with less participation generally show little or no change in body composition (19,25,42,62,67,84,85,87). Significant increases in Vo_2 max have been shown with 10 to 15 minutes of high intensity training (34,49,56,62,77,78), thus, if total body mass and FW reduction are not a consideration, then short duration, high intensity programs may be recommended for healthy, low risk (cardiovascular disease) persons.

4. The minimal threshold level for improvement in Vo_2 max is approximately 60% of the maximum heart rate reserve (50% of Vo_2 max) (33,37). Maximum heart rate reserve represents the percent difference between resting and maximum heart rate, added to the resting heart rate. The technique as described by Karvonen, Kentala, and Mustala (37), was validated by Davis and Convertino (14), and represents a heart rate of approximately 130 to 135 beats/minute for young persons. As a result of the aging curve for maximum heart rate, the absolute heart rate value (threshold

level) is inversely related to age, and can be as low as 110 to 120 beats/minute for older persons. Initial level of fitness is another important consideration in prescribing exercise (10,40,46,75,77). The person with a low fitness level can get a significant training effect with a sustained training heart rate as low as 110 to 120 beats/minute, while persons of higher fitness levels need a higher threshold of stimulation (26).

5. Intensity and duration of training are interrelated with the total amount of work accomplished being an important factor in improvement in fitness (2,7,12,40,61,62,76,78). Although more comprehensive inquiry is necessary, present evidence suggests that when exercise is performed above the minimal threshold of intensity, the total amount of work accomplished is the important factor in fitness development (2,7,12,61,62,76,79) and maintenance (68). That is, improvement will be similar for activities performed at a lower intensity-longer duration compared to higher intensity-shorter duration if the total energy cost of the activities are equal.

   If frequency, intensity, and duration of training are similar (total Kcal expenditure), the training result appears to be independent of the mode of aerobic activity (56,60,62,64). Therefore, a variety of endurance activities, e.g. listed above, may be used to derive the same training effect.

6. In order to maintain the training effect, exercise must be continued on a regular basis (2,6,11,21,44,73,74). A significant reduction in working capacity occurs after two weeks of detraining (73) with participants returning to near pretraining levels of fitness after 10 weeks (21) to 8 months of detraining (44). Fifty percent reduction in improvement of cardiorespiratory fitness has been shown after 4 to 12 weeks of detraining (21,41,73). More investigation is necessary to evaluate the rate of increase and decrease of fitness with varying training loads and reduction in training in relation to level of fitness, age, and length of time in training. Also, more information is needed to better identify the minimal level of work necessary to maintain fitness.

7. Endurance activities that require running and jumping generally cause significantly more debilitating injuries to beginning exercisers than other non-weight bearing activities (42,55,69). One study showed that beginning joggers had increased foot, leg, and knee injuries when training was performed more than 3 days per week and longer than 30 minutes duration per exercise session (69). Thus, caution should be taken when recommending the type of activity and exercise prescription for the beginning exerciser. Also, the increase of orthopedic injuries as related to overuse (marathon training) with chronic jogger-runners is apparent. Thus, there is a need for more inquiry into the effect that different types of activities and the quantity and quality of training has on short-term and long-term participation.

8. Most of the information concerning training described in this position statement has been conducted on men. The lack of information on women is apparent, but the available evidence indicates that women tend to adapt to endurance training in the same manner as men (8,22,89).

9. Age in itself does not appear to be a deterrent to endurance training. Although some earlier studies showed a lower training effect with middle-aged or elderly participants (4,17,34,83,86), more recent study shows the relative change in Vo_2 max to be similar to younger age groups (3,52,66,75,86). Although more investigation is necessary concerning the rate of improvement in Vo_2 max with age, at present it appears that elderly participants need longer periods of time to adapt to training (17,66). Earlier studies showing moderate to no improvement in Vo_2 max were conducted over a short time-span (4) or exercise was conducted at a moderate to low Kcal expenditure (17), thus making the interpretation of the results difficult.

   Although Vo_2 max decreases with age, and total body mass and FW increase with age, evidence suggests that this trend can be altered with endurance training (9,12,38,39,62). Also, 5 to 10 year follow-up studies where participants continued their training at a similar level showed maintenance of fitness (39,70). A study of older competitive runners showed decreases in Vo_2 max from the fourth to seventh decade of life, but also showed reductions in their training load (63). More inquiry into the relationship of long-term training (quantity and quality) for both competitors and non-competitors and physiological function with increasing age, is necessary before more definitive statements can be made.

10. An activity such as weight training should not be considered as a means of training for developing Vo_2 max, but has significant value for increasing muscular strength and endurance, and LBW (16,24,47,49,88). Recent studies evaluating circuit weight training (weight training conducted almost continuously with moderate weights, using 10 to 15 repetitions per exercise session with 15 to 30 seconds rest between bouts of activity) showed little to no improvements in working capacity and Vo_2 max (1,24,90).

Despite an abundance of information available concerning the training of the human organism, the lack of standardization of testing protocols and procedures, methodology in relation to training procedures and experimental design, a preciseness in the documentation and reporting of the quantity and quality of training prescribed, make interpretation difficult (62,67). Interpretation and comparison of results are also dependent on the initial level of fitness (18,74–76,81), length of time of the training experiment (20,57,58,61,62), and specificity of the testing and training (64). For example, data from training studies using subjects with varied levels of Vo_2 max, total body mass and FW have found changes to occur in relation to their initial values (5,15,48,50,51), i.e., the lower the initial Vo_2 max the larger the percent of improvement found, and the higher the FW the greater the reduction. Also, data evaluating trainability with age, comparison of the different magnitudes and quantities of effort, and comparison of the trainability of men and women may have been influenced by the initial fitness levels.

In view of the fact that improvement in the fitness variables discussed in this position statement continue over many months of training (12,38,39,62), it is reasonable to believe that short-term studies conducted over a few weeks have certain limitations. Middle-aged sedentary and older participants may take several weeks to adapt to the initial rigors of training, and thus need a longer adaptation period to get the full benefit from a program. How long a training experiment should be conducted is difficult to determine, but 15 to 20 weeks may be a good minimum standard. For example, two investigations conducted with middle-aged men who jogged either 2 or 4 days per week found both groups to improve in Vo_2 max. Mid-test results of the 16 and 20 week programs showed no difference between groups, while subsequent final testing found the 4 day per week group to improve significantly more (58,59). In a similar study with young college men, no differences in Vo_2 max were found among groups after 7 and 13 weeks of interval training (20). These latter findings and those of other investigators point to the limitations in interpreting results from investigations conducted over a short time-span (62,67).

In summary, frequency, intensity and duration of training have been found to be effective stimuli for producing a training effect. In general, the lower the stimuli, the lower the training effect (2,12,13,27,35,46, 77,78,90), and the greater the stimuli, the greater the effect (2,12,13,27,58,77,78). It has also been shown that endurance training less than two days per week, less than 50% of maximum oxygen uptake, and less than 10 minutes per day is inadequate for developing and maintaining fitness for healthy adults.

REFERENCES

1. Allen, T. E., R. J. Byrd, and D. P. Smith. Hemodynamic consequences of circuit weight training. *Res. Q.* 43:299–306, 1976.
2. American College of Sports Medicine. *Guidelines for Graded Exercise Testing and Exercise Prescription.* Philadelphia: Lea and Febiger, 1976.
3. Barry, A. J., J. W. Daly, E. D. R. Pruett, J. R. Steinmetz, H. F. Page, N. C. Birkhead, and K. Rodahl. The effects of physical conditioning on older individuals. I. Work capacity, circulatory-respiratory function, and work electrocardiogram. *J. Gerontol.* 21:182–191, 1966.
4. Bensetad, A. M. Trainability of old men. *Acta. Med. Scandinav.* 178:321–327, 1965.
5. Boileau, R. A., E. R. Buskirk, D. H. Horstman, J. Mendez, and W. C. Nicholas. Body composition changes in obese and lean men during physical conditioning. *Med. Sci. Sports* 3:183–189, 1971.
6. Brynteson, P., and W. E. Sinning. The effects of training frequencies on the retention of cardiovascular fitness. *Med. Sci. Sports* 5:29–33, 1973.
7. Burke, E. J., and B. D. Franks. Changes in Vo_2 max resulting from bicycle training at different intensities holding total mechanical work constant. *Res. Q.* 46:31–37, 1975.
8. Burke, E. J. Physiological effects of similar training programs in males and females. *Res. Q.* 48:510–517, 1977.
9. Carter, J. E. L., and W. H. Phillips. Structural changes in exercising middle-aged males during a 2-year period. *J. Appl. Physiol.* 27:787–794, 1969.
10. Crews, T. R., and J. A. Roberts. Effects of interaction of frequency and intensity of training. *Res. Q.* 47:48–55, 1976.
11. Cureton, T. K., and E. E. Phillips. Physical fitness changes in middle-aged men attributable to equal eight-week periods of training, non-training and retraining. *J. Sports Med. Phys. Fitness* 4:1–7, 1964.

12. Cureton, T. K. *The Physiological Effects of Exercise Programs upon Adults.* Springfield: Charles C. Thomas, Publisher, 1969.
13. Davies, C. T. M., and A. V. Knibbs. The training stimulus, the effects of intensity, duration and frequency of effort on maximum aerobic power output. *Int. Z. Angew. Physiol.* 29:299–305, 1971.
14. Davis, J. A., and V. A. Convertino. A comparison of heart rate methods for predicting endurance training intensity. *Med. Sci. Sports* 7:295–298, 1975.
15. Delorme, T. L. Restoration of muscle power by heavy resistance exercise. *J. Bone and Joint Surgery* 27:645–667, 1945.
16. Dempsey, J. A. Anthropometrical observations on obese and nonobese young men undergoing a program of vigorous physical exercise. *Res. Q.* 35:275–287, 1964.
17. DeVries, H. A. Physiological effects of an exercise training regimen upon men aged 52 to 88. *J. Gerontol.* 24:325–336, 1970.
18. Ekblom, B., P. O. Åstrand, B. Saltin, J. Sternberg, and B. Wallstrom. Effect of training on circulatory response to exercise. *J. Appl. Physiol.* 24:518–528, 1968.
19. Flint, M. M., B. L. Drinkwater, and S. M. Horvath. Effects of training on women's response to submaximal exercise. *Med. Sci. Sports* 6:89–94, 1974.
20. Fox, E. L., R. L. Bartels, C. E. Billings, R. O'Brien, R. Bason, and D. K. Mathews. Frequency and duration of interval training programs and changes in aerobic power. *J. Appl. Physiol.* 38:481–484, 1975.
21. Fringer, M. N., and A. G. Stull. Changes in cardiorespiratory parameters during periods of training and detraining in young female adults. *Med. Sci. Sports* 6:20–25, 1974.
22. Getchell, L. H., and J. C. Moore. Physical training: comparative responses of middle-aged adults. *Arch. Phys. Med. Rehab.* 56:250–254, 1975.
23. Gettman, L. R., M. L. Pollock, J. L. Durstine, A. Ward, J. Ayres, and A. C. Linnerud. Physiological responses of men to 1, 3, and 5 day per week training programs. *Res. Q.* 47:638–646, 1976.
24. Gettman, L. R., J. Ayres, M. L. Pollock, J. L. Durstine, and W. Grantham. Physiological effects of circuit strength training and jogging on adult men. *Arch. Phys. Med. Rehab.* In press.
25. Girandola, R. N. Body composition changes in women: Effects of high and low exercise intensity. *Arch. Phys. Med. Rehab.* 57:297–300, 1976.
26. Gledhill, N., and R. B. Eynon. The intensity of training. In: A. W. Taylor and M. L. Howell (editors). *Training Scientific Basis and Application.* Springfield: Charles C. Thomas, Publisher, pp. 97–102, 1972.
27. Golding, L. Effects of physical training upon total serum cholesterol levels. *Res. Q.* 32:499–505, 1961.
28. Goode, R. C., A. Virgin, T. T. Romet, P. Crawford, J. Duffin, T. Pallandi, and Z. Woch. Effects of a short period of physical activity in adolescent boys and girls. *Canad. J. Appl. Sports Sci.* 1:241–250, 1976.
29. Gwinup, G. Effect of exercise alone on the weight of obese women. *Arch. Int. Med.* 135:676–680, 1975.
30. Hanson, J. S., B. S. Tabakin, A. M. Levy, and W. Nedde. Long-term physical training and cardiovascular dynamics in middle-aged men. *Circ.* 38:783–799, 1968.
31. Hartley, L. H., G. Grimby, A. Kilbom, N. J. Nilsson, I. Åstrand, J. Bjure, B. Ekblom, and B. Saltin. Physical training in sedentary middle-aged and older men. *Scand. J. Clin. Lab. Invest.* 24:335–344, 1969.
32. Hill, J. S. The effects of frequency of exercise on cardiorespiratory fitness of adult men. M. S. Thesis, Univ. of Western Ontario, London, 1969.
33. Hollmann, W., and H. Venrath. Experimentelle Untersuchungen zur bedentung aines trainings unterhalb and oberhalb der dauerbeltz stungsgranze. In: Korbs (editor). *Carl Diem Festschrift.* W. u. a. Frankfurt/Wein, 1962.
34. Hollman, W. Changes in the capacity for maximal and continuous effort in relation to age. *Int. Res. Sport Phys. Ed.,* (E. Jokl and E. Simon, editors). Springfield: Charles C. Thomas, Publisher, 1964.
35. Huibregtse, W. H., H. H. Hartley, L. R. Jones, W. D. Doolittle, and T. L. Criblez. Improvement of aerobic work capacity following non-strenuous exercise. *Arch. Env. Health,* 27:12–15, 1973.
36. Ismail, A. H., D. Corrigan, and D. F. McLeod. Effect of an eight-month exercise program on selected physiological, biochemical, and audiological variables in adult men. *Brit. J. Sports Med.* 7:230–240, 1973.
37. Karvonen, M., K. Kentala, and O. Mustala. The effects of training heart rate: a longitudinal study. *Ann. Med. Exptl. Biol. Fenn.* 35:307–315, 1957.
38. Kasch, F. W., W. H. Phillips, J. E. L. Carter, and J. L. Boyer. Cardiovascular changes in middle-aged men during two years of training. *J. Appl. Physiol.* 314:53–57, 1972.
39. Kasch, F. W., and J. P. Wallace. Physiological variables during 10 years of endurance exercise. *Med. Sci. Sports* 8:5–8, 1976.
40. Kearney, J. T., A. G. Stull, J. L. Ewing, and J. W. Strein. Cardiorespiratory responses of sedentary college women as a function of training intensity. *J. Appl. Physiol.* 41:822–825, 1976.
41. Kendrick, Z. B., M. L. Pollock, T. N. Hickman, and H. S. Miller. Effects of training and detraining on cardiovascular efficiency. *Amer. Corr. Ther. J.* 25:79–83, 1971.
42. Kilbom, A., L. Hartley, B. Saltin, J. Bjure, G. Grimby, and I. Åstrand. Physical training in sedentary middle-aged and older men. *Scand. J. Clin. Lab. Invest.* 24:315–322, 1969.
43. Knehr, C. A., D. B. Dill, and W. Neufeld. Training and its effect on man at rest and at work. *Amer. J. Physiol.* 136:148–156, 1942.
44. Knuttgen, H. G., L. O. Nordesjo, B. Ollander, and B. Saltin. Physical conditioning through interval training with young male adults. *Med. Sci. Sports* 5:220–226, 1973.
45. Mann, G. V., L. H. Garrett, A. Farhi, H. Murray, T. F. Billings, F. Shute, and S. E. Schwarten. Exercise to prevent coronary heart disease. *Amer. J. Med.* 46:12–27, 1969.
46. Marigold, E. A. The effect of training at predetermined heart rate levels for sedentary college women. *Med. Sci. Sports* 6:14–19, 1974.
47. Mayhew, J. L., and P. M. Gross. Body composition changes in young women with high resistance weight training. *Res. Q.* 45:433–439, 1974.
48. Milesis, C. A., M. L. Pollock, M. D. Bah, J. J. Ayres, A. Ward, and A. C. Linnerud. Effects of different durations of training on cardiorespiratory function, body composition and serum lipids. *Res. Q.* 47:716–725, 1976.
49. Misner, J. E., R. A. Boileau, B. H. Massey, and J. H. Mayhew. Alterations in body composition of adult men during selected physical training programs. *J. Amer. Geriatr. Soc.* 22:33–38, 1974.
50. Moody, D. L., J. Kollias, and E. R. Buskirk. The effect of a moderate exercise program on body weight and skinfold thickness in overweight college women. *Med. Sci. Sports* 1:75–80, 1969.
51. Moody, D. L., J. H. Wilmore, R. N. Girandola, and J. P. Royce. The effects of a jogging program on the body composition of normal and obese high school girls. *Med. Sci. Sports* 4:210–213, 1972.
52. Myrhe, L., S. Robinson, A. Brown, and F. Pyke. Paper presented to the American College of Sports Medicine, Albuquerque, New Mexico, 1970.
53. Naughton, J., and F. Nagle. Peak oxygen intake during physical fitness program for middle-aged men. *JAMA* 191:899–901, 1965.
54. O'Hara, W., C. Allen, and R. J. Shephard. Loss of body weight and fat during exercise in a cold chamber. *Europ. J. Appl. Physiol.* 37:205–218, 1977.

55. Oja, P., P. Teraslinna, T. Partaner, and R. Karava. Feasibility of an 18 months' physical training program for middle-aged men and its effect on physical fitness. *Am. J. Public Health* 64:459–465, 1975.

56. Olree, H. D., B. Corbin, J. Penrod, and C. Smith. Methods of achieving and maintaining physical fitness for prolonged space flight. Final Progress Rep. to NASA, Grant No. NGR–04–002–004, 1969.

57. Oscai, L. B., T. Williams, and B. Hertig. Effects of exercise on blood volume. *J. Appl. Physiol.* 24:622–624, 1968.

58. Pollock, M. L., T. K. Cureton, and L. Greninger. Effects of frequency of training on working capacity, cardiovascular function, and body composition of adult men. *Med. Sci. Sports* 1:70–74, 1969.

59. Pollock, M. L., J. Tiffany, L. Gettman, R. Janeway, and H. Lofland. Effects of frequency of training on serum lipids, cardiovascular function, and body composition. In: *Exercise and Fitness* (B. D. Franks, ed.). Chicago: Athletic Institute, 1969, pp. 161–178.

60. Pollock, M. L., H. Miller, R. Janeway, A. C. Linnerud, B. Robertson, and R. Valentino. Effects of walking on body composition and cardiovascular function of middle-aged men. *J. Appl. Physiol.* 30:126–130, 1971.

61. Pollock, M. L., J. Broida, Z. Kendrick, H. S. Miller, R. Janeway, and A. C. Linnerud. Effects of training two days per week at different intensities on middle-aged men. *Med. Sci. Sports* 4:192–197, 1972.

62. Pollock, M. L. The quantification of endurance training programs. *Exercise and Sport Sciences Reviews,* (J. Wilmore, editor). New York: Academic Press, pp. 155–188, 1973.

63. Pollock, M. L., H. S. Miller, Jr., and J. Wilmore. Physiological characteristics of champion American track athletes 40 to 70 years of age. *J. Gerontol.* 29:645–649, 1974.

64. Pollock, M. L., J. Dimmick, H. S. Miller, Z. Kendrick, and A. C. Linnerud. Effects of mode of training on cardiovascular function and body composition of middle-aged men. *Med. Sci. Sports* 7:139–145, 1975.

65. Pollock, M. L., H. S. Miller, A. C. Linnerud, and K. H. Cooper. Frequency of training as a determinant for improvement in cardiovascular function and body composition of middle-aged men. *Arch. Phys. Med. Rehab.* 56:141–145, 1975.

66. Pollock, M. L., G. A. Dawson, H. S. Miller, Jr., A. Ward, D. Cooper, W. Headly, A. C. Linnerud, and M. M. Nomeir. Physiologic response of men 49 to 65 years of age to endurance training. *J. Amer. Geriatr. Soc.* 24:97–104, 1976.

67. Pollock, M. L., and A. Jackson. Body Composition: Measurement and changes resulting from physical training. Proceedings National College Physical Education Association for Men and Women, pp. 125–137, January, 1977.

68. Pollock, M. L., J. Ayres, and A. Ward. Cardiorespiratory fitness: Response to differing intensities and durations of training. *Arch. Phys. Med. Rehab.* 58:467–473, 1977.

69. Pollock, M. L., L. R. Gettman, C. A. Milesis, M. D. Bah, J. L. Durstine, and R. B. Johnson. Effects of frequency and duration of training on attrition and incidence of injury. *Med. Sci. Sports* 9:31–36, 1977.

70. Pollock, M. L., H. S. Miller, and P. M. Ribisl. Body composition and cardiorespiratory fitness in former athletes. *Phys. Sports Med.* In press, 1978.

71. Ribisl, P. M. Effects of training upon the maximal oxygen uptake of middle-aged men. *Int. Z. Angew. Physiol.* 26:272–278, 1969.

72. Robinson, S., and P. M. Harmon. Lactic acid mechanism and certain properties of blood in relation to training. *Amer. J. Physiol.* 132:757–769, 1941.

73. Roskamm, H. Optimum patterns of exercise for healthy adults. *Canad. Med. Ass. J.* 96:895–899, 1967.

74. Saltin, B., G. Blomqvist, J. Mitchell, R. L. Johnson, K. Wildenthal, and C. B. Chapman. Response to exercise after bed rest and after training. *Circ.* 37 and 38, Supp. 7, 1–78, 1968.

75. Saltin, B., L. Hartley, A. Kilbom, and I. Åstrand. Physical training in sedentary middle-aged and older men. *Scand. J. Clin. Lab. Invest.* 24:323–334, 1969.

76. Sharkey, B. J. Intensity and duration of training and the development of cardiorespiratory endurance. *Med. Sci. Sports* 2:197–202, 1970.

77. Shephard, R. J. Intensity, duration, and frequency of exercise as determinants of the response to a training regime. *Int. Z. Angew. Physiol.* 26:272–278, 1969.

78. Shephard, R. J. Future research on the quantifying of endurance training. *J. Human Ergology* 3:163–181, 1975.

79. Sidney, K. H., R. B. Eynon, and D. A. Cunningham. Effect of frequency of training of exercise upon physical working performance and selected variables representative of cardiorespiratory fitness. In: Training Scientific Basis and Application (A. W. Taylor, ed.) Springfield: Charles C. Thomas, Publishers, pp. 144–188, 1972.

80. Sidney, K. H., R. J. Shephard, and J. Harrison. Endurance training and body composition of the elderly. *Amer. J. Clin. Nutr.* 30:326–333, 1977.

81. Siegel, W., G. Blomqvist, and J. H. Mitchell. Effects of a quantitated physical training program on middle-aged sedentary males. *Circ.* 41:19, 1970.

82. Skinner, J., J. Holloszy, and T. Cureton. Effects of a program of endurance exercise on physical work capacity and anthropometric measurements of fifteen middle-aged men. *Amer. J. Cardiol.* 14:747–752, 1964.

83. Skinner, J. The cardiovascular system with aging and exercise. In: Brunner, D. and E. Jokl (editors). *Physical Activity and Aging.* Baltimore: University Park Press, 1970, pp. 100–108.

84. Smith, D. P., and F. W. Stransky. The effect of training and detraining on the body composition and cardiovascular response of young women to exercise. *J. Sports Med.* 16:112–120, 1976.

85. Terjung, R. L., K. M. Baldwin, J. Cooksey, B. Samson, and R. A. Sutter. Cardiovascular adaptation to twelve minutes of mild daily exercise in middle-aged sedentary men. *J. Amer. Geriatr. Soc.* 21:164–168, 1973.

86. Wilmore, J. H., J. Royce, R. N. Girandola, F. I. Katch, and V. L. Katch. Physiological alterations resulting from a 10-week jogging program. *Med. Sci. Sports* 2(1):7–14, 1970.

87. Wilmore, J. H., J. Royce, R. N. Girandola, F. I. Katch, and V. L. Katch. Body composition changes with a 10-week jogging program. *Med. Sci. Sports* 2:113–117, 1970.

88. Wilmore, J. H. Alterations in strength, body composition, and anthropometric measurements consequent to a 10-week weight training program. *Med. Sci. Sports* 6:133–138, 1974.

89. Wilmore, J. Inferiority of female athletes: myth or reality. *J. Sports Med.* 3:1–6, 1974.

90. Wilmore, J., R. B. Parr, P. A. Vodak, T. J. Barstow, T. V. Pipes, A. Ward, and P. Leslie. Strength, endurance, BMR, and body composition changes with circuit weight training (Abstract) *Med. Sci. Sports* 8:58–60, 1976.

American College of Sports Medicine Position Stand on Proper and Improper Weight Loss Programs

Millions of individuals are involved in weight reduction programs. With the number of undesirable weight loss programs available and a general misconception by many about weight loss, the need for guidelines for proper weight loss programs is apparent.

Based on the existing evidence concerning the effects of weight loss on health status, physiologic processes, and body composition parameters, the American College of Sports Medicine makes the following statements and recommendations for weight loss programs.

For the purposes of this position stand, body weight will be represented by two components, fat and fat-free (water, electrolytes, minerals, glycogen stores, muscular tissue, bone, etc.):

1. Prolonged fasting and diet programs that severely restrict caloric intake are scientifically undesirable and can be medically dangerous.

2. Fasting and diet programs that severely restrict caloric intake result in the loss of large amounts of water, electrolytes, minerals, glyocen stores, and other fat-free tissue (including proteins within fat-free tissues), with minimal amounts of fat loss.

3. Mild calorie restriction (500–1000 kcal less than the usual daily intake) results in a smaller loss of water, electrolytes, minerals, and other fat-free tissue, and is less likely to cause malnutrition.

4. Dynamic exercise of large muscles helps to maintain fat-free tissue, including muscle mass and bone density, and results in losses of body weight. Weight loss resulting from an increase in energy expenditure is primarily in the form of fat weight.

5. A nutritionally sound diet resulting in mild calorie restriction coupled with an endurance exercise program along with behavioral modification of existing eating habits is recommended for weight reduction. The rate of sustained weight loss should not exceed 1 kg (2 lb) per week.

6. To maintain proper weight control and optimal body fat levels, a lifetime commitment to proper eating habits and regular physical activity is required.

Research Background for the Position Stand

Each year millions of individuals undertake weight loss programs for a variety of reasons. It is well known that obesity is associated with a number of health-related problems (3,4,57). These problems include impairment of cardiac function due to an increase in the work of the heart (2) and to left ventricular dysfunction (1,40); hypertension (6,22,80); diabetes (83,97); renal disease (95); gall bladder disease (55, 72); respiratory dysfunction (19); joint diseases and gout (90); endometrial cancer (15); abnormal plasma lipid and lipoprotein concentrations (56, 74); problems in the administration of anesthetics during surgery (93); and impairment of physical working capacity (49). As a result, weight reduction is frequently advised by physicians for medical reasons. In addition, there are a vast number of individuals who are on weight reduction programs for aesthetic reasons.

It is estimated that 60–70 million American adults and at least 10 million American teenagers are overfat (49). Because millions of Americans have adopted unsupervised weight loss programs, it is the opinion of the American College of Sports Medicine that guidelines are needed for safe and effective weight loss programs. This position stand deals with desirable and undesirable weight loss programs. Desirable weight loss programs are defined as those that are nutritionally sound and result in maximal losses in fat weight and minimal losses of fat-free tissue. Undesirable weight loss programs are defined as those that are not nutritionally sound, that result in large losses of fat-free tissue, that pose potential serious medical complications, and that cannot be followed for long-term weight maintenance.

Therefore, a desirable weight loss program is one that:

1. Provides a caloric intake not lower than 1200 kcal $\cdot$ d^{-1} for normal adults in order to get a proper blend of foods to meet nutritional requirements. (Note: this requirement may change for children, older individuals, athletes, etc.)

2. Includes foods acceptable to the dieter from the viewpoints of socio-cultural background, usual habits, taste, cost, and ease in acquisition and preparation.

3. Provides a negative caloric balance (not to exceed 500–1000 kcal $\cdot$ d^{-1} lower than recommended), resulting in gradual weight loss without metabolic derangements. Maximal weight loss should be 1 kg $\cdot$ wk^{-1}.

4. Includes the use of behavior modification techniques to identify and eliminate dieting habits that contribute to improper nutrition.

5. Includes an endurance exercise program of at least 3 d/wk, 20–30 min in duration, at a minimum intensity of 60% of maximum heart rate (refer to ACSM Position Stand on the Recommended Quantity and Quality of Exercise for Developing and Maintaining Fitness in Healthy Adults, *Med. Sci. Sports* 10:vii, 1978).

6. Provides that the new eating and physical activity habits can be continued for life in order to maintain the achieved lower body weight.

1. Since the early work of Keys et al. (50) and Bloom (16), which indicated that marked reduction in caloric intake or fasting (starvation or semistarvation) rapidly reduced body weight, numerous fasting, modified fasting, and fad diet and weight loss programs have emerged. While these programs promise and generally cause rapid weight loss, they are associated with significant medical risks.

The medical risks associated with these types of diet and weight loss programs are numerous. Blood glucose concentrations have been shown to be markedly reduced in obese subjects who undergo fasting (18,32,74,84). Further, in obese non-diabetic subjects, fasting may result in impairment of glucose tolerance (10,52). Ketonuria begins within a few hours after fasting or low-carbohydrate diets are begun (53) and hyperuricemia is common among subjects who fast to reduce body weight (18). Fasting also results in high serum uric acid levels with decreased urinary output (59). Fasting and low-calorie diets also result in urinary nitrogen loss and a significant decrease in fat-free tissue (7,11,17,42,101; see section 2). In comparison to ingestion of a normal diet, fasting substantially elevates urinary excretion of potassium (10,32,37,52,53,78). This, coupled with the aforementioned nitrogen loss, suggests that the potassium loss is due to a loss of lean tissue (78). Other electrolytes, including sodium (32,53), calcium (30,84), magnesium (30,84), and phosphate (84) have been shown to be elevated in urine during prolonged fasting. Reductions in blood volume

and body fluids are also common with fasting and fad diets (18). This can be associated with weakness and fainting (32). Congestive heart failure and sudden death have been reported in subjects who fasted (48,79,80) or markedly restricted their caloric intake (79). Myocardial atrophy appears to contribute to sudden death (79). Sudden death may also occur during refeeding (25,79). Untreated fasting also has been reported to reduce serum iron binding capacity, resulting in anemia (47,73,89). Liver glycogen levels are depleted with fasting (38,60,63) and liver function (29,31,37,75,76,92) and gastrointestinal tract abnormalities (13,32,53,65,85,91) are associated with fasting. While fasting and calorically restricted diets have been shown to lower serum cholesterol levels (88,96), a large portion of the cholesterol reduction is a result of lowered HDL-cholesterol levels (88,96). Other risks associated with fasting and low-calorie diets include lactic acidosis (12,26), alopecia (73), hypoalaninemia (34), edema (23,78), anuria (101), hypotension (18,32,78), elevated serum bilirubin (8,9), nausea and vomiting (53), alterations in thyroxine metabolism (71,91), impaired serum triglyceride removal and production (86), and death (25,37,48,61,80).

2. The major objective of any weight reduction program is to lose body fat while maintaining fat-free tissue. The vast majority of research reveals that starvation and low-calorie diets result in large losses of water, electrolytes, and other fat-free tissue. One of the best controlled experiments was conducted from 1944 to 1946 at the Laboratory of Physiological Hygiene at the University of Minnesota (50). In this study subjects had their base-line caloric intake cut by 45% and body weight and body composition changes were followed for 24 wk. During the first 12 wk of semistarvation, body weight declined by 25.4 lb (11.5 kg) with only an 11.6-lb (5.3 kg) decline in body fat. During the second 12-wk period, body weight declined on additional 9.1 lb (4.1 kg) with only a 6.1-lb (2.8 kg) decrease in body fat. These data clearly demonstrate that fat-free tissue significantly contributes to weight loss from semistarvation. Similar results have been reported by several other investigators. Buskirk et al. (20) reported that the 13.5-kg weight loss in six

subjects on a low-calorie mixed diet averaged 76% fat and 24% fat-free tissue. Similarly, Passmore et al. (64) reported results of 78% of weight loss (15.3 kg) as fat and 22% as fat-free tissue in seven women who consumed a 400-kcal · d^{-1} diet for 45 d. Yang and Van Itallie (101) followed weight loss and body composition changes for the first 5 d of a weight loss program involving subjects consuming either an 800-kcal mixed diet, an 800-kcal ketogenic diet, or undergoing starvation. Subjects on the mixed diet lost 1.3 kg of weight (59% fat loss, 3.4% protein loss, 37.6% water loss), subjects on the ketogenic diet lost 2.3 kg of weight (33.2% fat, 3.8% protein, 63.0% water), and subjects on starvation regimens lost 3.8 kg of weight (32.3% fat, 6.5% protein, 61.2% water). Grande (41) and Grande et al. (43) reported similar findings with a 1000-kcal carbohydrate diet. It was further reported that water restriction combined with 1000-kcal · d^{-1} of carbohydrate resulted in greater water loss and less fat loss.

Recently, there has been some renewed speculation about the efficacy of the very-low-calorie diet (VLCD). Krotkiewski and associates (51) studied the effects on body weight and body composition after 3 wk on the so-called Cambridge diet. Two groups of obese middle-aged women were studied. One group had a VLCD only, while the second group had a VLCD combined with a 55-min/d, 3-d/wk exercise program. The VLCD-only group lost 6.2 kg in 3 wk, of which only 2.6 kg was fat loss, while the VLCD-plus-exercise group lost 6.8 kg in 3 wk with only a 1.9-kg body fat loss. Thus it can be seen that VLCD results in undesirable losses of body fat, and the addition of the normally protective effect of chronic exercise to VLCD does not reduce the catabolism of fat-free tissue. Further, with VLCD, a large reduction (29% in HDL-cholesterol is seen (94).

3. Even mild calorie restriction (reduction of 500–1000 kcal · d^{-1} from base-line caloric intake), when used alone as a tool for weight loss, results in the loss of moderate amounts of water and other fat-free tissue. In a study by Goldman et al. (39), 15 female subjects consumed a low-calorie mixed diet for 7–8 wk. Weight loss during this period averaged 6.43 kg (0.85 kg · wk^{-1}), 88.6% of which was

fat. The remaining 11.4% represented water and other fat-free tissue. Zuti and Golding (102) examined the effect of 500 kcal · d^{-1} calorie restriction on body composition changes in adult females. Over a 16-wk period the women lost approximately 5.2 kg; however, 1.1 kg of the weight loss (21%) was due to a loss of water and other fat-free tissue. More recently, Weltman et al. (96) examined the effects of 500 kcal · d^{-1} calorie restriction (from base-line levels) on body composition changes in sedentary middle-aged males. Over a 10-wk period subjects lost 5.95 kg, 4.03 kg (68%) of which was fat loss and 1.92 kg (32%) was loss of water and other fat-free tissue. Further, with calorie restriction only, these subjects exhibited a decrease in HDL-cholesterol. In the same study, the two other groups who exercised and/or dieted and exercised were able to maintain their HDL-cholesterol levels. Similar results for females have been presented by Thompson et al. (88). It should be noted that the decrease seen in HDL-cholesterol with weight loss may be an acute effect. There are data that indicate that stable weight loss has a beneficial effect on HDL-cholesterol (21,24,46,88).

Further, an additional problem associated with calorie restriction alone for effective weight loss is the fact that it is associated with a reduction in basal metabolic rate (5). Apparently exercise combined with calorie restriction can counter this response (14).

4. There are several studies that indicate that exercise helps maintain fat-free tissue while promoting fat loss. Total body weight and fat weight are generally reduced with endurance training programs (70) while fat-free weight remains constant (36,54,69,70,98) or increases slightly (62,96,102). Programs conducted at least 3 d/wk (66–69,98), of at least 20-min duration (58,69,98) and of sufficient intensity and duration to expend at least 300 kcal per exercise session have been suggested as a threshold level for total body weight and fat weight reduction (27,44,69,70). Increasing caloric expenditure above 300 kcal per exercise session and increasing the frequency of exercise sessions will enhance fat weight loss while sparing fat-free tissue (54,102). Leon et al. (54) had six obese male subjects walk vigorously for 90 min, 5 d/wk for 16 wk. Work output progressed weekly to an energy

expenditure of 1000–1200 kcal/session. At the end of 16 wk, subjects averaged 5.7 kg of weight loss with a 5.9-kg loss of fat weight and a 0.2-kg gain in fat-free tissue. Similarly, Zuti and Golding (102) followed the progress of adult women who expended 500 kcal/exercise session 5 d/wk for 16 wk of exercise. At the end of 16 wk the women lost 5.8 kg of fat and gained 0.9 kg of fat-free tissue.

5. Review of the literature cited above strongly indicates that optimal body composition changes occur with a combination of calorie restriction (while on a well-balanced diet) plus exercise. This combination promotes loss of fat weight while sparing fat-free tissue. Data of Zuti and Golding (102) and Weltman et al. (96) support this contention. Calorie restriction of 500 kcal · d^{-1} combined with 3–5 d of exercise requiring 300–500 kcal per exercise session results in favorable changes in body composition (96,102). Therefore, the optimal rate of weight loss should be between 0.45–1 kg (1–2 lb) per wk. This seems especially relevant in light of the data which indicates that rapid weight loss due to low caloric intake can be associated with sudden death (79). In order to institute a desirable pattern of calorie restriction plus exercise, behavior modification techniques should be incorporated to identify and eliminate habits contributing to obesity and/or overfatness (28,33,35,81,87,99,100).

6. The problem with losing weight is that, although many individuals succeed in doing so, they invariably put the weight on again (45). The goal of an effective weight loss regimen is not merely to lose weight. Weight control requires a lifelong commitment, an understanding of our eating habits and a willingness to change them. Frequent exercise is necessary, and accomplishment must be reinforced to sustain motivation. Crash dieting and other promised weight loss cures are ineffective (45).

REFERENCES

1. Alexander, J. K., and J. R. Pettigrove. Obesity and congestive heart failure. *Geriatrics* 22:101–108, 1967.
2. Alexander, J. K., and K. L. Peterson. Cardiovascular effects of weight reduction. *Circulation* 45:310–318, 1972.
3. Angel, A. Pathophysiologic changes in obesity. *Can. Med. Assoc. J.* 119:1401–1406, 1978.
4. Angel, A., and D. A. K. Roncari. Medical complications of obesity. *Can. Med. Assoc. J.* 119:1408–1411, 1978.
5. Appelbaum, M., J. Bostsarron, and D. Lacatis. Effect of caloric restriction and excessive caloric intake on energy expenditure. *Am. J. Clin. Nutr.* 24:1405–1409, 1971.
6. Bachman, L., V. Freschuss, D. Hallberg, and A. Melcher. Cardiovascular function in extreme obesity. *Acta Med. Scand.* 193:437–446, 1972.
7. Ball, M. F., J. J. Canary, and L. H. Kyle. Comparative effects of caloric restrictions and total starvation on body composition in obesity. *Ann. Intern. Med.* 67:60–67, 1967.
8. Barrett, P. V. D. Hyperbilirubinemia of fasting. *JAMA* 217:1349–1353, 1971.
9. Barrett, P. V. D. The effect of diet and fasting on the serum bilirubin concentration in the rat. *Gastroenterology* 60:572–576, 1971.
10. Beck, P., J. J. T. Koumans, C. A. Winterling, M. F. Stein, W. H. Daughaday, and D. M. Kipnis. Studies of insulin and growth hormone secretion in human obesity. *J. Lab. Clin. Med.* 64:654–667, 1964.
11. Benoit, F. L., R. L. Martin, and R. H. Watten. Changes in body composition during weight reduction in obesity. *Ann. Intern. Med.* 63:604–612, 1965.
12. Berger, H. Fatal lactic acidosis during "crash" reducing diet. *N.Y. State J. Med.* 67:2258–2263, 1967.
13. Billich, C., G. Bray, T. F. Gallagher, A. V. Hoffbrand, and R. Levitan. Absorptive capacity of the jejunum of obese and lean subjects; effect of fasting. *Arch. Intern. Med.* 130:377–387, 1972.
14. Bjorntorp, P., L. Sjostrom, and L. Sullivan. The role of physical exercise in the management of obesity. In: *The Treatment of Obesity,* J. F. Munro (Ed.). Lancaster, England: MTP Press, 1979.
15. Blitzer, P. H., E. C. Blitzer, and A. A. Rimm. Association between teenage obesity and cancer in 56,111 women. *Prev. Med.* 5:20–31, 1976.
16. Bloom, W. L. Fasting as an introduction to the treatment of obesity. *Metabolism* 8:214–220, 1959.
17. Bolinger, R. E., B. P. Lukert, R. W. Brown, L. Guevera, and R. Steinberg. Metabolic balances of obese subjects during fasting. *Arch. Intern. Med.* 118:3–8, 1966.
18. Bray, G. A., M. B. Davidson, and E. J. Drenick. Obesity: a serious symptom. *Ann. Intern. Med.* 77:779–805, 1972.
19. Burwell, C. S., E. D. Robin, R. D. Whaley, and A. G. Bickelmann. Extreme obesity associated with alveolar hypoventilation—a Pickwickian syndrome. *Am. J. Med.* 21:811–818, 1956.
20. Buskirk, E. R., R. H. Thompson, L. Lutwak, and G. D. Whedon. Energy balance of obese patients during weight reduction: influence of diet restriction and exercise. *Ann. NY Acad. Sci.* 110:918–940, 1963.
21. Caggiula, A. W., G. Christakis, M. Ferrand, et al. The multiple risk factors intervention trial. IV Intervention on blood lipids. *Prev. Med.* 10:443–475, 1981.
22. Chaing, B. M., L. V. Perlman, and F. H. Epstein. Overweight and hypertension: a review. *Circulation* 39:403–421, 1969.
23. Collison, D. R. Total fasting for up to 249 days. *Lancet* 1:112, 1967.
24. Contaldo, F., P. Strazullo, A. Postiglione, et al. Plasma high density lipoprotein in severe obesity after stable weight loss. *Atherosclerosis* 37:163–167, 1980.
25. Cruickshank, E. K. Protein malnutrition. In: Proceedings of a conference in Jamaica (1953), J. C. Waterlow (Ed.). Cambridge: University Press, 1955, p. 107.
26. Cubberley, P. T., S. A. Polster, and C. L. Shulman. Lactic acidosis and death after the treatment of obesity by fasting. *N. Engl. J. Med.* 272:628–633, 1965.
27. Cureton, T. K. *The Physiological Effects of Exercise Programs Upon Adults.* Springfield, IL: C. Thomas Company, 1969.
28. Dahlkoetter, J., E. J. Callahan, and J. Linton. Obesity and the unbalanced energy equation: exercise versus eating habit change. *J. Consult. Clin. Psychol.* 47:898–905, 1979.

29. Drenick. E.J. The relation of BSP retention during prolonged fasts to changes in plasma volume. *Metabolism* 17:522–527, 1968.

30. Drenick, E. J., I. F. Hunt, and M. E. Swendseid. Magnesium depletion during prolonged fasting in obese males. *J. Clin. Endocrinol. Metab.* 29:1341–1348, 1969.

31. Drenick, E. J., F. Simmons, and J. F. Murphy. Effect on hepatic morphology of treatment of obesity by fasting, reducing diets and small-bowel bypass. *N. Engl. J. Med.* 282:829–834, 1970.

32. Drenick, E. J., M. E. Swendseid, W. H. Blahd, and S. G. Tuttle. Prolonged starvation as treatment for severe obesity. *JAMA* 187:100–105, 1964.

33. Epstein, L. H., and R. R. Wing. Aerobic exercise and weight. *Addict. Behav.* 5:371–388, 1980.

34. Felig, P., O. E. Owen, J. Wahren, and G. F. Cahill, Jr. Amino acid metabolism during prolonged starvation. *J. Clin. Invest.* 48:584–594, 1969.

35. Ferguson, J. *Learning to Eat: Behavior Modification for Weight Control*. Palo Alto, CA: Bull Publishing, 1975.

36. Franklin, B., E. Buskirk, J. Hodgson, H. Gahagan, J. Kollias, and J. Mendez. Effects of physical conditioning on cardiorespiratory function, body composition and serum lipids in relatively normal-weight and obese middle-aged women. *Int. J. Obesity* 3:97–109, 1979.

37. Garnett, E. S., J. Ford, D. L. Barnard, R. A. Goodbody, and M. A. Woodehouse. Gross fragmentation of cardiac myofibrils after therapeutic starvation for obesity. *Lancet* 1:914, 1969.

38. Garrow, J. S. *Energy Balance and Obesity in Man*. New York: American Elsevier, 1974.

39. Goldman, R. F., B. Bullen, and C. Seltzer. Changes in specific gravity and body fat in overweight female adolescents as a result of weight reduction. *Ann. NY Acad. Sci.* 110:913–917, 1963.

40. Gordon, T., and W. B. Kannel. The effects of overweight on cardiovascular diseases. *Geriatrics* 28:80–88, 1973.

41. Grande, F. Nutrition and energy balance in body composition studies. In: *Techniques for Measuring Body Composition*, J. Brozek and A. Henschel (Eds.). Washington, DC: National Academy of Sciences—National Research Council, 1961. (Reprinted by the Office of Technical Services, U.S. Department of Commerce, Washington, DC as U.S. Government Research Report AD286, 1963, 560.)

42. Grande, F. Energy balance and body composition changes. *Ann. Intern. Med.* 68:467–480, 1968.

43. Grande, F., H. L. Taylor, J. T. Anderson, E. Buskirk, and A. Keys. Water exchange in men on a restricted water intake and a low calorie carbohydrate diet accompanied by physical work. *J. Appl. Physiol.* 12:202–210, 1958.

44. Gwinup, G. Effect of exercise alone on the weight of obese women. *Arch. Intern. Med.* 135:676–680, 1975.

45. Hafen, B. A. *Nutrition, Food and Weight Control*. Boston: Allyn and Bacon, 1981, pp. 271–289.

46. Hulley, S. B., R. Cohen, and G. Widdowson. Plasma high-density lipoprotein cholesterol level: influence of risk factor intervention. *JAMA* 238:2269–2271, 1977.

47. Jagenburg, R., and A. Svanborg. Self-induced protein-calorie malnutrition in a healthy adult male. *Acta Med. Scand.* 183:67–71, 1968.

48. Kahan, A. Death during therapeutic starvation. *Lancet* 1:1378–1379, 1968.

49. Katch, F. I., and W. B. McArdle. *Nutrition, Weight Control and Exercise*. Boston: Houghton Mifflin, 1977.

50. Keys, A., J. Brozek, A. Henshel, O. Mickelson, and H. L. Taylor. *The Biology of Human Starvation*. Minneapolis: University of Minnesota Press, 1950.

51. Krotkiewski, M., L. Toss, P. Bjorntorp, and G. Holm. The effect of a very-low-calorie diet with and without chronic exercise on thyroid and sex hormones, plasma proteins, oxygen uptake, insulin and c peptide concentrations in obese women. *Int. J. Obes.* 5:287–293, 1981.

52. Laszlo, J., R. F. Klein, and M. D. Bogdonoff. Prolonged starvation in obese patients, in vitro and in vivo effects. *Clin. Res.* 9:183, 1961. (Abstract)

53. Lawlor, T., and D. G. Wells. Metabolic hazards of fasting. *Am. J. Clin. Nutr.* 22:1142–1149, 1969.

54. Leon, A. S., J. Conrad, D. M. Hunninghake, and R. Serfass. Effects of a vigorous walking program on body composition, and carbohydrate and lipid metabolism of obese young men. *Am. J. Clin. Nutr.* 32:1776–1787, 1979.

55. Mabee, F. M., P. Meyer, L. DenBesten, and E. E. Mason. The mechanism of increased gallstone formation on obese human subjects. *Surgery* 79:460–468, 1978.

56. Matter, S., A. Weltman, and B. A. Stamford. Body fat content and serum lipid levels. *J. Am. Diet. Assoc.* 77:149–152, 1980.

57. McArdle, W. D., F. I. Katch, and V. L. Katch. *Exercise Physiology: Energy, Nutrition and Human Performance.* Philadelphia: Lea and Febiger, 1981.

58. Milesis, C. A., M. L. Pollock, M. D. Bah, J. J. Ayres, A. Ward, and A. C. Linerud. Effects of different durations of training on cardiorespiratory function, body composition and serum lipids. *Res. Q.* 47:716–725, 1976.

59. Murphy, R., and K. H. Shipman. Hyperuricemia during total fasting. *Arch. Intern. Med.* 112:954–959, 1963.

60. Nilsson, L. H., and E. Hultman. Total starvation or a carbohydrate-poor diet followed by carbohydrate refeeding. *Scand. J. Clin. Lab. Invest.* 32:325–330, 1973.

61. Norbury, F. B. Contraindication of long term fasting. *JAMA* 188:88, 1964.

62. O'Hara, W., C. Allen, and R. J. Shepard. Loss of body weight and fat during exercise in a cold chamber. *Eur. J. Appl. Physiol.* 37:205–218, 1977.

63. Oyama, J., J. A. Thomas, and R. L. Brant. Effect of starvation on glucose tolerance and serum insulin-like activity of Osborne-Mendel rats. *Diabetes* 12:332–334, 1963.

64. Passmore, R., J. A. Strong, and F. J. Ritchie. The chemical composition of the tissue lost by obese patients on a reducing regimen. *Br. J. Nutr.* 12:113–122, 1958.

65. Pittman, F. E. Primary malabsorption following extreme attempts to lose weight. *Gut* 7:154–158, 1966.

66. Pollock, M. L., T. K. Cureton, and L. Greninger. Effects of frequency of training on working capacity, cardiovascular function and body composition of adult men. *Med. Sci. Sports* 1:70–74, 1969.

67. Pollock, M. L., J. Tiffany, L. Gettman, R. Janeway, and H. Lofland. Effects of frequency of training on serum lipids, cardiovascular function and body composition. In: *Exercise and Fitness*, B. D. Franks (Ed.). Chicago: *Athletic Institute,* 1969, pp. 161–178.

68. Pollock, M. L., J. Broida, Z. Kendrick, H. S. Miller, Jr., R. Janeway, and A. C. Linnerud. Effects of training two days per week at different intensities on middle aged men. *Med. Sci. Sports* 4:192–197, 1972.

69. Pollock, M. L. The quantification of endurance training programs. *Exercise and Sports Sciences Reviews*, J. Wilmore (Ed.). New York: Academic Press, 1973, pp. 155–188.

70. Pollock, M. L., and A. Jackson. Body composition: measurement and changes resulting from physical training. In: *Proceedings National College Physical Education Association for Men and Women,* 1977, pp. 123–137.

71. Portnay, G. I., J. T. O'Brian, J. Bush, et al. The effect of starvation on the concentration and binding of thyroxine and triiodothyronine in serum and on the response to TRH. *J. Clin. Endocrinol. Metab.* 39:191–194, 1974.

72. Rimm, A. A., L. H. Werner, R. Bernstein, and B. VanYserloo. Disease and obesity in 73,532 women. *Obesity Bariatric Med.* 1:77–84, 1972.

73. Rooth, G., and S. Carlstrom. Therapeutic fasting. *Acta Med. Scand.* 187:455–463, 1970.

74. Rossner, S., and D. Hallberg. Serum lipoproteins in massive obesity. *Acta Med. Scand.* 204:103–110, 1978.

75. Rozental, P., C. Biara, H. Spencer, and H. J. Zimmerman. Liver morphology and function tests in obesity and during starvation. *Am. J. Dig. Dis.* 12:198–208, 1967.
76. Runcie, J. Urinary sodium and potassium excretion in fasting obese subjects. *Br. Med. J.* 3:432–435, 1970.
77. Runcie, J., and T. J. Thomson. Total fasting, hyperuricemia and gout. *Postgrad. Med. J.* 45:251–254, 1969.
78. Runcie, J., and T. J. Thomson. Prolonged starvation—a dangerous procedure? *Br. Med. J.* 3:432–435, 1970.
79. Sours, H. E., V. P. Frattali, C. D. Brand, et al. Sudden death associated with very low calorie weight reduction regimens. *Am. J. Clin. Nutr.* 34:453–461, 1981.
80. Spencer, I. O. B. Death during therapeutic starvation for obesity. *Lancet* 2:679–680, 1968.
81. Stalonas, P. M., W. G. Johnson, and M. Christ. Behavior modification for obesity: the evaluation of exercise, contingency, management, and program behavior. *J. Consult. Clin. Psychol.* 46:463–467, 1978.
82. Stamler, R., J. Stamler, W. F. Riedlinger, G. Algera, and R. H. Roberts. Weight and blood pressure. Findings in hypertension screening of 1 million Americans. *JAMA* 240:1607–1610, 1978.
83. Stein, J. S., and J. Hirsch. Obesity and pancreatic function. In: *Handbook of Physiology, Section 1. Endocrinology,* Vol. 1, D. Steener and N. Frankel (Eds.). Washington, DC: American Physiological Society, 1972.
84. Stewart, W. K., and L. W. Fleming. Features of a successful therapeutic fast of 382 days duration. *Postgrad. Med. J.* 49:203–209, 1973.
85. Stewart, J. S., D. L. Pollock, A. V. Hoffbrand, D. L. Mollin, and C. C. Booth. A study of proximal and distal intestinal structure and absorptive function in idiopathic steatorrhea. *Q.J. Med.* 36:425–444, 1967.
86. Streja, D. A., E. B. Marliss, and G. Steiner. The effects of prolonged fasting on plasma triglyceride kinetics in man. *Metabolism* 26:505–516, 1977.
87. Stuart, R. B., and B. Davis. *Slim Chance in a Fat World. Behavioral Control of Obesity.* Champaign, IL: Research Press, 1972.
88. Thompson, P. D., R. W. Jeffrey, R. R. Wing, and P. D. Wood. Unexpected decrease in plasma high density lipoprotein cholesterol with weight loss. *Am. J. Clin. Nutr.* 32:2016–2021, 1979.
89. Thomson, T. J., J. Runcie, and V. Miller. Treatment of obesity of total fasting up to 249 days. *Lancet* 2:992–996, 1966.
90. Thorn, G. W., M. M. Wintrobe, R.D. Adams, E. Braunwald, K. J. Isselbacher, and R. G. Petersdorf. *Harrison's Principles of Internal Medicine,* 8th Edition. New York: McGraw-Hill, 1977.
91. Vegenakis, A. G., A. Burger, G. I. Portnay, et al. Diversion of peripheral thyroxine metabolism from activating to inactivating pathways during complete fasting. *J. Clin. Endocrinol. Metab.* 41:191–194, 1975.
92. Verdy, M. B.S.P. retention during total fasting. *Metabolism* 15:769, 1966.
93. Warner, W. A., and L. P. Garrett. The obese patient and anesthesia. *JAMA* 205:102–103, 1968.
94. Wechsler, J. G., V. Hutt, H. Wenzel, H. Klor, and H. Ditschuneit. Lipids and lipoproteins during a very-low-calorie diet. *Int. J. Obes.* 5:325–331, 1981.
95. Weisinger, J. R., A. Seeman, M. G. Herrera, J. P. Assal, J. S. Soeldner, and R. E. Gleason. The nephrotic syndrome: a complication of massive obesity. *Ann. Intern. Med.* 80:332–341, 1974.
96. Weltman, A., S. Matter, and B. A. Stamford. Caloric restriction and/or mild exercise: effects on serum lipids and body composition. *Am. J. Clin. Nutr.* 33:1002–1009, 1980.
97. West, K. *Epidemiology of Diabetes and its Vascular Lesions.* New York: Elsevier, 1978.
98. Wilmore, J. H., J. Royce, R. N. Girandola, F. I. Katch, and V. L. Katch. Body composition changes with a 10 week jogging program. *Med. Sci. Sports* 2:113–117, 1970.
99. Wilson, G. T. Behavior modification and the treatment of obesity. In: *Obesity,* A. J. Stunkard (Ed.). Philadelphia: W. B. Saunders, 1980.
100. Wooley, S. C., O. W. Wooley, and S. R. Dyrenforth. Theoretical, practical and social issues in behavioral treatments of obesity. *J. Appl. Behav. Anal.* 12:3–25, 1979.
101. Yang, M., and T. B. Van Itallie. Metabolic responses of obese subjects to starvation and low calorie ketogenic and nonketogenic diets. *J. Clin. Invest.* 58:722–730, 1976.
102. Zuti, W. B., and L. A. Golding. Comparing diet and exercise as weight reduction tools. *Phys. Sportsmed.* 4(1):49–53, 1976.

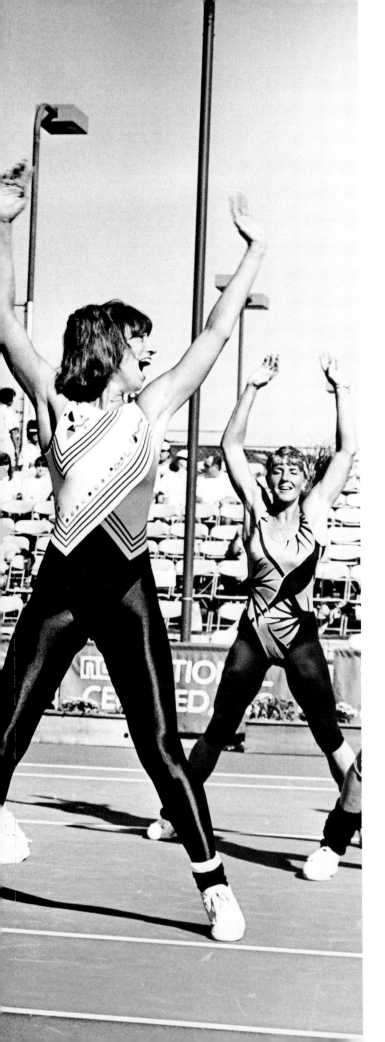

CALORIE EXPENDITURE PER MINUTE FOR SELECTED EXERCISES

It is important to remember that these values are for only the time engaged in the activity. For example, you may spend ninety minutes in the weight-training room, but only twelve minutes of that time might actually be spent in lifting weights. You would calculate the caloric expenditure for twelve minutes, not for ninety minutes. Remember also that in order to obtain a cardiovascular endurance training effect, the minimum duration is fifteen minutes of *continuous* activity.

Note: If an activity is not listed in the charts that follow, check figure 3.4 in chapter 3, which explains how to determine caloric expenditure from exercise heart rate.

Calorie Expenditure per Minute for Various Activities

	Body Weight																					
	90	99	108	117	125	134	143	152	161	170	178	187	196	205	213	222	231	240	249	257	266	275
Aerobic dance	6.8	7.4	8.1	8.8	9.4	10.1	10.7	11.4	12.1	12.8	13.4	14.0	14.7	15.4	16.0	16.7	17.3	18.0	18.7	19.3	20.0	20.6
Archery	3.1	3.4	3.7	4.0	4.5	4.6	4.9	5.2	5.5	5.8	6.1	6.4	6.7	7.0	7.3	7.6	7.9	8.2	8.5	8.8	9.1	9.4
Badminton (recreation)	3.4	3.8	4.1	4.4	4.8	5.1	5.4	5.6	6.1	6.4	6.8	7.1	7.4	7.8	8.1	8.3	8.8	9.1	9.4	9.8	10.1	10.4
Badminton (competition)	5.9	6.4	7.0	7.6	8.1	8.7	9.3	9.9	10.4	11.0	11.6	12.1	12.7	13.3	13.9	14.4	15.0	15.6	16.1	16.7	17.3	17.9
Baseball (player)	2.8	3.1	3.4	3.6	3.9	4.2	4.5	4.7	5.0	5.3	5.5	5.8	6.1	6.4	6.6	6.9	7.2	7.5	7.7	8.0	8.3	8.6
Baseball (pitcher)	3.5	3.9	4.3	4.6	5.0	5.3	5.7	6.0	6.4	6.7	7.1	7.4	7.8	8.1	8.5	8.8	9.2	9.5	9.9	10.2	10.6	10.9
Basketball (half-court)	2.5	3.3	3.5	3.8	4.1	4.4	4.7	4.9	5.3	5.6	5.9	6.2	6.4	6.7	7.0	7.3	7.5	7.6	8.2	8.5	8.8	9.0
Basketball (moderate)	4.2	4.6	5.0	5.5	5.9	6.3	6.7	7.1	7.5	7.9	8.3	8.8	9.2	9.6	10.0	10.4	10.8	11.2	11.6	12.1	12.5	12.9
Basketball (competition)	5.9	6.5	7.1	7.7	8.2	8.8	9.4	10.0	10.6	11.1	11.7	12.3	12.9	13.5	14.0	14.6	15.0	15.2	16.3	16.9	17.5	18.1
Bicycling (level) 5.5 mph	3.0	3.3	3.6	3.9	4.2	4.5	4.8	5.1	5.4	5.6	5.9	6.2	6.5	6.8	7.1	7.4	7.7	8.0	8.3	8.6	8.9	9.2
Bicycling (level) 13 mph	6.4	7.1	7.7	8.3	8.9	9.6	10.2	10.8	11.4	12.1	12.7	13.4	14.0	14.6	15.2	15.9	16.5	17.1	17.8	18.4	19.0	19.6
Bowling (nonstop)	4.0	4.4	4.8	5.2	5.6	5.9	6.3	6.7	7.1	7.5	7.9	8.3	8.7	9.1	9.5	9.8	10.2	10.6	11.0	11.4	11.8	12.2
Boxing (sparring)	3.0	3.3	3.6	3.9	4.2	4.5	4.8	5.1	5.4	5.6	5.9	6.2	6.5	6.8	7.1	7.4	7.7	8.0	8.3	8.6	8.9	9.2
Calisthenics	3.0	3.3	3.6	3.9	4.2	4.5	4.8	5.1	5.4	5.6	5.9	6.2	6.5	6.8	7.1	7.4	7.7	8.0	8.3	8.6	8.9	9.2
Canoeing, 2.5 mph	1.8	1.9	2.0	2.2	2.3	2.5	2.7	3.0	3.2	3.4	3.6	3.7	3.9	4.1	4.3	4.4	4.6	4.8	5.0	5.1	5.3	5.5
Canoeing, 4.0 mph	4.2	4.6	5.0	5.5	5.9	6.3	6.7	7.1	7.5	7.9	8.3	8.7	9.2	9.4	10.0	10.5	10.8	11.2	11.6	12.0	12.4	12.9
Dance, modern (moderate)	2.5	2.8	3.0	3.2	3.5	3.7	4.0	4.2	4.5	4.7	5.0	5.2	5.4	5.7	5.9	6.2	6.4	6.7	6.9	7.2	7.4	7.6
Dance, modern (vigorous)	3.4	3.7	4.1	4.4	4.7	5.1	5.4	5.7	6.1	6.4	6.7	7.1	7.4	7.7	8.1	8.4	8.7	9.1	9.4	9.7	10.1	10.4
Dance, fox-trot	2.7	2.9	3.2	3.4	3.7	4.0	4.2	4.5	4.7	5.0	5.3	5.5	5.8	6.0	6.3	6.6	6.8	7.1	7.3	7.6	7.9	8.1
Dance, rumba	4.2	4.6	5.0	5.4	5.8	6.2	6.6	7.0	7.4	7.8	8.2	8.6	9.0	9.4	9.8	10.2	10.6	11.0	11.5	11.9	12.3	12.6
Dance, square	4.1	4.5	4.9	5.3	5.7	6.1	6.5	6.9	7.3	7.8	8.1	8.5	8.9	9.3	9.7	10.1	10.5	10.9	11.3	11.7	12.1	12.4
Dance, waltz	3.1	3.4	3.7	4.0	4.3	4.6	4.9	5.2	5.5	5.8	6.1	6.4	6.7	7.0	7.3	7.6	7.9	8.2	8.5	8.8	9.1	9.4

Adapted from Physiological Measurements of Metabolic Functions in Man by C. Frank Consolazio, Robert E. Johnson, and Louis J. Pecora, pp. 331–32. Copyright 1963 by McGraw-Hill Book Company. Reprinted by permission of the publisher. Research completed at the Human Performance Laboratory, Brigham Young University, Provo, Utah.

Calorie Expenditure per Minute for Various Activities (continued)

Body Weight

	90	99	108	117	125	134	143	152	161	170	178	187	196	205	213	222	231	240	249	257	266	275
Fencing (moderate)	3.0	3.3	3.6	3.9	4.2	4.5	4.8	5.1	5.4	5.6	6.0	6.2	6.5	6.8	7.1	7.4	7.7	8.0	8.3	8.6	8.9	9.2
Fencing (vigorous)	6.2	6.8	7.4	8.0	8.6	9.2	9.8	10.4	11.0	11.6	12.2	12.8	13.4	14.0	14.6	15.2	15.8	16.4	17.0	17.6	18.2	18.8
Football (moderate)	3.0	3.3	3.6	4.0	4.2	4.5	4.8	5.1	5.4	5.7	6.0	6.2	6.5	6.8	7.1	7.4	7.7	8.0	8.3	8.6	8.9	9.2
Football (vigorous)	5.0	5.5	6.0	6.4	6.9	7.4	7.9	8.4	8.9	9.4	9.8	10.3	10.8	11.3	11.8	12.3	12.8	13.2	13.7	14.2	14.7	15.2
Golf, twosome	3.3	3.6	3.9	4.2	4.5	4.8	5.2	5.5	5.8	6.1	6.4	6.7	7.1	7.4	7.7	8.0	8.3	8.6	9.0	9.3	9.6	10.0
Golf, foursome	2.4	2.7	2.9	3.2	3.4	3.6	3.9	4.1	4.3	4.6	4.8	5.1	5.3	5.5	5.8	6.0	6.2	6.5	6.7	7.0	7.2	7.4
Handball	5.9	6.4	7.0	7.6	8.1	8.7	9.3	9.9	10.4	11.0	11.6	12.1	12.7	13.3	13.9	14.4	15.0	15.6	16.1	16.7	17.3	17.9
Hiking, 40 lb. pack, 3.0 mph	4.1	4.5	4.9	5.3	5.7	6.1	6.5	6.9	7.3	7.7	8.1	8.5	8.9	9.3	9.7	10.1	10.5	10.9	11.3	11.7	12.1	12.5
Horseback Riding (walk)	2.0	2.3	2.4	2.6	2.8	3.0	3.1	3.3	3.5	3.7	3.9	4.1	4.3	4.5	4.7	4.9	5.1	5.3	5.5	5.7	5.8	6.0
Horseback Riding (trot)	4.1	4.4	4.8	5.2	5.6	6.0	6.4	6.8	7.2	7.6	8.0	8.4	8.8	9.2	9.6	10.0	10.4	10.8	11.2	11.6	12.0	12.4
Horseshoe Pitching	2.1	2.3	2.5	2.7	3.0	3.3	3.4	3.6	3.8	4.0	4.2	4.4	4.6	4.8	5.0	5.2	5.4	5.6	5.8	6.0	6.3	6.5
Judo, Karate	7.7	8.5	9.2	10.0	10.7	11.5	12.2	13.0	13.7	14.5	15.2	16.0	16.7	17.5	18.2	19.0	19.7	20.5	21.2	22.0	22.7	23.5
Mountain Climbing	6.0	6.5	7.2	7.8	8.4	9.0	9.6	10.1	10.7	11.3	11.9	12.5	13.1	13.7	14.3	14.8	15.4	16.0	16.6	17.2	17.8	18.4
Pool, Billiards	1.1	1.2	1.3	1.4	1.5	1.6	1.7	1.8	1.9	2.0	2.1	2.2	2.4	2.5	2.6	2.7	2.8	2.9	3.0	3.1	3.2	3.3
Racquetball, Paddleball	5.9	6.4	7.0	7.6	8.1	8.7	9.3	9.9	10.4	11.0	11.6	12.1	12.7	13.3	13.9	14.4	15.0	15.6	16.1	16.7	17.3	17.9
Rope Jumping 110 rpm	5.8	6.4	7.0	7.6	8.1	8.6	9.2	9.8	10.4	11.0	11.5	12.1	12.6	13.2	13.7	14.3	14.9	15.5	16.1	16.6	17.2	17.7
Rope Jumping 120 rpm	5.6	6.1	6.7	7.2	7.7	8.3	8.8	9.4	9.9	10.5	11.0	11.5	12.1	12.6	13.1	13.7	14.3	14.8	15.4	15.9	16.4	17.0
Rope Jumping 130 rpm	5.2	5.7	6.2	6.6	7.2	7.7	8.3	8.8	9.3	9.8	10.3	10.8	11.3	11.8	12.3	12.8	13.3	13.8	14.4	14.8	15.3	15.9
Rowing (recreation)	3.0	3.3	3.6	3.9	4.2	4.5	4.8	5.1	5.4	5.6	6.0	6.2	6.5	6.8	7.1	7.5	7.7	8.0	8.3	8.6	8.9	9.2
Rowing (machine)	8.2	9.0	9.8	10.6	11.4	12.2	13.0	13.8	14.6	15.4	16.2	17.0	17.8	18.6	19.4	20.2	21.0	21.8	22.6	23.4	24.2	25.0
Running, 11-min mile, 5.5 mph	6.4	7.1	7.7	8.3	9.0	9.6	10.2	10.8	11.5	12.1	12.7	13.4	14.0	14.6	15.2	15.9	16.5	17.1	17.8	18.4	19.0	19.6

Calorie Expenditure per Minute for Various Activities (continued)

	Body Weight																					
	90	99	108	117	125	134	143	152	161	170	178	187	196	205	213	222	231	240	249	257	266	275
Running, 8.5-min. mile, 7 mph	8.4	9.2	10.0	10.8	11.7	12.5	13.3	14.1	14.9	15.7	16.6	17.4	18.2	19.0	19.8	20.7	21.5	22.3	23.1	23.9	24.8	25.6
Running, 7-min. mile, 9 mph	9.3	10.2	11.1	12.9	13.1	13.9	14.8	15.7	16.6	17.5	18.9	19.3	20.2	21.1	22.1	23.0	23.9	24.8	25.7	26.6	27.5	28.4
Running, 5-min. mile, 12 mph	11.8	13.0	14.1	15.3	16.4	17.6	18.7	19.9	21.0	22.2	23.3	24.5	25.6	26.8	27.9	29.1	30.2	31.4	32.5	33.7	34.9	36.0
Stationary Running, 140 counts/min.	14.6	16.1	17.5	18.9	20.4	21.8	23.2	24.6	26.1	27.5	28.9	30.4	31.8	33.2	34.6	36.1	37.5	38.9	40.4	41.8	43.2	44.6
Sprinting	13.8	15.2	16.6	17.9	19.2	20.5	21.9	23.3	24.7	26.1	27.3	28.7	30.0	31.4	32.7	34.0	35.4	36.8	38.2	39.4	40.3	42.2
Sailing	1.8	2.0	2.1	2.3	2.4	2.7	2.8	3.0	3.2	3.4	3.6	3.8	3.9	4.1	4.3	4.4	4.6	4.8	5.0	5.1	5.3	5.5
Skating (moderate)	3.4	3.8	4.1	4.4	4.8	5.1	5.4	5.8	6.1	6.4	6.8	7.1	7.4	7.8	8.1	8.3	8.8	9.1	9.4	9.8	10.1	10.4
Skating (vigorous)	6.2	6.8	7.4	8.0	8.6	9.2	9.8	10.4	11.0	11.6	12.2	12.8	13.4	14.0	14.6	15.2	15.8	16.4	17.0	17.6	18.2	18.8
Skiing (downhill)	5.8	6.4	6.9	7.5	8.1	8.6	9.2	9.8	10.3	10.9	11.4	12.0	12.6	13.1	13.7	14.3	14.8	15.4	16.0	16.5	17.1	17.7
Skiing (level, 5 mph)	7.0	7.7	8.4	9.1	9.8	10.5	11.1	11.8	12.5	13.2	13.9	14.6	15.2	15.9	16.6	17.3	18.0	18.7	19.4	20.0	20.7	21.4
Skiing (racing downhill)	9.9	10.9	11.9	12.9	13.7	14.7	15.7	16.7	17.7	18.7	19.6	20.6	21.6	22.6	23.4	24.4	25.4	26.4	27.4	28.3	29.3	30.2
Snowshoeing (2.3 mph)	3.7	4.1	4.5	4.8	5.2	5.5	5.9	6.3	6.7	7.0	7.4	7.8	8.1	8.5	8.8	9.2	9.6	9.9	10.3	10.6	11.0	11.4
Snowshoeing (2.5 mph)	5.4	5.9	6.5	7.0	7.5	8.0	8.6	9.1	9.7	10.2	10.7	11.2	11.8	12.3	12.8	13.3	13.9	14.4	14.9	15.4	16.0	16.5
Soccer	5.4	5.9	6.4	6.9	7.5	8.0	8.5	9.0	9.6	10.1	10.6	11.1	11.6	12.2	12.7	13.2	13.4	14.3	14.8	15.3	15.8	16.9
Squash	6.2	6.8	7.5	8.1	8.7	9.3	9.9	10.5	11.1	11.7	12.3	12.9	13.5	14.2	14.8	15.4	16.0	16.6	17.2	17.8	18.4	19.0
Stair Climbing and Descending																						
1 stair—25 trips/min.	4.1	4.5	4.9	5.3	5.6	6.0	6.4	6.8	7.2	7.7	8.0	8.4	8.8	9.2	9.6	10.0	10.4	10.8	11.2	11.6	12.0	12.4
1 stair—30 trips/min.	4.4	4.9	5.3	5.7	6.1	6.6	7.0	7.4	7.9	8.3	8.7	9.2	9.6	10.0	10.4	10.9	11.3	11.8	12.2	12.6	13.0	13.5
1 stair—35 trips/min.	5.0	5.5	6.0	6.6	7.0	7.5	8.0	8.5	9.0	9.5	10.0	10.5	11.0	11.5	11.9	12.4	12.9	13.4	13.9	14.4	14.9	15.4
3 stairs—12 trips/min.	4.8	5.2	5.7	6.2	6.6	7.1	7.6	8.1	8.5	9.0	9.4	9.9	10.4	10.9	11.3	11.8	12.2	12.7	13.2	13.6	14.1	14.6

Calorie Expenditure per Minute for Various Activities (continued)

	\multicolumn{22}{c}{Body Weight}																				
	90	99	108	117	125	134	143	152	161	170	178	187	196	205	213	222	231	240	249	257	266	275
3 stairs—15 trips/min.	5.8	6.3	6.9	7.5	8.0	8.6	9.2	9.8	10.3	10.9	11.4	12.0	12.5	13.1	13.6	14.2	14.8	15.4	15.9	16.4	17.0	17.6
3 stairs—18 trips/min.	6.8	7.4	8.1	8.8	9.4	10.1	10.7	11.4	12.1	12.8	13.4	14.0	14.7	15.4	16.0	16.7	17.3	18.0	18.7	19.3	20.0	20.6
5 stairs—8 trips/min.	4.9	5.3	5.8	6.3	6.8	7.2	7.7	8.2	8.7	9.2	9.6	10.1	10.6	11.1	11.5	12.0	12.5	13.0	13.4	13.9	14.4	14.9
5 stairs—10 trips/min.	6.0	6.6	7.2	7.8	8.4	9.0	9.6	10.2	10.8	11.4	11.9	12.5	13.1	13.7	14.3	14.9	15.5	16.1	16.7	17.2	17.8	18.4
5 stairs—12 trips/min.	6.8	7.5	8.2	8.9	9.5	10.2	10.9	11.6	12.2	12.9	13.5	14.2	14.9	15.6	16.2	16.9	17.6	18.2	18.9	19.5	20.2	20.9
7 stairs—6 trips/min.	5.1	5.6	6.2	6.7	7.1	7.7	8.2	8.7	9.2	9.7	10.1	10.7	11.2	11.7	12.1	12.7	13.2	13.7	14.2	14.6	15.2	15.7
7 stairs—7½ trips/min.	6.1	6.7	7.3	8.0	8.5	9.1	9.7	10.3	10.9	11.6	12.1	12.7	13.3	13.9	14.5	15.1	15.7	16.3	16.9	17.5	18.1	18.7
7 stairs—9 trips/min.	7.2	7.9	8.6	9.4	10.0	10.7	11.4	12.2	12.9	13.6	14.2	15.0	15.7	16.4	17.0	17.8	18.5	19.2	19.9	20.6	21.3	22.0
Swimming, pleasure 25 yds./min.	3.6	4.0	4.3	4.7	5.0	5.4	5.7	6.1	6.4	6.8	7.1	7.5	7.8	8.2	8.5	8.9	9.2	9.6	10.0	10.3	10.6	11.0
Swimming, back 20 yds./min.	2.3	2.6	2.8	3.0	3.2	3.5	3.7	3.9	4.1	4.2	4.6	4.8	5.0	5.3	5.5	5.7	6.0	6.2	6.4	6.6	6.9	7.1
Swimming, back 30 yds./min.	3.2	3.5	3.8	4.1	4.4	4.7	5.1	5.4	5.7	6.0	6.3	6.6	6.9	7.2	7.4	7.9	8.2	8.5	8.8	9.1	9.4	9.7
Swimming, back 40 yds./min.	5.0	5.5	5.8	6.5	7.0	7.5	7.9	8.5	8.9	9.4	9.9	10.4	10.9	11.4	11.9	12.3	12.8	13.3	13.8	14.3	14.8	15.3
Swimming, breast 20 yds./min.	2.9	3.2	3.4	3.8	4.0	4.3	4.6	4.9	5.1	5.4	5.7	6.0	6.3	6.5	6.8	7.1	7.4	7.7	7.9	8.2	8.5	8.8
Swimming, breast 30 yds./min.	4.3	4.8	5.2	5.7	6.0	6.4	6.9	7.3	7.7	8.1	8.6	9.0	9.4	9.9	10.3	10.8	11.1	11.5	11.9	12.4	13.0	13.3
Swimming, breast 40 yds./min.	5.8	6.3	6.9	7.5	8.0	8.6	9.2	9.7	10.3	10.8	11.4	12.0	12.5	13.1	13.7	14.2	14.8	15.4	15.9	16.5	17.0	17.6
Swimming, butterfly 50 yds./min.	7.0	7.7	8.4	9.1	9.8	10.5	11.1	11.9	12.5	13.2	13.9	14.6	15.2	15.9	16.6	17.3	18.0	18.7	19.4	20.0	20.7	21.4
Swimming, crawl 20 yds./min.	2.9	3.2	3.4	3.8	4.0	4.3	4.6	4.9	5.1	5.4	5.7	5.8	6.3	6.5	6.8	7.1	7.3	7.7	7.9	8.2	8.5	8.8

Calorie Expenditure per Minute for Various Activities (continued)

	Body Weight																					
	90	99	108	117	125	134	143	152	161	170	178	187	196	205	213	222	231	240	249	257	266	275
Swimming, crawl 45 yds./min.	5.2	5.8	6.3	6.8	7.3	7.8	8.3	8.8	9.3	9.8	10.4	10.9	11.4	11.9	12.4	12.9	13.4	13.9	14.4	15.0	15.5	16.0
Swimming, crawl 50 yds./min.	6.4	7.0	7.6	8.3	8.9	9.5	10.1	10.7	11.4	12.0	12.6	13.2	13.9	14.5	15.1	15.7	16.3	17.0	17.4	17.9	18.8	19.5
Table Tennis	2.3	2.6	2.8	3.0	3.2	3.5	3.7	3.9	4.1	4.2	4.6	4.8	5.0	5.3	5.5	5.7	6.0	6.2	6.4	6.6	6.9	7.1
Tennis (recreation)	4.2	4.6	5.0	5.4	5.8	6.2	6.6	7.0	7.4	7.8	8.2	8.6	9.0	9.4	9.8	10.2	10.6	11.0	11.5	11.9	12.3	12.6
Tennis (competition)	5.9	6.4	7.0	7.6	8.1	8.7	9.3	9.9	10.4	11.0	11.6	12.1	12.7	13.3	13.9	14.4	15.0	15.6	16.1	16.7	17.3	17.9
Timed Calisthenics	8.8	9.6	10.5	11.4	12.2	13.1	13.9	14.8	15.6	16.5	17.4	18.2	19.1	19.9	20.8	21.5	22.5	23.9	24.2	25.1	25.9	26.8
Volleyball (moderate)	3.4	3.8	4.0	4.4	4.8	5.1	5.4	5.8	6.1	6.4	6.8	7.1	7.4	7.8	8.1	8.3	8.8	9.1	9.4	9.8	10.1	10.4
Volleyball (vigorous)	5.9	6.4	7.0	7.6	8.1	8.7	9.3	9.9	10.4	11.0	11.6	12.1	12.7	13.3	13.9	14.4	15.0	15.6	16.1	16.7	17.3	17.9
Walking (2.0 mph)	2.1	2.3	2.5	2.7	2.9	3.1	3.3	3.5	3.7	4.0	4.2	4.4	4.6	4.8	5.0	5.2	5.4	5.6	5.8	6.0	6.2	6.4
Walking (4.5 mph)	4.0	4.4	4.7	5.1	5.5	5.9	6.3	6.7	7.1	7.5	7.8	8.2	8.6	9.0	9.4	9.8	10.1	10.6	10.9	11.3	11.7	12.0
Walking 110–120 steps/min.	3.1	3.4	3.7	4.0	4.3	4.7	5.0	5.3	5.6	5.9	6.2	6.5	6.8	7.1	7.4	7.7	8.0	8.3	8.6	8.9	9.2	9.5
Waterskiing	4.7	5.1	5.6	6.1	6.5	7.0	7.4	7.9	8.3	8.8	9.3	9.7	10.2	10.6	11.1	11.5	12.0	12.5	12.9	13.4	13.8	14.3
Weight Training	4.7	5.1	5.7	6.2	6.7	7.0	7.5	7.9	8.4	8.9	9.4	9.9	10.3	10.8	11.1	11.7	12.2	12.6	13.1	13.5	14.0	14.4
Wrestling	7.7	8.5	9.2	10.0	10.7	11.5	12.2	13.0	13.7	14.5	15.2	16.0	16.7	17.5	18.2	19.0	19.7	20.5	21.2	22.0	22.7	23.5
XBX, 5BX, Chart 1*	5.0	5.5	5.9	6.4	6.9	7.4	7.9	8.4	8.6	9.3	9.8	10.3	10.8	11.3	11.8	12.3	12.8	13.2	13.7	14.2	14.7	15.2
XBX, 5BX, Chart 2*	6.2	6.9	7.5	8.1	8.7	9.3	9.9	10.5	11.1	11.7	12.3	12.9	13.6	14.2	14.8	15.4	16.0	16.7	17.2	17.8	18.4	19.0
XBX, 5BX, Chart 3, 4*	8.8	9.6	10.5	11.4	12.2	13.1	13.9	14.8	15.6	16.5	17.4	18.2	19.1	19.9	20.8	21.6	22.5	23.4	24.2	25.1	25.9	26.8
5BX, Chart 5, 6*	10.0	10.9	11.9	12.9	13.9	14.9	15.8	16.8	17.8	18.7	19.7	20.7	21.7	22.6	23.6	24.6	25.5	26.7	27.4	28.1	29.4	30.1

*Canadian Ten Basic Exercise and Five Basic Exercise Programs in Royal Canadian Air Force, Royal Canadian Air Force Exercise Plans for Physical Fitness (New York: Essandess Special Editions), pp. 18, 24, 30, 36, 69, 71, 73, 75, 77, 79.

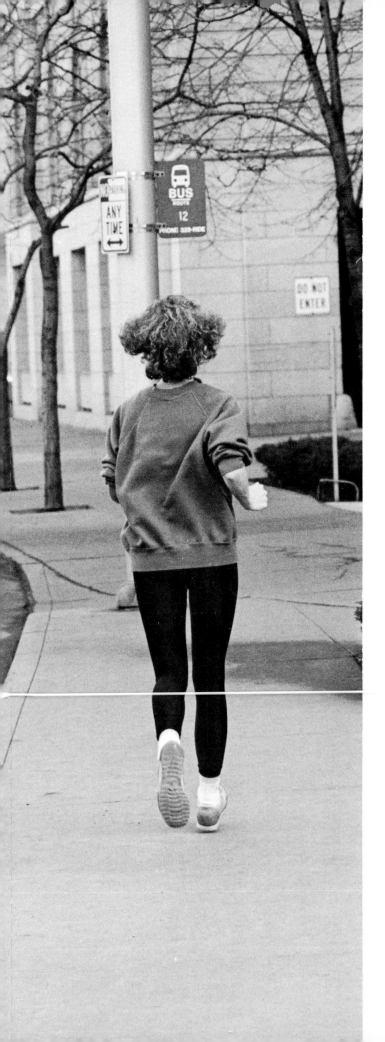

PROGRAM WORK SHEETS

Photocopies may be made of all work sheets in this section for distribution in the classroom or for use by students when they wish to fill out a work sheet more than once.

Cardiovascular Endurance Test Work Sheet

1. Name _____ Sex _____ Age _____

2. Medical Clearance: No Restrictions _____ Restrictions _____

3. Physical Condition: Unconditioned Beginner _____
   Conditioned Beginner _____

4. | **Physical Condition** | **Test Clearance** | **Suggestion** |
   |---|---|---|
   | No medical clearance | No | Get medical examination |
   | Unconditioned beginner | No | Complete beginner's program |
   | Conditioned beginner | Yes | |

   Test Clearance: Yes _____ No _____
   If no: Subject must have a medical exam _____
   Subject must complete beginner's program _____

5. Test: 1.5-mile run _____ 3-mile walk _____

6. When test will be held _____ Where _____

7. Time for 1.5-mile run _____ Time for 3-mile walk _____

8. Fitness Category: _____ I. Very Poor _____ III. Fair _____ V. Excellent
   _____ II. Poor _____ IV. Good _____ VI. Superior

(These tables give times in minutes and seconds.)

1.5-Mile Run Test
Age (years)

Fitness Category		13–19	20–29	30–39	40–49	50–59	60+
I. Very Poor	(men)	>15:31*	>16:01	>16:31	>17:31	>19:01	>20:01
	(women)	>18:31	>19:01	>19:31	>20:01	>20:31	>21:01
II. Poor	(men)	12:11–15:30	14:01–16:00	14:44–16:30	15:36–17:30	17:01–19:00	19:01–20:00
	(women)	16:55–18:30	18:31–19:00	19:01–19:30	19:31–20:00	20:01–20:30	20:31–21:00
III. Fair	(men)	10:49–12:10	12:01–14:00	12:31–14:45	13:01–15:35	14:31–17:00	16:16–19:00
	(women)	14:31–16:54	15:55–18:30	16:31–19:00	17:31–19:30	19:01–20:00	19:31–20:30
IV. Good	(men)	9:41–10:48	10:46–12:00	11:01–12:30	11:31–13:00	12:31–14:30	14:00–16:15
	(women)	12:30–14:30	13:31–15:54	14:31–16:30	15:56–17:30	16:31–19:00	17:31–19:30
V. Excellent	(men)	8:37– 9:40	9:45–10:45	10:00–11:00	10:30–11:30	11:00–12:30	11:15–13:59
	(women)	11:50–12:29	12:30–13:30	13:00–14:30	13:45–15:55	14:30–16:30	16:30–17:30
VI. Superior	(men)	< 8:37	< 9:45	<10:00	<10:30	<11:00	<11:15
	(women)	<11:50	<12:30	<13:00	<13:45	<14:30	<16:30

3-Mile Walking Test (No Running)
Age (years)

Fitness Category		13–19	20–29	30–39	40–49	50–59	60+
I. Very Poor	(men)	>45:00*	>46:00	>49:00	>52:00	>55:00	>60:00
	(women)	>47:00	>48:00	>51:00	>54:00	>57:00	>63:00
II. Poor	(men)	41:01–45:00	42:01–46:00	44:31–49:00	47:01–52:00	50:01–55:00	54:01–60:00
	(women)	43:01–47:00	44:01–48:00	46:31–51:00	49:01–54:00	52:01–57:00	57:01–63:00
III. Fair	(men)	37:31–41:00	38:31–42:00	40:01–44:30	42:01–47:00	45:01–50:00	48:01–54:00
	(women)	39:31–43:00	40:31–44:00	42:01–46:30	44:01–49:00	47:01–52:00	51:01–57:00
IV. Good	(men)	33:00–37:30	34:00–38:30	35:00–40:00	36:30–42:00	39:00–45:00	41:00–48:00
	(women)	35:00–39:30	36:00–40:30	37:30–42:00	39:00–44:00	42:00–47:00	45:00–51:00
V. Excellent	(men)	<33:00	<34:00	<35:00	<36:30	<39:00	<41:00
	(women)	<35:00	<36:00	<37:30	<39:00	<42:00	<45:00

Body Weight Work Sheet

1. Name _____ Sex _____ Date _____

2. Current Weight _____   Age _____

3. Skinfold Measurements

   Children: Triceps _____ Subscapula _____

   Men: Chest _____ Abdomen _____ Thigh _____

   Women: Triceps _____ Thigh _____ Iliac Crest _____

   Sum of Skinfolds _____

4. Body Measurements

   Men: Weight _____ Waist _____

   Women: Hip _____ Height _____

5. Percent Body Fat _____

6. Percent Body Fat Rating Scale

		Men (%)	Women (%)
_____	Very Lean	10 and below	13 and below
_____	Lean	11–14	14–17
_____	Moderate Fat	15–17	18–23
_____	Fat	18–21	24–28
_____	High Fat	22+	29+

Determining Selected Target Weight

7. Current fat weight (current body weight $\times$ item 5) _____
   (Round to nearest whole number.)

8. Current lean body weight (current body weight $-$ item 7) _____

9. Desired percent body fat (select from item 6) _____

10. Estimated target weight [item 8 $\div$ (1.00 $-$ item 9)] _____
    (Round to nearest whole number.)

11. Estimated pounds to gain or lose (item 2 $-$ item 10) _____

Strength Appraisal Work Sheet

1. Name _____ Sex _____

2. Body Weight _____

3. Test Administration

Determine the recommended percentage of total body weight for each exercise. Perform as many repetitions as you can, up to the listed maximum, through a full range of motion. See chapter 7 for a description of the exercises.

Exercise	Fraction of Body Weight (Male)	(Female)	Weight	Reps.	Points	Fitness Category
Arm Curl	.35	.18	_____	_____	_____	_____
Bench Press	.75	.45	_____	_____	_____	_____
Lat Machine Pulldown	.70	.45	_____	_____	_____	_____
Quad Lift	.65	.50	_____	_____	_____	_____
Leg Curl	.32	.25	_____	_____	_____	_____
Curl-Up	.16	.10	_____	_____	_____	_____

4. Fitness Category Chart

Exercise and Repetitions

Fitness Category	Points	Arm Curl Male	Female	Bench Press Male	Female	Lat Machine Pulldown Male	Female
Very Poor	5	2 or less	2 or less	0	0	3 or less	2 or less
Poor	7	3–4	3–5	1–2	1	4–5	3–5
Fair	9	5–7	6–7	3–6	2–4	6–8	6–8
Good	11	8–9	8–11	7–10	5–9	9–10	9–10
Very Good	13	10–14	12–15	11–15	11–15	11–15	11–15
Excellent	15	15–20	16–20	16–20	16–20	16–24	16–24
Superior	17	21+	21+	21+	21+	25+	25+

		Quad Lift Male	Female	Leg Curl Male	Female	Curl-Up Male	Female
Very Poor	5	3 or less	1 or less	1 or less	0	1 or less	0
Poor	7	4–6	2–4	2–3	1–2	2	1
Fair	9	7–9	5–7	4–7	3–4	3–7	2–3
Good	11	10–12	8–9	8–10	5–6	8–11	4–5
Very Good	13	13–14	10–12	11–14	7–9	12–16	6–13
Excellent	15	15–19	13–19	15–19	10–16	17–25	14–26
Superior	17	20+	20+	20+	17+	26+	27+

5. Overall Strength Score

_____

(Total all of the points in the selected exercises)

6. Strength Fitness Category (Check one)

Strength score		Category
Less than 42	_____	I. Very Poor
42–53	_____	II. Poor
54–65	_____	III. Fair
66–77	_____	IV. Good
78–89	_____	V. Very Good
90–101	_____	VI. Excellent
More than 101	_____	VII. Superior

Strength test. *(Adapted from test developed by W. W. K. Hoeger and D. R. Hopkins and used with their permission.)*

Flexibility Appraisal Work Sheet

1. Name _____ Sex _____

Test Administration

2. Sit-and-Reach _____

3. Flexibility Fitness Category

Score		Category
11 or less	_____	I. Very Poor
12–13	_____	II. Poor
14–16	_____	III. Fair
17–19	_____	IV. Good
20–21	_____	V. Very Good
22–23	_____	VI. Excellent
24 or more	_____	VII. Superior

4. Shoulder Lift _____
   (Inches raised)

5. Flexibility Fitness Category

Score		Category
10 or less	_____	I. Very Poor
11–14	_____	II. Poor
15–18	_____	III. Fair
19–21	_____	IV. Good
22–24	_____	V. Very Good
25–26	_____	VI. Excellent
27 or more	_____	VII. Superior

Cardiovascular Endurance Program Work Sheet

1. Name _____ Date _____
2. Weight _____ Age _____
3. Medical Clearance: No Restrictions _____   Restrictions _____

4. Fitness Category	Minimum Caloric Expenditure per Exercise Session	Exercise Intensity Cals./Min.	Minimum Number of Days to Exercise Each Week
_____ 0. Beginner	75	5	3-5
_____ I. Very Poor	100	5	3-5
_____ II. Poor	150	5-10	3-5
_____ III. Fair	200	5-10	3-5
_____ IV. Good	300+	10+	3-5
_____ V. Excellent	300+	10+	3-5
_____ VI. Superior	300+	10+	3-5

5. Exercise preference _____ Rate _____
6. Calories expended per minute (from Appendix B) _____
7. Recommended caloric expenditure per session (from item 4) _____
8. Number of minutes to exercise each day (item 7 ÷ item 6) _____
   Note: This should always be a minimum of 15 continuous minutes to obtain training effect. (Round off to nearest whole number.)
9. Recommended exercise heart rate training zone: _____ to _____

Age	Maximal Heart Rate	Target Zone 70%	Target Zone 85%	Age	Maximal Heart Rate	Target Zone 70%	Target Zone 85%
10	210	147	179	45	175	123	149
15	205	144	174	50	170	119	145
20	200	140	170	55	165	116	140
25	195	137	166	60	160	112	136
30	190	133	162	65	155	109	132
35	185	130	157	70	150	105	128
40	180	126	153	75	145	102	123

Cardiovascular Endurance Program

Week	Days	Exercise	Duration of Activity

Cardiovascular Endurance Program Contract

1. Name _____ Age _____

2. Beginning Fitness Category: ___ 0. Beginner ___ II. Poor ___ IV. Good ___ VI. Superior
   ___ I. Very Poor ___ III. Fair ___ V. Excellent

3. Desired cardiovascular exercise(s): _____

4. Recommended exercise heart rate training zone: _____ to _____

Week	Days	Exercise	Rate	Duration
1				
2				
3				
4				
5				
6				
7				
8				
9				
10				

Signature: _____

Contract approval date: _____ Approved by: _____

Progress check date: _____ Approved by: _____

Contract completion date: _____ Approved by: _____

Cardiovascular Endurance Progress Log

Name _____ Age _____

Beginning cardiovascular endurance level _____

Exercise(s): _____ Exercise heart rate training zone: _____ to _____

| Week | Date | Day | Exercise | Rate | | Duration |
				Time	Distance	

Dietary Evaluation Work Sheet

Name _____ Date _____

Do you use iodized salt? yes _____   no _____

Food Eaten	Amount	Protein	Calcium	Iron	Vitamin A	Thiamine	Riboflavin	Vitamin C (ascorbic acid)
Totals								
Ratings								

Weight-Control Work Sheet

1. Name _____ Age _____ Sex _____ Date _____

2. Weight _____ Target Weight _____ Exercise Heart Rate Training Zone: _____ to _____

3. Medical Clearance: No Restrictions _____ Restrictions _____

4. **Fitness Category**

	Minimum Caloric Expenditure per Exercise Session	Suggested Exercise Intensity (Cals./ Min.)	Minimum Number of Days of Exercise Each Week
___ 0. Beginner	75	5	3-5
___ I. Very Poor	100	5	3-5
___ II. Poor	150	5-10	3-5
___ III. Fair	200	5-10	3-5
___ IV. Good	300+	10+	3-5
___ V. Excellent	300+	10+	3-5
___ VI. Superior	300+	10+	3-5

5. Exercise preference _____ Rate _____

6. Calories expended per minute (from Appendix B) _____

7. Recommended caloric expenditure per session (from item 4) _____

8. Number of minutes to exercise each day (item 7 ÷ item 6) _____
   Note: This should always be a minimum of 15 continuous minutes to obtain training effect. (Round off to nearest whole number.)

9. Number of days to exercise each week _____

10. Number of calories expended in exercise each week (line 7 × line 9) _____

11. Average number of calories expended daily in exercise (line 10 ÷ 7 days) _____
    (Round off answer to nearest whole number.)

Determining Caloric Intake

12. Typical daily caloric intake (Current weight × 15 cals.) _____

13. Caloric reduction per day to lose two pounds per week ___−1,000_____

14. Total daily caloric intake, without exercise, to lose two pounds per week _____
    (line 12 — line 13)

15. Daily caloric intake to lose two pounds per week, including exercise (line 14 + line 11). This figure should not be below 1,200 for women or 1,500 for men. (Always round answer to the *lowest* 100 calories.)

    _____

16. Maintaining body weight (target weight × 15 cals.) _____

Weight-Control Program Contract

1. Name _____ Age _____ Sex _____

2. Present weight _____ Pounds to be lost _____ Target weight _____ Fitness category _____

3. Desired exercise(s) _____

4. Exercise heart rate training zone: _____ to _____

Week	Exercise	Duration	Weekly Exercise Periods	Weight to Be Lost (lbs.)	Desired Caloric Intake
1				2	
2				2	
3				2	
4				2	
5				2	
6				2	
7				2	
8				2	
9				2	

Contract approval date: _____ Approved by: _____

Reassessment date: _____ Approved by: _____

Contract completion date: _____ Approved by: _____

Weight-Control Program Progress Log

Name ———— Age ———— Sex ————

Current weight ———— Pounds to be lost ———— Target weight ———— Fitness category ————

Exercise(s) ———————— Exercise heart rate training zone: ———— to ————

Week	Day and Date	Exercise	Duration		Caloric Intake	Weight
			Time	Distance		

Strength Program Work Sheet

1. Name: _____ Date: _____

2. Program Preference: Weight Training _____   Timed Calisthenics _____

3. Exercise Days for Weight Training: M   T   W   Th   F   S

   Exercise Days for Timed Calisthenics: 5 days per week

4. Strength Fitness Category: ___ 0. Beginner   ___ II. Poor   ___ IV. Good   ___ VI. Excellent
   ___ I. Very Poor   ___ III. Fair   ___ V. Very Good   ___ VII. Superior

5. Rest Periods:

   Weight Training: 90 seconds or alternating exercise _____

   Timed Calisthenics: 10 seconds and 2 minutes _____

I. WEIGHT TRAINING*

Body Parts	Exercise	Exercise Preference	Sets	Repetitions	Resistance
Shoulders	1, 2, 3		3	10	
Abdomen	10		3	30	
Chest	6, 7, 9		3	10	
Hamstrings	11		3	10	
Quadriceps	12, 13		3	10	
Legs (calves)	14		3	10	
Back	5, 1, 8		3	10	
Biceps	4, 2, 5		3	10	
Triceps	7, 1, 3, 6		3	10	

*Arabic numerals refer to charts in the weight-training program.

II. TIMED CALISTHENICS†

Body Parts	Exercise	Exercise Preference			
Shoulders	IV	four-count burpee			
Abdomen	VI	curl-up			
Chest	VII	push-up			
Hamstrings	II	treadmill			
Quadriceps	I, V	run in place/shuffle			
Legs (calves)	III	high jumper			
Triceps	VII	push-up			

†Roman numerals refer to charts in the timed calisthenics program.

Strength Program Contract

1. Name _____ Age _____ Sex _____

2. Strength Fitness Category: __ 0. Beginner __ II. Poor __ IV. Good __ VI. Excellent
                               __ I. Very Poor __ III. Fair __ V. Very Good __ VII. Superior

3. Body Measurements: Weight _____ Waist _____ Chest _____

       Hips _____ Biceps: Right _____ Left _____

       Calf: Right _____ Left _____

4. Selected Program: Weight Training _____ Days _____

              Timed Calisthenics _____

5. Number of Weeks for Program _____

Signature: _____

Contract approval date: _____ Approved by: _____

Reassessment check date: _____ Approved by: _____

Contract completion date: _____ Approved by: _____

Strength Program Progress Log

Name _____   Beginning Strength Category _____

Date	Day	Exercise	TIMED CALISTHENICS								WEIGHT TRAINING													
			I	II	III	IV	V	VI	VII	VIII	1	2	3	4	5	6	7	8	9	10	11	12	13	14
		Reps																							
		Resistance																							
		Reps																							
		Resistance																							
		Reps																							
		Resistance																							
		Reps																							
		Resistance																							
		Reps																							
		Resistance																							
		Reps																							
		Resistance																							
		Reps																							
		Resistance																							
		Reps																							
		Resistance																							
		Reps																							
		Resistance																							
		Reps																							
		Resistance																							
		Reps																							
		Resistance																							
		Reps																							
		Resistance																							

Flexibility Program Work Sheet

1. Name _____ Date _____

2. Flexibility Fitness Category

    A. Sit-and-Reach _____

    B. Shoulder Lift _____

3. Exercise Days for Flexibility: Daily

FLEXIBILITY

Body Parts	Exercise	Exercise Preference	Sets	Repetitions
Low back muscles	C D E		1	10
Hamstrings	A B		1	10
Trunk rotators	F G		1	10
Hip flexors	H I		1	10
Pectoral muscles	K L		1	10
Heel cords	M N		1	10
Pelvic muscles	J		1	10

*Letters refer to charts in the flexibility program.

Flexibility Program Contract

1. Name _____ Age _____ Sex _____

2. Flexibility Fitness Category

   A. Sit-and-Reach _____

   B. Shoulder Lift _____

3. Number of Weeks for Program _____

Signature _____

Contract approval date _____ Approved by _____

Reassessment check date _____ Approved by _____

Contract completion date _____ Approved by _____

Flexibility Program Progress Log

Name _____

Beginning Flexibility Category

A. Sit-and-Reach _____

B. Shoulder Lift _____

Flexibility Exercises

Date	Day	A	B	C	D	E	F	G	H	I	J	K	L	M

GLOSSARY

aerobic with the use of oxygen.

alveoli tiny air sacs in the lungs used to exchange gases.

amino acids the chemical units used to construct protein.

anaerobic without the use of oxygen.

angina pectoris an uncomfortable sensation of pressure or pain in the chest area caused by the heart muscle not getting enough oxygen through its blood supply.

anorexia nervosa a serious illness of deliberate self-starvation with profound psychiatric and physical components.

anxiety a feeling of uncertainty and apprehension that can interfere with thinking and other normal mental processes.

arteriosclerosis a general term for various types of arterial problems associated with rigidity of the arterial wall—also known as "hardening of the arteries."

atherosclerosis a disease of the coronary arteries in which the arterial opening becomes narrower due to deposits of fat, cholesterol, and other substances on the inner lining of the artery.

caloric expenditure number of calories expended for engaging in any activity.

calorie a measure of heat used to explain the potential energy value of food. Food is measured in large calories or kilocalories (kcals).

capillaries the smallest blood vessels of the circulatory system. They are used to exchange substances such as oxygen, carbon dioxide, and nutrients at the cellular level.

carbohydrate a type of food that is used as energy in the body.

cardiovascular endurance the ability of the heart, lungs, and circulatory system to provide the cells of the body with the substances necessary to perform work for long periods of time.

cellulite a term for fatty deposits that cause the skin to have a puckered appearance similar to an orange peel. This type of fat is no different from any other type of fat in the body.

cholesterol a fatlike substance found in the tissues and circulatory system.

circuit training an organized course of exercise at a series of exercise stations placed around a

ballistic stretch a fast, jerky, bobbing type of stretching movement.

barbell a six-foot bar with metal plates attached.

beta-endorphins chemicals produced by the body that reduce pain and may contribute to the aspect of "feeling better" when exercising.

blitz method a strength-training method to train just one body part in order to obtain maximum size and muscle definition.

bulimia an eating disorder, characterized by periods of voracious eating binges, followed by purging the food in order to prevent a weight gain.

burns using sets of rapid half contractions in strength training.

the circulatory system to aid in the flow of blood.

complex carbohydrates a form of carbohydrate, such as starch, found in vegetables, fruits, and cereals.

conditioned beginner an individual who has been engaging in a continuous, large muscle activity for fifteen or more minutes and for three or more days per week for at least four weeks.

cool down the time utilized for the body to recover from the stress of exercise.

coronary occlusion a narrowing of a coronary blood vessel that restricts the flow of blood.

coronary thrombosis a coronary occlusion caused by a blood clot that blocks the flow of blood to some part of the heart muscle.

depression associated with feelings of hopelessness and a reduction of the mental processes and other body functions.

dumbbell a hand weight.

duration the amount of time each exercise bout requires.

electrocardiogram (EKG) a graphic tracing of an electrical current produced by the contraction of the heart muscle.

essential amino acids amino acids that the human body cannot construct and must come from outside sources in the diet.

fat a type of food used as a form of stored energy in the body. It is also used to transport fat-soluble vitamins (A, D, E, K), provide cushioning for organs, and to insulate the body.

fiber an inert material found in certain foods that adds bulk to the diet and may help prevent colon problems.

flexibility the range of movement in a joint.

food exchanges six food groups used to plan menus: vegetables, breads, meats, milks, fruits, and fats.

forced reps. a strength-training method where a partner assists the lifter to do more repetitions than can be done alone.

free weights the use of barbells and dumbbells as strength-training equipment.

frequency number of times an exercise is done each week.

guestimate a method to determine the resistance to use in strength training.

heart attack a result of disease brought about by an adverse condition of the coronary arteries that supply the heart muscle with blood.

heart disease a disease that affects the tissues of the heart and is the most common cause of death in the United States.

heart rate training zone range of heart rate that will bring about cardiovascular endurance training effects. It is in a zone that is between 70–85 percent of the maximal heart rate.

hemoglobin a substance in red blood cells that is used to transport oxygen.

high-density lipoprotein cholesterol (HDL-C) contains high amounts of protein in relationship to cholesterol. It may help prevent the formation of plaque.

hydrostatic weighing a procedure of weighing a person underwater to determine the amount of body fat.

hypertension high blood pressure.

hypertrophy increase in cell size.

hypokinetic disease a disease that is related to or caused by a lack of physical activity.

intensity how stressful the exercise is.

interval training repeated periods of physical training interspersed with recovery periods.

isokinetic resistance an attempt to produce a maximal resistance to all joint angles through a range of motion. Requires a special machine to provide the resistance and control the speed of movement.

isometric contraction muscle contraction with little or no movement.

isotonic contraction muscle contraction with movement.

lean body weight the weight of the body when the percent body fat has been subtracted. It consists primarily of muscle, bone, and connective tissue.

left atrium a chamber of the heart that pumps blood to the left ventricle.

left ventricle a chamber of the heart that pumps blood to the working tissues of the body.

lipoproteins chemical units composed of triglycerides, cholesterol, and phospholipids that are attached to a protein carrier and used to transport fats and cholesterol in the blood.

low-density lipoprotein cholesterol (LDL-C) contains high amounts of cholesterol. It may contribute to the formation of plaque.

maximal heart rate highest heart rate or pulse rate an individual can attain. It can be estimated by subtracting a person's age from 220.

maximum resistance maximum weight lifted for one repetition of an exercise.

meditation the act of clearing the mind of stimuli that might be causing stress and tension within the body.

minerals used to provide hardness to body tissues and to control chemical functions in the body.

mode type of activity selected for a fitness program.

muscle-bound a decrease in flexibility. It is not caused by participation in a proper strength-training program.

muscle mass amount of muscle tissue in the body.

muscle pump forcing blood into the muscle area to increase muscular size.

muscular endurance ability to perform repeated muscle movements for a given period of time.

muscular strength ability to exert force against resistance.

myocardial infarct a heart attack brought about by an occlusion of blood to the heart muscle.

nutrients chemical substances obtained from food during digestion that build and maintain body cells, regulate body processes, and supply energy.

obese a person with an excess accumulation of body fat. Obesity for men is about 20 percent body fat and for women is about 28 percent body fat.

omega-3 fatty acids an unsaturated fat found in certain fish oils that may be helpful in lowering the likelihood of heart disease.

overload principle subjecting selected systems of the body to loads greater than they are accustomed to.

overweight someone who weighs 10 percent or more above a desired weight.

percent body fat the amount of fat in the body expressed as a percentage of the total body weight.

physical fitness a state of well-being with attributes that contribute to: (1) performing daily activities with vigor; (2) having minimal risk of health problems that are related to lack of exercise; and (3) providing a fitness base for participation in a variety of physical activities.

substances on the inner lining of arteries that cause the arterial opening to become narrower and thus restrict blood flow.

preexhaustion a strength-training method where stronger muscle groups are trained to exhaustion before exercising the weaker muscle groups.

progressive resistance increasing the resistance of an exercise as strength improves.

proprioceptive-neuromuscular-facilitation (PNF) a stretching procedure that utilizes a partner to assist in the flexibility routine and involves the contraction and relaxation of both the muscles being stretched and the opposing muscles.

protein used to build and rebuild body tissues and regulate chemical functions in the body.

pulse rate number of heart beats per minute.

pyramid system a type of strength training that consists of adding weight until only one complete repetition can be accomplished.

range of motion distance through which a limb can travel at a given point.

recovery period rest interval time between sets.

repetitions number of times an exercise is repeated.

resistance the amount of weight moved by a muscle contraction.

right atrium a chamber of the heart that pumps blood to the right ventricle.

right ventricle a chamber of the heart that pumps blood to the lungs.

risk factors factors that contribute to the cause of heart disease. Primary risk factors include hypertension, high blood lipids, smoking, EKG abnormalities, overfatness, diabetes, stress, diet, sedentary life-style, family history, sex, and age.

saturated fats fatty acid molecules that cannot accept any hydrogen atoms into their structure.

set a given number of repetitions.

set point a theory that suggests there is a regulatory center in the brain containing a mechanism that regulates food intake and body weight.

shin splints an inflammation of the muscles and/or tendons of the lower leg brought about by continual shock to the lower extremities.

simple carbohydrates usually known as sugars and found in foods with a high sugar content.

skinfold sites.

skinfold measurements a procedure to determine the amount of body fat by measuring the thickness of the skin at selected body sites.

specific overload specific body systems respond to specific loads and thus an overload for one system may be different from an overload for another system.

split routine a strength-training program that trains different groups of body parts on alternate days.

spot reducing A myth that proposes people can lose fat from specific areas of the body. A person will lose fat from the entire body on a fat-reduction program, with the greater percentage of fat lost from areas where there is a greater amount of fat.

spotting the use of a partner or partners to assist in an exercise program.

static stretch a slow, sustained type of stretching movement.

strength the ability to exert force against resistance.

stress the nonspecific response of the human organism to any demand that is placed on it or the rate of wear and tear on the body.

stretch stress that point in the stretching movement where a person feels some discomfort.

stroke volume the amount of blood ejected with each beat of the heart.

super multiple set system a method of strength training in which the lifter completes all of the sets for a given muscle group and then completes the same number of sets for the opposite muscle group.

supersets a system of strength training in which an exercise set for a particular muscle group is followed immediately by an exercise set for the antagonist (opposite) muscle group.

target weight the weight to achieve for a selected percent body fat.

thrombus a blood clot that is the result of the formation of plaque.

timed calisthenics a training program using the weight of the body to develop both strength and cardiovascular endurance.

triglyceride consists of three fatty acid molecules attached to a glycerol molecule.

United States Recommended Daily Allowance (U.S. RDA) a recommendation made for the amount of selected nutrients that a person should have in the daily diet.

unsaturated fats fatty acid molecules that can accept one or more hydrogen atoms into their structure.

variable resistance the use of a special machine that does not control speed of movement, but attempts to provide a maximal resistance to all joint angles through a range of motion.

vitamins used to control chemical functions in the body.

warm-up the act of increasing the body temperature in order to improve the efficiency of the various body systems.

BIBLIOGRAPHY

Allen, Roger J. *Human Stress: Its Nature and Control.* Minneapolis, Minnesota: Burgess Publishing Company, 1983.

Allsen, Philip E. *Conditioning and Physical Fitness—Current Answers to Relevant Questions.* Dubuque, Iowa: William C. Brown Company Publishers, 1978.

Allsen, Philip E. *Strength Training—Beginners, Bodybuilders, and Athletes.* Glenview, Illinois: Scott, Foresman and Company, 1987.

Anderson, Bob. *Stretching.* Bolinas, California: Shelter Publications, 1980.

Arnow, L. Earle. *Food Power—A Doctor's Guide to Common Sense Nutrition.* Chicago, Illinois: Nelson-Hall Company, 1972.

Åstrand, Per-Olof, and Rodahl Kaare. *Textbook of Work Physiology-Physiological Bases of Exercise.* New York, New York: McGraw-Hill Book Company, 1977.

Beaulieu, John. *Stretching for All Sports.* Pasadena, California: The Athletic Press, 1980.

Benson, Herbert. *The Relaxation Response.* New York, New York: Avon Books, 1975.

Bogert, L. Jean, George M. Briggs, and Doris H. Calloway. Nutrition and Physical Fitness. 8th ed., Philadelphia, Pennsylvania: W. B. Saunders Company, 1966.

Cooper, Kenneth H. *The Aerobics Way.* New York, New York: M. Evans and Company, Inc., 1977.

Cooper, Kenneth H. *The Aerobics Program for Total Well-being.* New York, New York: Bantam Books, 1982.

Corbin, Charles B., and Ruth Lindsey. *Concepts of Physical Fitness.* Dubuque, Iowa: William C. Brown Company Publishers, 1987.

Cundiff, David E., and Paul Brynteson. *Health Fitness—Guide to a Life-style.* Dubuque, Iowa: Kendall/Hunt Publishing Company,

Cureton, Thomas K. *Physical Fitness and Dynamic Health.* New York, New York: Oral Press, Inc., 1965.

Cureton, Thomas K. *The Physiological Effects of Exercise Programs on Adults.* Springfield, Illinois: Charles C. Thomas, Publisher, 1971.

DeVries, Herbert A. *Physiology of Exercise for Physical Education and Athletics.* Dubuque, Iowa: William C. Brown Company Publishers, 1980.

DiGennaro, Joseph. *The New Physical Fitness—Exercise for Everybody.* Englewood, Colorado: Morton Publishing Company, 1983.

Edwards, LaVell, and Chuck Stiggins. *Total Conditioning—The BYU Football Way.* Champaign, Illinois: Leisure Press, 1985.

Fisher, A. Garth, and Philip E. Allsen. *Jogging.* Dubuque, Iowa: William C. Brown Company Publishers, 1987.

Fox, Edward L., Timothy E. Kirby, and Ann Roberts Fox. *Bases of Fitness.* New York, New York: Macmillan Publishing Company, 1987.

Getchell, Bud. *Physical Fitness—A Way of Life.* New York, New York: John Wiley and Sons, 1983.

Greenberg, Jerold S., and David Paman. *Physical Fitness—A Wellness Approach.* Englewood Cliffs, New Jersey: Prentice-Hall, Inc. 1986.

Hockey, Robert V. *Physical Fitness: The Pathway to Healthful Living.* St. Louis, Missouri: Times Mirror-Mosby College Publishing, 1985.

Hoeger, Werner W. K. *Lifetime Physical Fitness and Wellness.* Englewood, Colorado: Morton Publishing, 1986.

Katch, Frank I., and William D. McArdle. *Nutrition, Weight Control, and Exercise.* Philadelphia, Pennsylvania: Lea and Febiger, 1983.

Konshi, Frank. *Exercise Equivalents of Foods.* Carbondale, Illinois: Southern Illinois University Press, 1974.

Kraus, Hans, and Wilhelm Roaab. *Hypokinetic Disease.* Springfield, Illinois: Charles C. Thomas Publisher, 1961.

Kusinitz, Ivan, and Fine Morton. *Your Guide to Getting Fat.* Palo Alto, California: Mayfield Publishing Company, 1987.

LaMott, Kenneth. *Escape From Stress.* New York, New York: Berkeley Windhover Books, 1975.

Mayer, Jean. *Overweight: Causes, Cost, and Control.* Englewood Cliffs, New Jersey: Prentice-Hall, Inc., 1968.

McGlynn, George. *Dynamic Fitness—A Practical Approach.* Dubuque, Iowa: William C. Brown Company Publishers, 1987.

Miller, David K., and T. Earl Allen. *Fitness, A Lifetime Commitment.* Edma, Minnesota: Burgess Publishing, 1986.

Nash, Joyce D., and Linda Ormiston Long. *Taking Charge of Your Weight and Well-being.* Palo Alto, California: Bull Publishing Company, 1978.

Parizkova, Jana, and V. A. Rogozkin. *Nutrition, Physical Fitness, and Health.* Baltimore, Maryland: University Park Press, 1978.

Pollock, Michael, Jack H. Wilmore, and Samuel M. Fox. *Health and Fitness Through Physical Activity.* New York, New York: John Wiley and Sons, 1978.

Rathbone, Josephine L. *Relaxation*. Philadelphia, Pennsylvania: Lea and Febiger, 1969.

Rosato, Frank D. *Fitness and Wellness—The Physical Connection*. New York, New York: West Publishing Company, 1986.

Seefeldt, Vern. *Physical Activity and Well-being*. Reston, Virginia: American Alliance for Health, Physical Education, Recreation, and Dance, 1986.

Selye, Hans. *The Stress of Life*. New York, New York: McGraw-Hill Book Company, 1956.

Sharkey, Brian J. *Physiology of Fitness*. Champaign, Illinois: Human Kinetics Publishers, Inc., 1984.

Shephard, Roy J. *Economic Benefits of Enhanced Fitness*. Champaign, Illinois: Human Kinetics Publishers, Inc., 1986.

Smith, Everett L., and Robert C. Serfass. *Exercise and Aging: The Scientific Basis*. Hillside, New Jersey: Enslow Publishers, 1981.

Stone, William J., and William A. Kroll. *Sports Conditioning and Weight Training: Programs for Athletic Competition*. Boston, Massachusetts: Allyn and Bacon, Inc., 1986.

Storlie, Jean, and Henry A. Jordan. *Nutrition and Exercise in Obesity Management*. New York, New York: Medical and Scientific Book—Spectrum Publications, Inc., 1984.

Stull, Alan G., and Thomas K. Cureton. *Encyclopedia of Physical Education, Fitness, and Sports*. Salt Lake City, Utah: Brighton Publishing Company, 1980.

Vodak, Paul. *Exercise—The Why and the How*. Palo Alto, California: 1980.

Westcott, Wayne L. *Strength Fitness—Physiological Principles and Training Techniques*. Boston, Massachusetts: Allyn and Bacon, Inc. 1983.

Williams, Melvin H. *Nutrition for Fitness and Sport*. Dubuque, Iowa: William C. Brown Company Publishers, 1983.

Williams, Melvin H. *Nutritional Aspects of Human Physical and Athletic Performance*. Springfield, Illinois: Charles C. Thomas Publisher, 1976.

Williams, Melvin H. *Lifetime Physical Fitness, A Personal Choice*. Dubuque, Iowa: William C. Brown Company Publishers, 1985.

Williams, Melvin H. *Ergogenic Aids in Sport*. Champaign, Illinois: Human Kinetics Publishers, 1983.

Wilmore, Jack H. *Sensible Fitness*. Champaign, Illinois: Leisure Press, 1986.

INDEX